Multilingual Perspec
on Child Language
Disorders

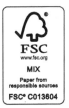

FSC
www.fsc.org
MIX
Paper from
responsible sources
FSC® C013604

COMMUNICATION DISORDERS ACROSS LANGUAGES

Series Editors: **Dr Nicole Müller** and **Dr Martin Ball,** *Linköping University, Sweden.*

While the majority of work in communication disorders has focused on English, there has been a growing trend in recent years for the publication of information on languages other than English. However, much of this is scattered through a large number of journals in the field of speech pathology/ communication disorders, and therefore, not always readily available to the practitioner, researcher and student. It is the aim of this series to bring together into book form surveys of existing studies on specific languages, together with new materials for the language(s) in question. We also have launched a series of companion volumes dedicated to issues related to the cross-linguistic study of communication disorders. The series does not include English (as so much work is readily available), but covers a wide number of other languages (usually separately, though sometimes two or more similar languages may be grouped together where warranted by the amount of published work currently available). We have been able to publish volumes on Finnish, Spanish, Chinese and Turkish, and books on multilingual aspects of stuttering, aphasia, and speech disorders, with several others in preparation.

Full details of all the books in this series and of all our other publications can be found on http://www.multilingual-matters.com, or by writing to Multilingual Matters, St Nicholas House, 31-34 High Street, Bristol BS1 2AW, UK.

COMMUNICATION DISORDERS ACROSS LANGUAGES: 14

Multilingual Perspectives on Child Language Disorders

Edited by
Janet L. Patterson and Barbara L. Rodríguez

MULTILINGUAL MATTERS
Bristol • Buffalo • Toronto

Library of Congress Cataloging in Publication Data
A catalog record for this book is available from the Library of Congress.
Names: Patterson, Janet L., 1955- editor. | Rodríguez, Barbara L., editor.
Title: Multilingual Perspectives on Child Language Disorders/Edited by
Janet L. Patterson and Barbara L. Rodríguez.
Description: Bristol : Multilingual Matters, [2016] |
Series: Communication Disorders Across Languages: 14 |
Includes bibliographical references and index.
Identifiers: LCCN 2015029085 | ISBN 9781783094721 (hbk : alk. paper) | ISBN
    9781783094714 (pbk : alk. paper) | ISBN 9781783094738 (ebook)
Subjects: LCSH: Language disorders in children. | Language acquisition. |
    Bilingualism. | Multilingual communication.
Classification: LCC RJ496.L35 M85 2016 | DDC 618.92/855–dc23 LC record available at
http://lccn.loc.gov/2015029085

British Library Cataloguing in Publication Data
A catalogue entry for this book is available from the British Library.

ISBN-13: 978-1-78309-472-1 (hbk)
ISBN-13: 978-1-78309-471-4 (pbk)

Multilingual Matters
UK: St Nicholas House, 31-34 High Street, Bristol BS1 2AW, UK.
USA: UTP, 2250 Military Road, Tonawanda, NY 14150, USA.
Canada: UTP, 5201 Dufferin Street, North York, Ontario M3H 5T8, Canada.

Website: www.multilingual-matters.com
Twitter: Multi_Ling_Mat
Facebook: https://www.facebook.com/multilingualmatters
Blog: www.channelviewpublications.wordpress.com

The policy of Multilingual Matters/Channel View Publications is to use papers that are natural, renewable and recyclable products, made from wood grown in sustainable forests. In the manufacturing process of our books, and to further support our policy, preference is given to printers that have FSC and PEFC Chain of Custody certification. The FSC and/or PEFC logos will appear on those books where full certification has been granted to the printer concerned.

Typeset by Deanta Global Publishing Services Limited.
Printed and bound in Great Britain by the CPI Books Group.

Contents

Acknowledgments

First and foremost, thank you to the authors for contributing to this book. It has been a pleasure to work with all of you. Many thanks to Philip Dale and to Melissa Axelrod for helpful suggestions and feedback on the introductory chapter. Thanks also to Jennifer Romero, Marcella Baileys, Abigail Fajardo, Anna Lundborg, Samantha Strong and Bryan Ho for their tireless attention to detail, including reference checking and formatting. We appreciate the help and feedback provided by the series editors, Martin Ball and Nicole Müller, as well as the patience and cheerful helpfulness of the Multilingual Matters editorial staff, especially Kim Eggleton.

Janet would like to thank her family and Willow for their encouragement and support over the years. She especially thanks Pete for always supporting her endeavors and Moises for his patience during this book and other projects.

Barbara would especially like to thank Ray and Lauren for their unending support, encouragement and patience while working on this book and throughout her professional career. She also wishes to acknowledge her parents – Albert and Consuelo – who sacrificed much for their children's success and will always be in her heart.

Contributors

Truman Coggins is a professor at the University of Washington and a research affiliate in the Eunice Kennedy Shriver Intellectual and Developmental Disabilities Research Center at the Center on Human Development and Disability. Dr Coggins is an ASHA fellow whose research interests focus on communication disorders in a social context.

Elizabeth Kay-Raining Bird (Mandy) is a professor in the School of Human Communication Disorders at Dalhousie University in Halifax, Nova Scotia, Canada. Her research and teaching are in the areas of child language development and disorders, particularly individuals with developmental disabilities and issues of cultural and linguistic diversity.

Nita Madhani is an experienced bilingual speech and language therapist and is head of children's therapy services for the North East London Foundation Trust in Redbridge. She continues to work with and develop therapy services that meet the cultural and linguistic needs of local communities. Nita has developed pilot service models for children and young people with complex needs and adults with acquired difficulties from diverse communities that have been adapted widely within other areas of the UK.

Stefka H. Marinova-Todd is an associate professor at the School of Audiology and Speech Sciences at the University of British Columbia in Vancouver, Canada. Her current research is focused on the language and cognitive abilities of typically developing children and children with ASD, and on the language and literacy development of children and adults who are learning English as a second language.

İlknur Maviş is a professor (PhD) at Anadolu University, Faculty of Health Sciences, Department of Speech and Language Pathology. She has published research on typically developing children and language development, acquired and primary language disorders. She is known internationally for research on aphasia and its characteristics in Turkish. She has developed the first standardized test in Aphasia Assessment in Turkish (ADD). She has supervised a great number of MSc and PhD theses on language disorders and SLI.

Pat Mirenda is a professor in the Department of Educational & Counseling Psychology and Special Education and director of the Centre for Interdisciplinary Research and Collaboration in Autism at the University of British Columbia. She is a board-certified behavior analyst and teaches courses on augmentative communication, autism and positive behavior supports. She is a fellow of both the American Speech-Language-Hearing Association (ASHA) and the International Society for Augmentative and Alternative Communication (ISAAC). Her current research includes a Canada-wide study of developmental trajectories in children with autism and a study of bilingualism in children with autism and other developmental disabilities.

Janet L. Patterson is an associate professor of speech and hearing sciences at the University of New Mexico. Her teaching and research interests are in child language development and disorders, with a focus on multilingual children. Her experiences as a speech-language pathologist motivated her research on typical language acquisition in young children with bilingual experience and on developing more accurate screening tools for identifying language disorders in young bilingual children.

Barbara L. Rodríguez is a professor in the Department of Speech and Hearing Sciences at the University of New Mexico. Dr Rodriguez's research and teaching interests are in bilingual language acquisition. Her recent research has focused on language and literacy development in bilingual (English/Spanish), cultural and environmental influences on the language development of children from diverse backgrounds and speech/language assessment and screening of bilingual (English/Spanish) and monolingual Spanish-speaking children. She served as associate editor for the *American Journal of Speech-Language Pathology* and volunteered service to ASHA on the multicultural issues board and the special interest group focusing on cultural and linguistic diverse populations.

Vesna Stojanovik is associate professor of clinical linguistics at the School of Psychology and Clinical Language Sciences at the University of Reading. Her research focus is language and communication development in children affected by genetic disorders, such as those with Williams and those with Down syndrome. She has also conducted research in prosodic abilities in children with Williams and Down syndrome and coedited a book, together with Jane Setter: *Prosody in Atypical Populations: Assessment and Remediation* (2011). Vesna has been the chair of the British Association of Clinical Linguistics since 2008.

Jane Stokes is a senior lecturer in speech and language therapy at the University of Greenwich in the UK. She has worked as a speech and language therapist in London and Hong Kong. She has always enjoyed clinical work with children and adults with communication difficulties and managing teams in linguistically and culturally diverse communities. Throughout her career, she has been committed to joint work with people who share her enthusiasm for continuous improvement of the services provided to children and families who speak languages other than English.

Elin Thordardottir is a professor at the School of Communication Sciences and Disorders at McGill University in Montreal, director of research at CRIR-Institut Raymond Dewar in Montreal and researcher at Reykjavikur Akademian in Iceland. Her research focuses on language development and language disorders in children who speak French, English and Icelandic, as well as in bilingual children and second language learners. She is a certified speech-language pathologist.

John C. Thorne is a lecturer at the University of Washington, a clinician with the Fetal Alcohol Syndrome Diagnostic & Prevention Network, and the head of speech-language pathology at the Center on Human Development & Disability in Seattle. Since earning his PhD at the University of Washington, his research has focused on developing rigorous tools for measuring later-developing aspects of communicative discourse in school-aged children with neurodevelopmental disability.

Carol K.S. To is associate professor and the director of clinical education in the Division of Speech and Hearing Sciences at The University of Hong Kong. She researches and teaches in the areas of pediatric communication disorders with particular interest in children with speech sound disorders and autism spectrum disorders.

Seyhun Topbaş pioneered the first graduate and undergraduate speech-language pathology programs at Anadolu University in Turkey and is one of the founders of the Association of the Speech and Language Pathology Profession in Turkey. She is currently head of the Department of Speech and Language Therapy at İstanbul Medipol University. Dr Topbaş has published many articles in international journals and books, developed tests on speech sound disorders and language impairments and coauthored a book, *Communication Disorders in Turkish*. She has served on the ASHA International Issues Board and the Cultural and Linguistic Considerations Across the Discipline convention committee, and she is on the editorial board of the ICPLA and APSSLH journals.

1 Child Language Disorders Across Languages, Cultural Contexts and Syndromes

Janet L. Patterson

This book is about children with language disorders who speak languages other than or in addition to English. The authors address a wide range of clinical and theoretical questions. For example, what do we know about the course of development in bilingual children with Down syndrome (DS)? What language measures are available for French-speaking children? For Turkish-speaking children? How can we deliver early intervention services effectively to a Gujarati-speaking family living in London? Is the profile of strengths and weaknesses in Williams syndrome (WS) similar across languages?

The rich and increasing body of cross-linguistic research on specific language impairment (SLI) illustrates the value of a multilinguistic perspective for theory testing and development, as well as for clinical applications (e.g. Leonard, 2009, 2014; Paradis, 2010). This book extends a multilinguistic perspective to a wider range of child language disorders. This volume is organized in two sections. The chapters in the first section of the book focus on language disorders associated with four different syndromes in multilingual populations and contexts. The chapters in the second section of the book are language-specific, although the issues they address are relevant across languages and cultural contexts.

In the section on language impairments associated with specific syndromes, the first two chapters provide research reviews and clinical implications for bilingual children with autism spectrum disorders (ASD; Marinova-Todd and Mirenda, Chapter 2) and DS (Kay-Raining Bird, Chapter 3). These two chapters address important clinical and theoretical questions such as 'Is learning two languages harder than learning one language for children with language disorders?', 'What language(s) should be included in intervention?' and 'Is the profile of typical strengths and weaknesses and the rate of language development different for bilingual children versus monolingual children with syndromes such as ASD or DS?'. In Chapter 4, Thorne and Coggins provide information on language and communication impairments among children with fetal alcohol spectrum disorders (FASD), assessment tools and intervention. Stojanovik reviews the literature on language and communication difficulties in Williams syndrome (WS) among English-speaking children and children who speak other languages (Chapter 5). The chapters on FASD and WS include discussions of assessment and intervention implications for children with these syndromes, regardless of the language(s) they speak.

The language-specific section of the book starts with To's chapter (Chapter 6) on language impairment in Cantonese Chinese-speaking children. Her chapter includes information on Cantonese oral and written language; manifestations of language impairment in Chinese children with SLI, dyslexia and ASD; and clinical resources and guidelines for assessment and intervention. Although the clinical tools and strategies that To discusses specifically address Cantonese-speaking children, she and the authors of the other chapters in this section discuss assessment and intervention issues and strategies that are relevant to children with language disorders more generally. Stokes and Madhani (Chapter 7) present a framework for providing early intervention services and they demonstrate its application to working in London with children and families who speak North Indian languages (Panjabi, Gujarati and Bengali). Their chapter includes information on cultural and linguistic considerations for families from northern India, widely applicable clinical strategies for working with families in multilingual contexts and a case example to demonstrate the strategies. In Chapter 8, Elin Thordardottir provides a wealth of information on language development, primary language impairment (PLI) and assessment tools for French-speaking preschool and early school-age children, and she discusses important issues in developing and using valid assessment tools for monolingual versus bilingual children. Topbaş and Maviş (Chapter 9) focus on the development of Turkish language assessment tools and, more generally, the importance of developing valid language measures for identifying children with PLI or SLI. Without such tools, Topbaş and Maviş point out that children with SLI may not be provided with appropriate services since their needs will not be identified on the basis of associated cognitive, motoric or sensory impairments. In Chapter 10, Rodríguez focuses on dialectal differences in Spanish and the importance of taking linguistic variation into account in language assessment.

Multiple Dimensions of Diversity

An understanding of the ways in which language disorders are manifested across languages enhances our understanding of the nature of language disorders and how to better serve children and families from diverse cultural and linguistic backgrounds. This book includes cross-linguistic information on patterns of language growth and weaknesses among children with SLI, and among children with language impairments associated with other developmental difficulties and diagnoses. Thus, the diversity in this book extends to variation within and across clinical populations as well as across languages and cultures.

Although there are many language-specific and culture-specific facts, details, assessment tools and intervention recommendations included in this volume, this book is intended to provide a foundation for working with multilingual children and families in general, including those who speak languages not specifically addressed in this book. Examining language disorders in widely divergent circumstances (different languages, monolingual versus bilingual, different cultural contexts and different diagnoses and developmental disabilities) gives us a perspective on the range of considerations necessary for clinical practice when we work with children who speak languages other than those specifically addressed in this book. An understanding of diversity among children with language disorders is a key not only to understanding what is language-specific and culture-specific, but also to identifying commonalities across languages and across cultural and clinical contexts.

Diversity in languages

An encyclopedic knowledge of all of the world languages isn't necessary or feasible for clinicians and researchers. However, an understanding that what is true of one's native language(s) is not necessarily true of other languages and a familiarity with some of the ways in which languages vary provide a foundation for good clinical practice and research. Cross-linguistic research allows us to examine how language works in general, without depending on assumptions based on our understanding of a particular language. As Slobin (1985) pointed out in a classic series on language acquisition in 15 languages, cross-linguistic research is essential for identifying universal aspects and principles of language acquisition. Subsequently, there was a growing recognition of the importance of cross-linguistic research for clinical work and for identifying and testing theories about underlying mechanisms involved in language breakdown in aphasia (e.g. Bates *et al.*, 1991) and on the nature of SLI (e.g. Leonard, 1990, 2009, 2014). Cross-linguistic research on child language disorders associated with other diagnoses such as WS, DS, FASD and ASD can further our understanding of commonalities and differences in language development in diverse circumstances and populations.

The languages represented in this book vary widely in their structural characteristics. Three points of divergence are noted in particular here: word order, morphological typology and writing systems.

The most common word order across languages is subject-object-verb (SOV) and the second most common is subject-verb-object (SVO), the basic word order of English. As shown in Table 1.1, SOV is the basic word order of Turkish and of the North Indian languages, Panjabi, Gujarati and Bengali, languages discussed in two chapters in this book. Three chapters focus on languages in which SVO is the basic word order (Cantonese, French and Spanish). The flexibility of word order and the degree to which the subject must be stated also vary across languages. In some languages, grammatical relations – the 'who does what to whom' information – are indicated by verbal affixes rather than solely by word order. In those languages, the subject may be omitted and word order may vary for pragmatic purposes, such as for focus or emphasis. In contrast, in languages such as English in which grammatical relations are indicated largely through word order, there is less variation from SVO word order and subjects are almost always stated in declarative statements.

Morphological typology, the classification of languages according to the way morphemes are put together to form words, is quite varied in the languages considered in this volume. Linguists generally classify languages as being either analytic (isolating) or synthetic. Analytic languages, like Mandarin and Cantonese, construct sentences through the use of isolated morphemes, without the use of affixes. Synthetic languages, in contrast, express meanings by combining free and bound morphemes. Synthetic languages may be agglutinating, like Turkish, where the affixes can easily be separated from the stems to which they are attached, and each affix generally conveys only one meaning. For example, *ellerimde* (in my hands) includes four morphemes: *el* (hand) + *ler* (plural) + *im* (my) + *de* (in). Another kind of synthetic language is fusional, where affixes and the bases to which they are attached are fused together in pronunciation and therefore are not easily separated from one another. In addition, there is generally a fusion of meanings that are represented by the affixes in such languages. As an example, verb forms in Spanish are marked for a range of inflectional categories, including person, number, tense and aspect in a

Table 1.1 Selected grammatical characteristics of English and other languages in this book

Language	Basic word order	Noun case marking	Gender marking on nouns	Gender-specific third-person pronouns
Cantonese	SVO	No	No	No
English	SVO	No	No	Yes; singular only
French	SVO	No	Yes	Yes
Gujarati, Panjabi, Bengali	SOV	Yes	Yes No	No
Spanish	SVO	No	Yes	Yes
Turkish	SOV	Yes	No	No

single affix. For the verb, *hablar* (to speak/talk), *hablo* (I speak) and *hablaron* (they spoke), the *-o* in *hablo* conveys first-person singular, present tense, and *-aron* indicates third-person plural, past perfective.

The meanings expressed by affixes also differ across languages. In contrast with English, which has a sparse inflectional morphology, French and Spanish are moderately inflected, with specific inflections for verb tense, aspect and person, as well as number and gender marking and agreement in noun phrases (see Table 1.1). However, in contrast with Spanish, spoken French has many homophones for forms that differ in written language. For example, Elin Thordardottir (Chapter 8) points out that the spoken verb forms in *j'aime* (I love), *tu aimes* (you love), *il aime* (he loves) and *ils/ells aiment* (they love) are all homophones, although they differ in written form.

Turkish and the North Indian languages, Bengali, Gujarati and Panjabi, have multiple suffixes that are added to root nouns and verbs. Nouns are marked for case; for example, a suffix indicates whether a noun is a direct object (accusative case) or an indirect object (dative case). However, the specific types of suffixes vary across these languages. For example, Turkish does not mark gender with different forms for nouns, but two of the North Indian languages do.

As a final example of cross-linguistic variation in grammatical morphology, gender marking differs across languages for pronouns as well as nouns (and for other forms, as well). As shown in Table 1.1, English differentiates gender only in third-person singular pronouns (*he, she, it*), French and Spanish mark gender in third-person singular *and* plural pronouns, while Cantonese, Turkish and the North Indian languages do not differentiate gender in third-person pronouns (i.e. a single pronoun is used where English would differentiate *he, she* and *it*).

In addition to crosslinguistic differences, another important consideration is variation across dialects or varieties of languages. Rodríguez (Chapter 10) provides examples of phonological, morphological and syntactic variation in two varieties of Spanish that are widely spoken in the United States.

Diversity in written language systems is also found among the languages discussed in this book. In contrast with the alphabetic writing systems of English, French, Spanish, North Indian languages and Turkish, the written language used by Cantonese speakers is a logographic system, Modern Standard Chinese. To's chapter on Cantonese illustrates variation in writing systems that can occur even within a language or language group. Because Modern Standard Chinese corresponds more closely to the spoken form of Mandarin than to Cantonese, Cantonese-speaking children experience a great difference between written and oral language when learning to read than Mandarin-speaking children do. Another difference in Mandarin- and Cantonese-speaking children's experience is the use of an alphabetic system, Pinyin, which is taught to beginning readers in mainland China, but not in Hong Kong.

Among the languages with alphabetic writing systems, there is diversity in the scripts used. Latin scripts are used for English, French, Spanish and modern Turkish, but the degree of phonetic transparency or correspondence between spoken and written forms varies; for example, Spanish written forms correspond more closely to the pronunciation of spoken forms than English and French. Devanagari scripts are used for many languages, including Bengali, Gujarati and Panjabi. Although they vary in some details, Devanagari scripts are written from left to right and most consonants have an 'inherent' following vowel, 'a' (Bright, 1996; Cardona, 1987; Klaiman, 1987). Other post-consonantal vowels are indicated with diacritic symbols added to the consonant, and vowels also can be indicated with independent symbols as needed, such as in word-initial contexts.

The details and range of variation across languages can seem overwhelming, even based on the small sample of cross-linguistic differences described here. Stokes and Madhani discuss the challenges clinicians face in working with multilingual populations and they provide a framework for working with children and families in early intervention when the clinician is not familiar with the languages and cultural backgrounds of the families that he or she serves. To's chapter on Cantonese-speaking children with language impairments, Elin Thordardottir's chapter on PLI in French-speaking children and Stojanovik's review of cross-linguistic research on WS illustrate how our understanding of the nature of language impairments is broadened through research with languages other than English.

Diversity: Monolingual and multilingual experiences

Another aspect of linguistic diversity is the number of languages individuals hear and use. Although many children are monolingual, a sizeable minority or even the majority of children in many countries and communities are multilingual, speaking two or more languages. As Kay-Raining Bird (Chapter 3) points out, bilinguals (and, more generally, multilinguals) differ not only in the languages they hear and speak, and how much they use each language, but also on a multitude of other variables. She illustrates the varied multilingual experiences of children with case examples of four multilingual children with DS and presents evidence of similar outcomes for bilingual and monolingual children with DS. Marinova-Todd and Mirenda (Chapter 2) present emerging evidence that there are similar outcomes in the early language development of bilingual and monolingual children with ASD. The similarity between monolinguals and bilinguals in early developmental profiles and outcomes in children with ASD and DS merits highlighting since the common practice of advising families to use only one language assumes (incorrectly) that multilingualism is problematic for children with language disorders. Marinova-Todd and Mirenda review recent research indicating that there may be important *negative* results and implications when families of children with ASD are advised to use only one language. Stokes and Madhani (Chapter 7) take a broad perspective, viewing multilingualism as one of many variables incorporated in family-centered services for young children. They highlight the dynamic and changing language contexts that young children experience in multilingual families and communities, and they present a framework for collaborating with parents to consider all languages the child experiences in intervention planning and strategies.

Cultural diversity

Cultural considerations are essential to a multilingual perspective. The authors of the chapters in this book address various cultural factors and their clinical implications, including (1) the use of culturally appropriate materials and activities in assessment and intervention; (2) relationships among cultural values, family roles and assessment and intervention activities; and (3) intervention approaches that address the multiple, complex and dynamic cultural systems that multilingual children with language disorders experience.

Assessment stimuli and materials that are congruent with children's life experiences are recommended so that interpretation of children's performance on language tests and in language samples can focus to a greater extent on the linguistic aspects of their performance. Elin Thordardottir points out that differences in the life experiences of European and North American French-speaking children (in addition to the linguistic differences in varieties of French spoken in Canada and France) are important considerations in selecting, developing and adapting language assessment tools for francophone children (Chapter 8). For example, if a French–Canadian child scores low on a European French picture vocabulary test, the low score could be due to lack of familiarity with some of the objects and events depicted, or due to vocabulary deficits or to a combination of factors. Turning to intervention, although providing new experiences can be valuable, use of intervention activities that are culturally congruent with child and family experiences may allow children (and their parents) to focus to a greater extent on linguistic input and expectations, and less on learning about unfamiliar materials and how to use them. Stokes and Madhani (Chapter 7) discuss the importance of drawing on community resources to develop culturally and locally appropriate materials and activities and they provide an illustration in their case example, a preschool child in a Gujarati family of North Indian heritage living in London.

Congruence with family roles is another consideration in assessment and intervention activities. For example, direct participation in play activities is not typical of parent–child interactions in some cultures, so language sampling and intervention contexts may need to be adjusted to be culturally appropriate. To (Chapter 6) discusses links between cultural values and child socialization practices, explaining how family roles and expectations for child behaviors in traditional Cantonese families relate to Confucian philosophy, and she discusses how these roles and expectations may relate to parent and child interactions in assessment and intervention interactions.

Cultures are complex and dynamic, shifting across contexts and changing over time. In the case of Chinese children, To suggests that Western influences and also Chinese policies and practices regarding family size may result in variation in child socialization practices. At the level of day-to-day experience, multilingual children must negotiate multiple, complex and dynamic social environments. Supporting skills and participation in complex social worlds is essential for multilingual children with FASD, as Thorne and Coggins (Chapter 4) point out. Although the intervention approaches they discuss are specific to children with FASD, their families and their teachers, many of the intervention principles apply to children with other social, language and developmental disorders. Finally, because languages and cultures are dynamic, Stokes and Madhani urge us to use information on typical cultural practices and language features in this book and in other resources as a starting point, rather than as a set of expectations, when working with individual families.

Strengths and weaknesses across and within clinical groups

Particular patterns of strengths and weaknesses are associated with many diagnoses or clinical groups, although heterogeneity within clinical groups is widely recognized. Thorne and Coggins (Chapter 4) report that language is commonly affected in children with FASD, with impairments in various areas of language occurring in about a quarter of children diagnosed with FASD. Children with DS typically have a greater degree of language impairment compared to their non-verbal cognitive development, but the degree of impairments varies widely (Kay-Raining Bird, Chapter 3). Although language has been identified as a relative strength in WS, Stojanovik (Chapter 5) presents evidence of variability and of several areas of language and communication weaknesses in this population. Social communication is a core area of deficiency in individuals diagnosed with ASD, but the range of variation is wide, from individuals with little or no functional communication to individuals who are verbal but have significant pragmatic difficulties (Marinova-Todd and Mirenda, Chapter 2).

Language profiles across clinical groups

We turn now to a summary of specific areas of strength and weaknesses in language and communication associated with different disorders.

Typical areas of strength and weakness in morphosyntax, pragmatics and lexical development associated with various clinical groups are briefly summarized in this section, based on the research reported and reviewed in several chapters in this book.

Expressive morphosyntax is generally an area of weakness compared to other language areas for children with DS as well as children with SLI. In contrast, regular grammatical morphology is not an area of weakness and may be an area of relative strength in children with WS.

Pragmatics is a core area of difficulty in individuals with ASD, which by definition involves deficits in social communication skills. On the other hand, pragmatics generally has been identified as an area of strength in WS compared to ASD. However, although individuals with WS are often characterized as gregarious, research has documented difficulty in some pragmatic areas, including responding to requests for clarification and providing information appropriate to listener perspective. Similarly, although there is great variation among children with FASD, older children with FASD may have difficulty with complex social uses of language and discourse demands, including taking listener perspective into account.

Turning to lexical development, receptive vocabulary (as measured by standardized vocabulary tests) is generally an area of relative strength in DS and WS, and vocabulary is relatively robust in FASD as well. Although mean scores on receptive vocabulary tests are lower among children with SLI than among typically developing children, many children with SLI have receptive vocabulary scores within the average range (Gray et al., 1999). In general, it appears that receptive vocabulary, as measured by single-word picture-pointing tasks, is relatively strong in most clinical groups with language impairment. However, other aspects of lexical and semantic development are affected to a greater extent in some clinical groups. In ASD, lexical development is generally a strength, but mental state terms are an area of specific relative weakness (Marinova-Todd and Mirenda, Chapter 2), while children with SLI use less diverse vocabulary in language samples than same-age peers, and controls matched on mean length of utterance (MLU; Elin Thordardottir, Chapter 8).

In the area of literacy, To (Chapter 6) reviews research on Cantonese-speaking children with dyslexia, focusing on the relationship between phonological awareness skills and reading (word recognition). Although research in this area is limited, findings indicate that the relationship differs depending on the type of writing system and the degree to which written forms correspond to spoken forms (phonetic transparency). Furthermore, several chapters present evidence that the relationship between phonological awareness skills and reading may differ in children with ASD and typically developing children, and perhaps in other clinical populations such as WS and DS, although, again, the research to date is limited.

Language profiles within clinical groups

Studies of children who speak one or more languages other than English indicate that within clinical populations, phenotypic characteristics are broadly similar, although the details may vary. As noted previously, bilingual children with SLI, with DS and with ASD have similar early language profiles compared to monolinguals with the same disorders, and they have similar areas of strength and weakness. For example, Kay-Raining Bird (Chapter 3) notes that French–English bilingual children with DS have greater difficulty with expressive morphosyntax than other language domains in both languages, as do monolingual children across a variety of languages.

At a more detailed level, the manifestations of language disorders vary across languages. For example, in contrast with the particular difficulty that English-speaking preschool children with SLI have with marking verb tense and number, Spanish-speaking children with SLI also have difficulty with noun phrase morphology, including the use of articles and article–noun agreement in gender and number (Restrepo & Gutiérrez-Clellen, 2012; Rodríguez, Chapter 10, this volume). In Turkish-speaking children with language impairment, noun case inflections and verb tense markers are affected (Topbaş and Maviş, Chapter 9).

Patterns of errors among older and younger children also differ across languages. In contrast with English-speaking preschool children with SLI, Elin Thordardottir (2014a) found that French-speaking preschool children with SLI used present, past and future tense forms and they made few morphological errors on these verb forms. She notes that higher error rates on verb inflections have been reported in older French-speaking children with SLI, even on simple verb forms, perhaps due to older children using and selecting verb forms out of a larger set of options that includes complex verb forms such as the pluperfect (an English example would be *I had eaten*). She suggests an additional or alternate reason is that older children are using verb forms in more complex sentences.

When compared with inflected languages, what does SLI look like in a language with minimal bound morphology such as Cantonese? Cantonese-speaking children with SLI have difficulty with aspect markers (To, Chapter 5). To reports that children with SLI used fewer aspect markers than controls in one study, and they used aspect markers in more restricted contexts than typically developing children matched for language level in another study. In other words, in addition to delays in acquiring language forms, children with SLI used forms (specifically, aspect markers) that were in their repertoire in fewer contexts. Other qualitative differences, such as error patterns that differ from those seen in typical development, are reported in studies of Turkish-speaking children with SLI (Topbaş and Maviş, Chapter 9) for some grammatical forms. These findings from analytic (Cantonese) and synthetic (Turkish) languages indicate that it is important to consider qualitative as well as quantitative differences in the use of grammatical morphemes in children with SLI.

Lexical diversity in children with SLI has been examined in several languages. Children with SLI use fewer different words in language samples compared to their age peers, and in some studies, their vocabulary use is less diverse when compared to younger, typically developing children at a similar overall language level (most often matched on MLU). The authors of chapters in this book review evidence of reduced lexical diversity in children with SLI who speak English, Turkish, French and Cantonese. However, there are cross-linguistic differences within lexical categories. For example, To reviews research indicating that Cantonese-speaking children with SLI have similar diversity in verbs compared to typically developing children at a similar language level, unlike findings of reduced diversity in verbs for English-speaking children with SLI.

Broadly similar patterns of strength and weakness across languages with differences occurring in the specific manifestations of language impairment occur not only in SLI, but also among children with other disorders. For example, pragmatics is consistently an area of difficulty in ASD even though the linguistic mechanisms and non-verbal aspects of communication vary across languages and cultures. To explains that irony is conveyed through the use of sentence-final particles (SFP) that signal pragmatic intent and also through prosody in Cantonese. She reports that older Cantonese-speaking children with ASD have difficulty with identifying irony when either or both types of cues are available (SFP and/ or prosodic).

Taking both clinical and linguistic diversity into account, it appears that for broadly defined language areas, patterns of strength and weakness within clinical populations are sufficiently robust that similar findings are reported across languages, although the specific manifestations do vary across languages.

Diversity in clinical practices and contexts

A final area of diversity to consider is differences across clinical contexts. It is important to recognize that terminology differs across languages and cultures. Instead of standardizing terms in this book, for the most part the terms in each chapter are those that are used in the authors' cultural and clinical contexts. For example, some chapters refer to speech-language pathologists (SLPs) while others refer to speech-language therapists (SLTs); some refer to SLI, but PLI is also used. Elin Thordardottir discusses the overlap and the differences between PLI and the French term *dysphasie*, and she points out the research and clinical implications when there are differences in diagnostic categories across languages and cultures.

In addition to differences in terminology, there are significant differences across the clinical and social contexts represented in this book. For example, Topbaş and Maviş highlight the importance of valid language measures for identifying children with SLI as a step toward accessing intervention mandated recently by public policy in Turkey. In another chapter, Stokes and Madhani discuss early intervention and care pathways within the British health and educational systems, pointing out the importance of considering the interface between non-Western families and early intervention services.

There is tremendous diversity in the topics addressed in this book, including a wide range of clinical and educational contexts, languages, cultures and developmental disorders. However, there also are common themes in assessment and intervention.

Assessment

What language skills should be considered in assessment? What language measures are available and what is the evidence of their validity? How do we meet the challenges of language assessment for children who are bilingual or multilingual? These are some of the pressing questions that the authors in this volume address.

What skills should be included in language assessment?

The need for comprehensive assessment is highlighted in the chapters on WS and on FASD. Stojanovik (Chapter 5) reports that in spite of the commonly noted gregarious nature associated with WS and initial characterizations of language as an area of strength in WS, subsequent research indicates many individuals with WS have delays in language and communication as well as some areas of particular weakness, including figurative language and providing sufficient information for listener needs. In view of these findings, and in view of the heterogeneity in language, literacy and related areas of development in individuals with WS, Stojanovik points out the importance of comprehensive assessments for identifying language intervention needs for individuals with WS. Thorne and Coggins (Chapter 4) point out that assessment in the school-age years may identify areas of language and communication difficulty that were not evident at younger ages. Some children with FASD may not evidence language and social communication difficulties until there are expectations for more complex language use and understanding in the school-age years. Therefore, periodic monitoring of children who are at high risk for language impairment may be advisable, even if no delays were present in earlier development. The need for comprehensive assessments with changes in areas evaluated over time also applies to other language disorders. For example, even though the most salient difficulties in SLI are in morphosyntax and lexical development, pragmatic and social communication difficulties also occur (Brinton & Fujiki, 1999; Conti-Ramsden & Botting, 2004) and older children with persisting language impairments may have difficulty with written language and the language demands of the classroom, even when they no longer have noticeable oral language impairments (Nelson, 2010).

A comprehensive approach to language assessment for multilingual children requires an understanding of cross-linguistic differences in language structure. The 'same' finding may be very different as to whether it indicates typical development or possible impairment. For example, a child's typical sentence length in words has a different meaning in synthetic languages in which words are typically multimorphemic versus a sparsely inflected language such as English. Stokes and Madhani present an example from a North Indian language, pointing out that characterizing a child as 'having two word combinations' could result in an underestimation of morphosyntactic development.

The relationship between mean length of utterance in morphemes (MLU-M) and in words (MLU-W) is affected by language typology. For example, Topbaş and Maviş report that the mean MLU for children age 4;2 (±6 months) in the Turkish Systematic Analysis of Language Transcript (SALT) database is approximately 2.5 in words and approximately 4.6 in morphemes. In contrast, the SALT database for English-speaking children at the same age indicates an average MLU of approximately 3.4 in words and approximately 3.7 in morphemes (SALT, 2012). Although it is a rough comparison, the cross-linguistic variation in MLU-W and MLU-M and the difference between them appear to follow an expected pattern based on the degree of inflection for each language – a larger difference between MLU-W and MLU-M in a highly inflected language (Turkish) and a smaller difference between MLU-W and MLU-M in a sparsely inflected language (English). The variation in MLU-M and MLU-W across languages also illustrates the importance of language-specific normative data; what would be a low MLU-W for an English-speaking child might be well within the average range for a Turkish-speaking child.

Specific structures and types of error patterns also vary across languages. Therefore, language measures should address structures and error patterns that are relevant for the child's language(s). As noted previously, in contrast with English-speaking children, errors may occur more often in noun phrase morphology in Turkish-speaking and Spanish-speaking children, and aspect markers may be an important assessment focus for Cantonese-speaking children. Another example is SFPs, which have no direct parallel in English. SFPs are an important means of conveying pragmatic information in Cantonese and many other Asian languages, including Japanese (Katagiri, 2007), and they should be included in the assessment of children who speak Cantonese and other languages that include these elements.

Assessment tools

Comprehensive assessments should employ several types of tools and varied sources of information. Parent interviews, observations of children in authentic contexts, language sampling, use of appropriate standardized tests when they are available, probes and dynamic assessment (DA) all yield different types of information. For example, the weaknesses in figurative language and in providing information appropriate to listener perspectives reported in studies of individuals with WS may not be evident in conversational and narrative language samples (Stojanovik, Chapter 5), but deficiencies in these areas can have a significant impact on the effectiveness of communication. Use of probes (tasks designed to assess particular skills) may be necessary to assess skills that do not necessarily appear frequently in naturalistic language samples.

The types of tools that are most helpful depend on the child's age, the clinical context and the assessment questions to be addressed. As Kay-Raining Bird (Chapter 3) notes, there may be little need to use standardized, norm-referenced language tests with children with DS since diagnosis is rarely an assessment question for the SLP/SLT to address in this population and intervention needs are best determined based on other types of assessment (Paul & Norbury, 2012). In contrast, normative data are useful in identifying children with SLI, an issue that Topbaş and Maviş highlight in Chapter 9. In early intervention, parent interviews and observations of the child are the key components in the approach that Stokes and Madhani present for conducting assessments designed to identify and provide intervention in areas of need (Chapter 7).

Several authors note the challenges in developing standardized, norm-referenced tests for children who speak languages other than English. Tests that have been translated from one language to another (e.g. from English to French) have multiple problems. As Elin Thordardottir points out, even if standardized tests are renormed after translation, the language structures and content that are addressed are those that are relevant to English, rather than the language the child speaks. Furthermore, even tools that have been appropriately adapted and renormed or have been developed and normed specifically in other languages have unknown qualities for diagnostic purposes. Elin Thordardottir and Topbaş and Maviş remind us that the diagnostic accuracy (e.g. sensitivity and specificity) of measures is a key consideration for any tool used for diagnostic purposes. The diagnostic accuracy of many adapted and renormed tools is unknown, and test scores must be interpreted with particular caution.

Although language samples are widely recommended as a major assessment tool, language sample measures and analyses are subject to the same concerns about validity and diagnostic accuracy as standardized tests. The language sampling context must be considered for cultural congruence, as To points out when discussing the assessment of children from Chinese-speaking families. Measures must be adapted or developed to focus on linguistic features that are germane to the language in question and adequate norms are needed for quantitative measures such as MLU and number of different words (NDW). Good examples of this type of work are the adaptations of SALT for French-speaking children (Elin Thordardottir, Chapter 8) and for Turkish-speaking children (Topbaş and Maviş, Chapter 9). Although children with SLI have lower scores on most of these measures compared to their peers, the authors note that their diagnostic accuracy needs to be established. Determining the diagnostic accuracy of language measures is complex; for example, Elin Thordardottir reports that in a study of French-speaking children, a low MLU indicated a high likelihood of language impairment, but not all children with language impairment had low MLUs.

This highlights the importance of multiple measures in language assessment (Paul & Norbury, 2012). Diagnostic accuracy is optimal when highly sensitive and specific measures are combined, as indicated by research on diagnostic accuracy for measures for French-speaking children (Elin Thordardottir, Chapter 8) and Spanish-speaking children (Restrepo, 1998). Although the accuracy of specific language measures and combinations of measures is not established for many children from culturally and linguistically diverse backgrounds, research currently does provide a basis for selecting diagnostic measures for some languages and ages.

Although the chapters in this book provide a wealth of resources for assessment in several different languages, there are many languages and many unique circumstances for which developmental data and assessment tools are lacking. Therefore, alternative approaches such as DA or using processing measures that may require less language-specific information are also included in the authors' recommendations.

Assessment of children who speak two or more languages

This book includes chapters that address both senses of multilingual considerations – cross-linguistic considerations for monolingual speakers, and also research and clinical strategies focusing on children who speak more than one language. Because there is limited work addressing children who speak more than two languages, most information to date concerns bilingual children. Properly identifying measures and strategies for monolingual versus bilingual/multilingual assessment is essential, not only for the appropriate assessment of multilingual children, but also for ensuring accurate assessment of monolingual children (Elin Thordardottir, Chapter 8).

There is tremendous variation among bilingual children's experiences. One broad difference is in the timing of children's exposure to the two languages. Simultaneous bilinguals are exposed to two languages in infancy, while preschool and school-age sequential bilinguals begin learning a second language after first language acquisition has begun. Although the circumstances of bilingual children's language development differ, diagnostic assessments of bilingual children, whether they are simultaneous or sequential learners, must take the children's knowledge in each language into account for two reasons. First, bilingual children with language impairment have difficulty with both languages (Paradis *et al.*, 2011). For example, language impairment would be ruled out in a sequential bilingual with typical development in the first language. Second, considering the child's skills in only one language will underestimate the multilingual child's overall language knowledge (Patterson, 1998; Pearson, 2013; Peña *et al.*, 2011). As an example, consider the vocabulary development of a typically developing Canadian child, John. John is from an English-speaking home and has been educated in French throughout his primary school years. Although John has equivalent terms in French and English for some items, he knows some words only in English, and other words only in French, with no equivalent English word in his vocabulary. This 'distributed knowledge' in which there is overlapping but not identical vocabulary across the child's languages is typical of bilingual development (Bedore *et al.*, 2005; Core *et al.*, 2013; Umbel *et al.*, 1992). Due to the distributed nature of lexical development in bilinguals, single language measures will underestimate a multilingual child's vocabulary development. In John's case, his score on an English vocabulary test will not reflect words he knows in French from his school experience. Even though his home language is English, John may appear to have vocabulary delays if his performance on single language (English) testing is compared to monolingual children for whom English is the home language and the language used in school.

In order to measure overall vocabulary knowledge in bilinguals, researchers and clinicians have combined children's vocabulary scores for the two languages. Combined vocabulary scores can be calculated in two ways – total vocabulary (TV) and total conceptual vocabulary (TCV; Core *et al.*, 2013; Patterson & Pearson, 2012; Pearson *et al.*, 1993). For example, in order to characterize John's overall vocabulary quantitatively, we could calculate TV by simply counting the total number of words he knows in each language and adding them together for a combined score. In contrast, for TCV we would measure the number of concepts included in his lexicon, regardless of whether the words he knows for each concept are in French, English or both (TCV). However, TCV scoring is not always straightforward because it requires identifying 'translation equivalents', something that isn't possible for some words. We could also use 'conceptual scoring' (Bedore *et al.*, 2005) for other language tasks, crediting any semantically correct response, whether it is in French or English. For example, if John is asked what the opposite of *hot* is, *froid* (cold) would be scored as correct when using conceptual scoring.

What is the 'better' measure – TV or conceptual scoring methods such as TCV? For very young children, TV may be the more representative measure of lexical growth and it may be a more accurate basis for identifying possible delay (Patterson & Pearson, 2012). Core *et al.* (2013) found that TV scores for bilingual 2-year-olds resulted in vocabulary scores that were similar to those of monolingual children and that growth rates based on TV were similar in bilingual and monolingual children. In contrast, bilingual children's TCV scores were lower than monolingual children's scores.

Results from another recent study (Gross *et al.*, 2014) also indicate that TCV scores on vocabulary measures should be interpreted with caution for the diagnosis of language impairment. Gross *et al.* reported mixed findings on the use of TCV for 5- to 7-year-olds on receptive and expressive vocabulary measures. They administered single language vocabulary tests to bilingual children and then readministered items that children missed in the other language, scoring items correct if they got them correct in either language (TCV). Although conceptual scoring resulted in fewer bilingual children having receptive and expressive vocabulary scores below the average range when their performance was compared to monolingual norms, the bilingual children's expressive TCV scores were still lower than the scores of monolingual children, and receptive vocabulary scores were lower than monolingual scores for sequential bilinguals. Because vocabulary development is related to socioeconomic status in typically developing bilingual and monolingual children, the Gross *et al.* study was particularly informative because it controlled for socioeconomic status in the analyses.

In spite of the limitations of TCV on vocabulary measures, conceptual scoring may provide an appropriate representation of older bilingual children's skills on more complex semantic tasks (Bedore *et al.*, 2005). Skills such as semantic categorization and word definition strategies transfer from one language to the other among bilingual children (e.g. Ordóñez *et al.*, 2002), presumably due to *common underlying proficiency* – language knowledge that is not language-specific (Cummins, 1991). Due to common underlying proficiency, bilingual or multilingual children do not have to learn all language skills (e.g. semantic categorization) anew for each language. Evidence for common underlying proficiency is strongest for academic language skills (Paradis *et al.*, 2011) and conceptual scoring may be more appropriate for these types of tasks.

What about morphosyntactic development? In general, basic milestones such as word combinations appear to occur in at least one language at about the same age in monolingual and bilingual children (Patterson, 1998; Pearson, 2013). For example, most bilingual children are combining words in one or more languages by 18–24 months of age. However, as illustrated with the languages represented in this book, many morphosyntactic structures differ greatly across languages and therefore must be considered on a language-specific basis. Furthermore, the circumstances of acquisition are important to consider in evaluating morphosyntactic development. For example, the course of morphosyntactic development may differ for young simultaneous bilingual children who have been exposed to two languages since birth versus sequential bilinguals who are monolingual for several years and then begin learning a second language upon entering school.

The evidence is now clear that young simultaneous bilingual children have separate grammatical systems for the two languages from the earliest stages of development and that morphosyntactic development generally follows the same path as that of monolingual children in each language (Elin Thordardottir, 2014a), although with some subtle cross-linguistic influences (Paradis *et al.*, 2011). Elin Thordardottir's (2014a) study of French–English simultaneous bilingual children also showed that morphosyntactic development in children with approximately equal experience with the two languages was similar to that of monolingual peers, but that for children with unequal exposure, grammatical development lagged in the language with which children had less experience. Thus, based on the data available to date, morphosyntactic development in simultaneous bilingual children is expected to be *generally* similar to that of monolingual peers in *at least one language* (but not necessarily in both languages).

Second language learners typically require several years to master certain grammatical structures in their second language, especially for forms that differ from the morphosyntactic features of their first language (Paradis *et al.*, 2011). The morphosyntax of the first language will be similar to that of monolinguals, although in situations where children's language experience shifts to being primarily in the second language, there may be a plateau or some degree of attrition (Anderson, 2012).

Pragmatics is another area in which there are many commonalities but also differences between multilinguals and monolinguals. For example, children from bilingual homes and communities often code-switch, using both languages with other bilingual speakers for many purposes, including pragmatic effects such as expressing closeness (Paradis *et al.*, 2011). As Stokes and Madhani point out, code-switching with other bilingual speakers is a skill, not an indication of deficiency.

Although consideration of all languages a multilingual child speaks is necessary for diagnostic evaluations, the issue of normative samples is very complex for multilinguals (Pearson, 2013). Given the diversity in multilingual children's circumstances, it is particularly challenging to identify peers in order to determine if language is progressing as expected – a child who is a simultaneous learner of Spanish and English is very different from a child who learns Cantonese at home and then learns French in school. Although some bilingual tests have been developed for specific populations (e.g. the

Bilingual English–Spanish Assessment in the United States, Peña *et al.*, 2014), it isn't feasible to develop norms for every language combination. Therefore, alternative assessment approaches are needed.

Alternative assessment includes a broad range of approaches, including language-processing tasks and DA. Non-word repetition (NWR), a language-processing task in which children are asked to repeat nonsense words of increasing length, has been advocated for use with multilingual populations. The advantage of NWR is that accuracy of response does not depend upon the child's knowledge of specific vocabulary. However, because there are language-specific influences on children's performance on NWR, language-specific stimuli and norms have been developed for a variety of languages including English, French, Greek, Italian and Spanish (Windsor *et al.*, 2010). For bilingual children, the diagnostic accuracy of NWR has varied widely across studies. Elin Thordardottir (2014b) reported 85% sensitivity and 79% specificity for NWR in French among French–English simultaneous bilingual children. Gutierrez-Clellen and Simon-Cerejido (2010) found that considering performance on NWR in both languages for Spanish–English sequential bilinguals resulted in higher specificity than single language NWR performance, even for NWR in the child's stronger language. That is, fewer typically developing bilingual children were misidentified as having a language impairment if the criterion was scoring low on *both* the English NWR and the Spanish NWR tasks. However, in their study, the sensitivity of NWR scores was low, indicating a likelihood of underidentification of language impairment. Rodriguez (Chapter 10) reports that the sensitivity of NWR varies with young Spanish-speaking children, depending on the scoring method used. Overall, NWR shows promise as a diagnostic tool, but diagnostic accuracy varies across studies.

In contrast with NWR and other approaches, which seek to reduce the role of language-specific knowledge, children are taught new language skills in DA, in which the focus is not on what the child already knows, but on the child's response to instruction. In general, DA measures focus on the child's responses during instruction and/or the child's ability to transfer newly learned skills to untaught instances, although the teaching frameworks and measures used in DA vary widely (Patterson *et al.*, 2013). Although the literature is limited, there is evidence of acceptable diagnostic accuracy for DA in children from culturally and linguistically diverse backgrounds on a variety of tasks, including novel word learning in preschool children (Kapatzoglou *et al.*, 2012) and producing narratives in school-age children (Peña *et al.*, 2006).

In summary, in addition to the guidelines and resources for the assessment of children who speak languages other than English provided by the authors of chapters in this book, additional considerations are necessary when assessing bilingual (and by extension, multilingual) children. It is important that assessments include all languages with which a child has significant experience. Because the performance of multilingual children is not accurately portrayed by comparing their performance to monolingual norms for diagnostic purposes, tools developed for bilingual/multilingual children are needed, including alternative assessment approaches, and the use of multiple sources of information and tools is necessary.

Intervention

Providing appropriate intervention services to multilingual children and their families requires the integration of clinical and family perspectives with evidence from research (van Kleeck *et al.*, 2010). However, there is limited research on many aspects of language intervention, particularly for children from multilingual backgrounds. The authors in this book provide evidence-based intervention recommendations and strategies for putting widely recognized principles of intervention into practice with multilingual populations by considering family, community and wider cultural contexts. Thorne and Coggins (Chapter 4) highlight the importance of using evidence-based approaches to intervention whenever possible, and they review research on the efficacy of several intervention programs and methods for children with FASD. They also discuss the importance of environmental modifications, and involving and educating parents and teachers of children with FASD so that they can understand and more effectively support children in complex social and linguistic situations.

Linguistic and cultural considerations

Providing appropriate intervention services requires that we target linguistically and culturally relevant skills for multilingual children. Intervention with multilingual children will be misguided if we focus on parallels to English language structures and the pragmatic conventions of particular English-speaking communities, a point that Elin Thordardottir (Chapter 8) makes in discussing the need for language measures that are appropriate to particular language(s) that children and their families speak. For example, case marking on nouns is an important feature of many languages, including Turkish, but English-based assessment tools are not designed to focus on noun case markings. Therefore, Topbaş and Maviş (Chapter 9) have designed and used assessment tools that focus on forms that are important in Turkish, including children's use of case markers, such as the accusative (indicating the noun is the direct object) and the dative suffix (indicating the noun is the indirect object or something given).

Because assessments that are appropriate for the child's language(s) will inform clinicians about the child's strengths and weaknesses in areas relevant to the languages she or he is acquiring, language-appropriate measures are a key to intervention planning. In addition, because forms vary across dialects, it is important to also consider the specific variety of the language spoken, as Rodríguez (Chapter 10) points out in her discussion of dialectal differences in Puerto Rican and Mexican varieties of Spanish.

Cultural factors and family perspectives also are essential in designing intervention plans that are relevant and appropriate for children and families. Identifying important daily activities, potential barriers to participating in those activities and the skills necessary to effectively communicate in family, community and school contexts requires considering cultural and family-specific factors (Westby, 2009). For school-age children, cultural variation in teacher expectations and strategies, as well as children's background and experiences are important considerations in planning intervention to support children's success in school (Westby, 2006).

Differences within broadly defined cultural and linguistic groups are important to consider in order to provide services appropriate to individual children and families. For example, there is extensive variability in cultural beliefs, practices, values and educational experiences among Spanish-speaking families in the United States (Rodriguez & Olswang, 2002). To (Chapter 6) discusses assessment and intervention implications for families with traditional Chinese roles while also noting that cultural change over time may occur due to modifications in larger societal policies and practices. Given the variability and change in cultural systems, how should clinicians incorporate cultural considerations when working with individual families? Stokes and Madhani (Chapter 7) present a framework for determining the focus of intervention within a family-centered approach to early intervention and they illustrate with a case example of a young child in a Gujarati-speaking family living in London.

Collaborative service delivery

Even multilingual SLPs and other multilingual professionals will not be able to speak the language of every child and family needing services. Fortunately, recommended practices for language intervention are collaborative in nature for monolingual as well as multilingual children (ASHA, 2010; Damico et al., 1996; Patterson, 2012; Woods et al., 2011). Through collaboration with teachers, parents, siblings, peers and others, SLP services address language learning and language use in children's daily lives, regardless of the language(s) of the child and family. However, collaborative strategies and roles in intervention will vary. In some families, parents may become the primary agents of language intervention with young children and may provide significant support for schoolwork. However, in other families, this may not be congruent with family roles and values, and other family members such as older siblings, grandparents or aunts and uncles may have an important role (Rodriguez, Chapter 10; Westby, 2009). In preschool and school settings, paraprofessionals who speak the child's language are often a key resource, as are the child's typically developing peers (Kohnert, 2013).

In addition to working with a variety of collaborators to deliver services, it may be necessary to adapt intervention approaches for cultural congruence. For instance, adult responsivity, which includes specific strategies such as 'following the child's lead', has been demonstrated to have positive effects on communication and language development (e.g. Brady *et al.*, 2014). Following the child's lead is an important principle that is widely implemented in early intervention, but because it may not be a good fit with many families' expectations for the roles of children and adults, adaptations may be needed (To, Chapter 6; van Kleeck, 1994; Westby, 2009). Providing preschool children with experiences with decontextualized language use is another area in which research-based recommendations may need to be adapted for some families. For families in which early literacy activities and decontextualized language experiences are limited, van Kleeck (2013) suggests that instead of asking families to alter interaction patterns within their existing routines, they recommend that the family *add* routines that are explicitly presented to prepare children for school. This would maintain the family's style of interaction in daily life while also providing experiences with decontextualized and early literacy use. Van Kleeck's suggestions illustrate an integrated approach to evidence-based practice, starting with research-based evidence of the importance of early literacy and decontextualized language experiences, and making recommendations that are based on the clinician's knowledge of cultural and linguistic diversity, while taking individual family's lives and preferences into account.

Languages and targets of intervention for bilingual and multilingual children

What language(s) should be supported and included in intervention for bilingual and multilingual children with language disorders? Because there is very little research on intervention with children who speak three or more languages, it is currently necessary to rely primarily on what is known about intervention with bilingual children as a guideline for working with multilingual children. The literature indicates that both (or all) languages with which the child has significant experience should be supported in intervention. Children with language disorders can and do become bilingual and the degree of delay and general profiles of strengths and weaknesses are similar in bilingual and monolingual children with language disorders, including children with DS (Kay-Raining Bird, Chapter 3) and children with ASD (Marinova-Todd and Mirenda, Chapter 2). Marinova-Todd and Mirenda discuss the potential negative effects of the advice to use only one language with children with ASD; advice which is frequently given to families in spite of the research evidence. Language intervention that includes both languages results in equal or superior progress in the child's second language as well as advances in the child's first language compared to monolingual intervention for typically developing sequential bilingual preschoolers (Lugo-Neris *et al.*, 2010) and bilingual preschool children with language impairment (Pham *et al.*, 2013; Restrepo *et al.*, 2013). Stokes and Madhani (Chapter 7) point out that speech-language therapists may need to educate families on the evidence that a bilingual approach to intervention is effective so that families can make informed choices.

What do we target in each language when working with bilingual (and multilingual) children? Kohnert (2013: 189) states that '…if we want children to develop the skills necessary to be successful communicators in their different language environments, we should provide appropriate scaffolding and explicitly incorporate both languages and different settings…'. Widespread generalization of skills from one language to another without support in each language is unlikely to occur in children with language disorders. Even typically developing bilingual school-age children need training to use knowledge of a word in one language to infer the meaning of a related word in the other language, such as the English word 'amorous' and Spanish 'amor' (Carlo *et al.*, 2004). However, there is some evidence that for sequential bilingual children, teaching a word in the stronger language first results in faster learning of the word in the second language (Perozzi & Sanchez, 1992) and providing elaborative information in children's first language improves learning target words in the second language among typically developing preschool children (Lugo-Neris *et al.*, 2010). Thus, although there is no evidence of 'automatic' generalization from one language to the other, teaching in both languages benefits both the first and second languages in preschool and school-age bilinguals. In some instances, the amount of teaching needed in the second language may be relatively minimal for more advanced semantic skills such as including superordinate terms when defining words (e.g. a rose is a type of flower). In such cases, children may not need to learn the strategy anew for each language, even though they need language-specific vocabulary and forms to do the task in each language.

In the area of morphosyntax, it is possible that intervention targeting forms in one language may enhance or hasten learning of similar forms in another language. However, specific forms such as verb markers are not acquired at the same time in both languages in French–English simultaneous learners, indicating a lack of transfer across languages in typical development (Elin Thordardottir, 2014b). Although it is possible that in limited situations, with some supports, transfer might occur for very similar intervention targets, such as learning noun plural –s in

Spanish facilitating learning noun plural –s in English, there is little or no research on this issue for morphosyntactic forms. Furthermore, there are many forms that are not similar across languages, even for fairly closely related languages, and in many language pairs there are very few closely related forms. Even in languages such as Spanish and English, which have many similarities, many morphosyntactic aspects of each language are not shared and these may be important to target. Thus, a bilingual assessment is needed to identify appropriate targets for each language and, more generally, to formulate a complete intervention plan.

Intervention targeting narratives illustrates both language-general and language-specific considerations. Gutierrez-Clellen (2012) points out that learning skills such as providing sufficient background knowledge for listeners or readers, including narrative elements such as settings, problems and goal-directed actions in stories, and making chronological sequences clear, will probably transfer broadly to telling narratives in any language, although the specific linguistic means for doing so will differ from one language to the next. For example, children must learn how to introduce characters and how to refer to them subsequently, regardless of the language of narration. However, in English pronouns often are used to refer to characters after they are first mentioned, but in Spanish subject ellipsis is often appropriate after a character is introduced, depending on the context. Furthermore, there are cross-cultural differences in narrative conventions, so some children may need to learn different storytelling conventions for school and for home and other community settings (Westby, 2009). Thus, a complete intervention plan targeting narratives for a bilingual child would support storytelling in both languages in relevant settings, although some skills will transfer from one language and one setting to the next. Almost certainly, collaboration with family and school personnel will be needed to support narrative development in ways that are appropriate to each language and for the important settings in a child's life. More generally, as many authors have noted (e.g. Damico *et al.*, 1996; Kohnert, 2013), collaboration in creating and implementing intervention is essential for providing appropriate services to children from diverse cultural and linguistic backgrounds.

Concluding Remarks

Providing appropriate clinical services and conducting meaningful research require breadth of perspective and consideration of specific cultural, linguistic and individual circumstances. We hope that the information on diverse languages, cultures, clinical populations and clinical contexts presented in this volume will stimulate thoughtful clinical practices and further research in language disorders in multilingual populations.

References

American Speech-Language-Hearing Association (ASHA) (2010) Roles and responsibilities of speech-language pathologists in schools (Professional Issues Statement). See www.asha.org/policy (accessed 15 May 2015).

Anderson, R.T. (2012) First language loss in Spanish-speaking children: Patterns of loss and implications for clinical practice. In B. Goldstein (ed.) *Bilingual Language Development and Disorders in Spanish-English Speakers* (2nd edn; pp. 193–212). Baltimore, MD: Brookes.

Bates, E., Wulfeck, B. and MacWhinney, B. (1991) Cross-linguistic research in aphasia: An overview. *Brain and Language* 41, 123–148.

Bedore, L.D., Peña, E.M., Garcia, M. and Cortez, C. (2005) Conceptual versus monolingual scoring: When does it make a difference? *Language, Speech, and Hearing Services in Schools* 36, 188–200.

Brady, L., Warren, S.F., Fleming, K., Keller, J. and Sterling, A. (2014) Effect of sustained maternal responsivity on later vocabulary development in children with Fragile X syndrome. *Journal of Speech, Language, and Hearing Research* 57, 212–226.

Bright, W (1996) The Devanagari script. In P. Daniels and W. Bright (eds) *The World's Writing Systems* (pp. 384–390). Oxford: Oxford University Press.

Brinton, B. and Fujiki, M. (1999) Social interactional behaviors of children with specific language impairment. *Topics in Language Disorders* 19, 49–69.

Cardona, G. (1990) Sanskrit. In B. Comrie (ed.) *The World's Major Languages* (pp. 448–469). New York: Oxford University Press.

Carlo, M.S., August, D., McLaughlin, B., Snow, C.E., Dressler, C. and Lippman, D.N. (2004) Closing the gap: Addressing the vocabulary needs of English-language learners in bilingual and mainstream classrooms. *Reading Research Quarterly* 39, 188–215.

Conti-Ramsden, G. and Botting, N. (2004) Social difficulties and victimization in children with at 11 years of age. *Journal of Speech, Language, and Hearing Research* 47, 145–161.

Core, C., Hoff, E., Rumiche, R. and Señor, M. (2013) Total and conceptual vocabulary in Spanish-English bilinguals from 22 to 30 months: Implications for assessment. *Journal of Speech, Language, and Hearing Research* 56, 1637–1649.

Cummins, J. (1991) Interdependence of first and second language proficiency in bilingual children. In E. Bialystok (ed.) *Language Processing in Bilingual Children* (pp. 70–89). New York: Cambridge University Press.

Damico, J.S., Smith, M. and Augustine, L.E. (1996) Multicultural populations and language disorders. In M. Smith and J.S. Damico (eds) *Childhood Language Disorders* (pp. 272–299). New York: Thieme.

Elin Thordardottir (2014a) The relationship between bilingual exposure and morphosyntactic development. *International Journal of Speech-Language Pathology* 17 (2), 97–114. DOI: 10.3109/17549507.2014.923509.

Elin Thordardottir (2014b) The typical development of simultaneous bilinguals. In T. Grüter and J. Paradis (eds) *Input and Experience in Bilingual Development* (pp. 141–160). Philadelphia, PA: John Benjamins.

Gray, S., Plante, E., Vance, R. and Henrichsen, M. (1999) The diagnostic accuracy of four vocabulary tests administered to preschool-age children. *Language, Speech, and Hearing Services in Schools* 30, 196–206.

Gross, M., Buac, M. and Kaushanskaya, M. (2014) Conceptual scoring of receptive and expressive vocabulary measures in simultaneous and sequential bilingual children. *American Journal of Speech-Language Pathology* 23 (4), 574–586. DOI 10.1044/2014_AJSLP-13-0026.

Gutierrez-Clellen, V.F. (2012) Narrative development and disorders in bilingual children. In B. Goldstein (ed.) *Bilingual Language Development and Disorders in Spanish-English Speakers* (2nd edn; pp. 233–249). Baltimore, MD: Brookes.

Gutierrez-Clellen, V.F. and Simon-Cerejido, G. (2010) Using nonword repetition tasks for the identification of language impairment in Spanish-English-speaking children: Does the language of assessment matter? *Learning Disabilities Research and Practice* 25, 48–58.

Katagiri, Y. (2007) Dialogue functions of Japanese sentence-final particles 'Yo' and 'Ne'. *Journal of Pragmatics* 39, 1313–1323.

Katpantzoglou, M., Restrepo, M.A. and Thompson, M.S. (2012) Dynamic assessment of word learning skills: Identifying language impairment in bilingual children. *Language, Speech, and Hearing Services in Schools* 43, 81–96.

Klaiman, M.H. (1990) Bengali. In B. Comrie (ed.) *The World's Major Languages* (pp. 490–513). New York: Oxford University Press.

Kohnert, K. (2013) *Language Disorders in Bilingual Children and Adults* (2nd edn). San Diego, CA: Plural Publishing.

Leonard, L. (1990) The cross-linguistic study of language-impaired children. In J. Miller (ed.) *Research on Child Language Disorders* (pp. 379–386). Austin, TX: Pro-Ed.

Leonard, L. (2009) Cross-linguistic studies of language disorders. In R. Schwartz (ed.) *Handbook of Child Language Disorders* (pp. 308–324). New York: Psychology Press.

Leonard, L. (2014) *Children with Specific Language Impairment* (2nd edn). Cambridge, MA: MIT Press.

Lugo-Neris, M.J., Jackson, C.W. and Goldstein, H. (2010) Facilitating vocabulary acquisition of young English language learners. *Language, Speech, and Hearing Services in Schools* 41, 314–327.

Nelson, N.W. (2010) *Language and Literacy Disorders: Infancy through Adolescence*. Boston, MA: Allyn & Bacon.

Ordóñez, C.L., Carlo, M.S., Snow, C.E. and McLaughlin, B. (2002) Depth and breadth of vocabulary in two languages: Which vocabulary skills transfer? *Journal of Educational Psychology* 94, 719–728.

Paradis, J. (2010) The interface between bilingual development and specific language impairment. *Applied Psycholinguistics* 31, 227–252.

Paradis, J., Genesee, F. and Crago, M.B. (2011) *Dual Language Development and Disorders* (2nd edn). Baltimore, MD: Brookes.

Patterson, J.L. (1998) Expressive vocabulary development and word combinations of Spanish-English bilingual children. *American Journal of Speech-Language Pathology* 7 (4), 46–56.

Patterson, J.L. (2012) Teacher perceptions of preschool children's communication in a bilingual setting. *Journal of Interactional Research in Communication Disorders* 3, 71–90.

Patterson, J.L. and Pearson, B.Z. (2012) Bilingual lexical development, assessment, and intervention. In B. Goldstein (ed.) *Bilingual Language Development and Disorders in Spanish-English Speakers* (2nd edn; pp. 113–129). Baltimore, MD: Brookes.

Patterson, J.L., Rodríguez, B.L. and Dale, P.S. (2013) Response to dynamic language tasks among typically developing Latino preschool children with bilingual experience. *American Journal of Speech-Language Pathology* 22, 103–112.

Paul, R. and Norbury, C. (2012) *Language Disorders from Infancy through Adolescence*. St. Louis, MO: Elsevier.

Pearson, B.Z. (2013) Distinguishing the bilingual as a late talker from the late talker who is bilingual. In L.A. Rescorla and P.S. Dale (eds) *Late Talkers: Language Development, Interventions, and Outcomes* (pp. 67–87). Baltimore, MD: Brookes.

Pearson, B.Z., Fernández, S. and Oller, D.K. (1993) Lexical development in bilingual infants and toddlers: Comparison to monolingual norms. *Language Learning* 43, 93–120.

Peña, E.D., Gillam, R.B., Bedore, L.M. and Bohman, T.M. (2011) Risk for poor performance on a language screening measure for bilingual preschoolers and kindergarteners. *American Journal of Speech-Language Pathology* 20, 302–314.

Peña, E.D., Gillam, R.B., Malek, M., Ruiz-Felter, R., Resendiz, M., Fiestas, C. and Sabel, T. (2006) Dynamic assessment of school-age children's narrative ability: An experimental investigation of classification accuracy. *Journal of Speech, Language, and Hearing Research* 49, 1037–1057.

Peña, E.D., Gutiérrez-Clellen, V.F., Iglesias, A., Goldstein, B.A. and Bedore, L.M. (2014) *BESA: Bilingual English-Spanish Assessment*. San Rafael, CA: AR-Clinical Publications.

Perozzi, J. and Sanchez, M. (1992) The effect of instruction in L1 on receptive acquisition of L2 for bilingual children with language delay. *Language, Speech, and Hearing Services in Schools* 23, 348–352.

Pham, G., Kohnert, K. and Mann, D. (2011) Addressing clinician–client mismatch: A preliminary intervention study with a bilingual Vietnamese–English preschooler. *Language, Speech, and Hearing Services in Schools* 42, 408–422.

Restrepo, M.A. (1998) Identifiers of predominantly Spanish-speaking children with language impairment. *Journal of Speech, Language, and Hearing Research* 46, 1398–1411.

Restrepo, M.A. and Gutiérrez-Clellen, V.F. (2012) Grammatical impairments in bilingual children. In B. Goldstein (ed.) *Bilingual Language Development and Disorders in Spanish-English Speakers* (2nd edn; pp. 213–232). Baltimore, MD: Brookes.

Restrepo, M.A., Morgan, G.P. and Thompson, M.S. (2013) The efficacy of a vocabulary intervention for dual-language learners with language impairment. *Journal of Speech, Language, and Hearing Research* 56, 748–765.

Rodríguez, B. and Olswang, L.B. (2002) Cultural diversity is more than group differences: An example from the Hispanic community. *Contemporary Issues in Communication Science and Disorders* 29, 154–164.

SALT (2012) Systematic Analysis of Language Transcripts (SALT). (Computer software.) Madison, WI: SALT Software.

Slobin, D.I. (1985) Cross-linguistic evidence for the language-making capacity. In D. Slobin (ed.) *The Crosslinguistic Study of Language Acquisition, Vol. 2: Theoretical Issues* (pp. 1157–1256). Hillsdale, NJ: Lawrence Erlbaum Associates.

Umbel, V.M., Pearson, B.Z., Fernández, M.C. and Oller, K.D. (1992) Measuring bilingual children's receptive vocabularies. *Child Development* 63, 1012–1020.

van Kleeck, A. (1994) Potential cultural bias in training parents as conversational partners with their language-delayed children. *American Journal of Speech-Language Pathology* 3, 67–78.

van Kleeck, A. (2013) Guiding parents from diverse cultural backgrounds to promote language skills in preschoolers with language disorders: Two challenges and proposed solutions for them. *Perspectives on Language Learning and Education* August, 78–85.

van Kleeck, A., Schwartz, A.L., Fey, M., Kaiser, A., Miller, J. and Weitzman, E. (2010) Should we use telegraphic or grammatical input in the early stages of language development with children who have language impairments? A meta-analysis of the research and expert opinion. *American Journal of Speech-Language Pathology* 19, 3–21.

Westby, C. (2006) There's more to passing than knowing the answers: Learning to do school. In T. Ukrainetz (ed.) *Contextualized Language Intervention* (pp. 319–387). Eau Claire, WI: Thinking Publications.

Westby, C. (2009) Considerations in working successfully with culturally/linguistically diverse families in assessment and intervention of communication disorders. *Seminars in Speech and Language* 30, 279–289.

Windsor, J., Kohnert, K., Lobitz, K. and Pham, G. (2010) Cross-language nonword repetition by bilingual and monolingual children. *American Journal of Speech-Language Pathology* 19, 298–310.

Woods, J.J., Wilcox, M.J., Friedman, M. and Murch, T. (2011) Collaborative consultation in natural environments: Strategies to enhance family-centered supports and services. *Language, Speech, and Hearing Services in Schools* 42, 379–392.

Part 1

Language Disorders in Specific Clinical Populations

2 Language and Communication Abilities of Bilingual Children with Autism Spectrum Disorders

Stefka H. Marinova-Todd and
Pat Mirenda

Introduction

More than half of the world's population uses two or more languages (Grosjean, 2010). In Canada, 20% of the population speaks a language in addition to one of the two official languages, French and English, in their homes (Statistics Canada, 2011). As bilingualism becomes more prevalent, so does the research in language development comparing monolingual and bilingual children (Scheele *et al.*, 2010). The number of children diagnosed with autism spectrum disorder (ASD) is also on the rise. As of 2012, it was estimated that the prevalence rate of ASD was 1 in every 88 people (Centers for Disease Control and Prevention, 2012). However, little research has focused on the effect of bilingualism on the language development of children with ASD or other developmental disabilities.

Families of children with ASD who are exposed to two or more languages are often advised by child development professionals to speak only one language to their child (Kremer-Sadlik, 2005; Yu, 2013). This recommendation is usually based on the belief that exposing children with ASD to two languages will have a negative impact on their language development, as they already experience significant challenges in this area (Hambly & Fombonne, 2012; Yu, 2013). However, previous research examining the effects of bilingualism on the language development of children with language impairments associated with other developmental disabilities (e.g. specific language impairment, Down syndrome) has found that bilingual exposure does not have a negative impact on their development and that these children have the capacity to become bilingual (Kay-Raining Bird *et al.*, 2005; Paradis *et al.*, 2003). Similarly, a small number of recent studies on bilingual populations with ASD have shown the same trend (Hambly & Fombonne, 2012; Ohashi *et al.*, 2012; Petersen *et al.*, 2012). Because the amount of research on bilingual populations is very limited, additional research in this area is needed in order to better understand the effect of bilingual exposure and to provide high-quality therapy to children in this population.

Autism spectrum disorder

In the *Diagnostic and Statistical Manual of Mental Disorders*, 5th edition (DSM-5; American Psychiatric Association, 2013), the term *autism spectrum disorder* was introduced to consolidate several diagnostic categories defined in the previous DSM. These categories included autistic disorder, pervasive developmental disorder-not otherwise specified (PDD-NOS), Asperger's disorder and childhood disintegrative disorder. In addition, the DSM-5 also introduced a new set of diagnostic criteria for ASD, including the presence of symptoms in early childhood and a requirement that symptoms be severe enough to impair daily functioning. Perhaps more importantly, social and communication symptoms – previously considered separately – were combined into one category with three symptom subgroups, all three of which must be present for a diagnosis. They include (a) deficits in *social-emotional reciprocity* (e.g. ranging from total lack of social initiation to a failure to engage in normal back-and-forth conversations); (b) deficits in *non-verbal communicative behaviors used for social interaction* (ranging from total lack of facial expression or gestures to poorly integrated verbal and non-verbal communication); and (c) deficits in *developing and maintaining relationships appropriate to developmental level* (ranging from an apparent absence of interest in people to difficulties adjusting behavior to suit different social contexts). Finally, symptoms related to repetitive patterns of behavior, interests or activities are described in four subgroups, at least two of which must be present for a diagnosis. The subgroups include (a) stereotyped or repetitive motor movements, use of objects or speech (e.g. echolalia, idiosyncratic phrases); (b) excessive adherence to routines, ritualized patterns of verbal or non-verbal behavior or excessive resistance to change; (c) highly restricted, fixated interests that are abnormal in intensity or focus; and (d) hyper- or hyporeactivity to sensory input or unusual interest in sensory aspects of an environment. All four criteria – symptoms evident in early childhood; severity sufficient to impact daily functioning; symptoms present in all three social communication subgroups; and symptoms present in at least two of the four restricted, repetitive behavior subgroups – are required for a diagnosis of ASD. If an individual meets the first three ASD criteria but not the fourth (i.e. restricted, repetitive behavior), he or she can be assigned a diagnosis that is new to the DSM-5: social communication disorder (SCD).

Language and Communication Patterns Among English-Speaking Children with ASD

There is a significant body of evidence regarding the communication abilities of monolingual English-speaking children with ASD. Overall, research has shown that many children with ASD begin speaking late and develop speech at a significantly slower rate than typically developing (TD) children (Tager-Flusberg *et al.*, 2005). There is a significant correlation between IQ and language outcomes in children with ASD, although higher levels of non-verbal IQ are not always associated with higher-level language skills (Howlin *et al.*, 2004). A small percentage of children with ASD (estimates range from 10% to 25%; Mirenda *et al.*, 2013) never acquire functional speech or language. In this section, we briefly review some of the research that has examined the language and communication abilities of children with ASD, specifically in terms of lexical development, narrative skills and preliteracy skills such as phonological awareness (PA).

Lexical development

The developmental course for individuals with ASD, particularly in the domain of lexical development, appears similar to that of TD children. For some children with ASD (i.e. those with IQ scores that are close to 100 or above; Baron-Cohen *et al.*, 2005), vocabulary is an area of strength, as they tend to achieve high scores on standardized vocabulary assessments (Tager-Flusberg *et al.*, 2005). However, the acquisition of words that map onto mental state concepts and socio-emotional terms tend to pose greater difficulties in this population (Tager-Flusberg *et al.*, 2005). In addition, errors with temporal and spatial expressions (e.g. now/later, this/that, here/there) are relatively common (Perkins *et al.*, 2006), as are pronoun reversal errors (e.g. I/you; Tager-Flusberg *et al.*, 2005). These errors are generally seen as a difficulty with *deixis* – a term derived from the Greek word for pointing and indicating. Hobson *et al.* (2010: 403) described deictic words as 'person-centered', in that their meanings 'are related to the vantage points of the speaker who utters the terms and the listener who interprets them'. Recent research suggests that many of the lexical/semantic errors that are common in individuals with ASD stem from a delay in their acquisition of theory of mind – the ability to understand that others experience mental states that are different from one's own (Hale & Tager-Flusberg, 2005; Tager-Flusberg, 2007).

Narrative ability

Narrative abilities have been studied more extensively in this population as storytelling provides an insight into how children with ASD use language for communicative purposes. Previous research has shown that children with ASD who are verbal tend to have relatively intact, although often delayed, lexical, phonological, morphological and syntactic development, but have significant pragmatic deficits, such as rigid speech, difficulty organizing discourse and limited conversation skills (Diehl *et al.*, 2006; Tager-Flusberg *et al.*, 2005). Therefore, narratives provide a good venue for investigating the nature of the linguistic, social and cognitive deficits typically associated with autism (e.g. Capps *et al.*, 2000; Loveland *et al.*, 1990; Norbury & Bishop, 2003; Tager-Flusberg, 1995). Moreover, an analysis of narratives can provide an insight into the theory of mind hypothesis of autism, as described previously (e.g. Loveland & Tunali, 1993; Tager-Flusberg, 1995). Telling a story requires the narrator not only to tell the listener what happens in the story, but also to understand and interpret characters' mental states and ensure that the listener understands the story and is engaged in it.

There is limited but growing research evidence on the narrative abilities of children with ASD. Research to date has focused on basic measures of story length, narrative structure, cohesion and evaluation, and on narrative performance in relation to theory of mind. Generally, children with ASD are more likely to exhibit pragmatic violations and to include 'bizarre' or inappropriate information in their stories; they are also less likely to take their listeners' perspectives into account (Loveland *et al.*, 1990; Loveland & Tunali, 1993; Norbury & Bishop, 2003). Findings from a few studies suggest that individuals with ASD might be deficient not only in their awareness of listeners' needs, but also in their awareness of the cultural perspectives that often underlie the telling of stories (Bruner & Feldman, 1993; Loveland *et al.*, 1990; Loveland & Tunali, 1993). The relationship between narrative ability and cognitive ability is unclear, as few studies have examined narratives both in children with limited cognitive abilities (e.g. Capps *et al.*, 2000; Tager-Flusberg, 1995) and children who are more able (e.g. Losh & Capps, 2003; Norbury & Bishop, 2003).

Phonological awareness

PA consists of a subset of metalinguistic skills that result in the ability to identify and manipulate individual phonemes and syllabic structures in a spoken language (Nagy, 2007). PA skills have been shown to play an important role in the process of learning to read and write in an alphabetic system (Adams, 1992; Liberman *et al.*, 1989). Moreover, PA has been established as an essential precursor to the development of both reading (Bradley & Bryant, 1983; Stanovich, 1985) and spelling (Ehri, 2000; Treiman, 1984).

Several studies of monolingual children with ASD have included PA tasks as one component of a reading assessment and have revealed somewhat conflicting results. Heimann *et al.* (1995) were primarily interested in the effects of computer-aided instruction on teaching reading and writing. Their sample included 11 Swedish children with ASD, 9 children with mixed disabilities and 10 TD children, with chronological ages from 6 to 13 years. As part of their measures, they included an experimental task of PA, namely sound blending. Results indicated that, perhaps not surprisingly, the children in both disability groups had significantly lower PA scores than TD children, both before and after intervention. Similarly, a study by Gabig (2010) aimed to examine whether the strong association between PA skills and early word reading observed in TD children is similarly present in young children with ASD. Her sample included 14 children with ASD between the ages of 5 and 7 years 11 months, and 10 TD children who were matched on chronological age to the children with ASD. As a measure of PA, two subtests of the Comprehensive Test of Phonological Processing (CTOPP; Wagner *et al.*, 1999) were used, namely elision (i.e. sound and syllable deletion) and sound blending (i.e. sound and syllable combination). In addition, the children were also given standardized measures of word and non-word reading. The results revealed that the children with ASD had scores on the PA tasks that were significantly below those of the control group, although their word reading skills were equivalent to those of the control group.

Based on the two studies presented above, it appears that PA is an area of weakness for children with ASD, although it does not seem to affect their reading skills to the same extent as in TD children. In other words, children with ASD who score low on PA tasks are still able to perform at the same levels as age-matched TD children on reading tasks.

A different set of studies showed that there is an association between PA and reading ability in children with ASD. Newman *et al.* (2007: 761) were primarily interested in understanding the reading profile of individuals with ASD and hyperlexia, which they defined as a 'discrepancy between word-level decoding and comprehension'. They compared PA and other reading-related skills of individuals with ASD and hyperlexia ($n = 20$), ASD without hyperlexia ($n = 20$) and TD children ($n = 18$). Participants in the first two groups were matched by gender and chronological age (which ranged from 3 to 19 years) and the children in the control group were matched by single-word reading ability. As a measure of PA, they used the sound awareness subtest from the Woodcock–Johnson Tests of Achievement–III (Woodcock *et al.*, 2001) which includes tasks of rhyming, sound deletion, sound substitution and sound reversal within words. While the results showed that the participants with ASD and hyperlexia performed as well on the PA tasks as those in the control group and better than those without hyperlexia, the authors noted that the very young age of five of the hyperlexic children (age 5 and under) prevented accurate assessment of their skills in this area. Nonetheless, the overall results were echoed in two recent studies conducted in the United Kingdom (White et al., 2006) and Sweden (Åsberg & Dahlgren-Sandberg, 2012). Among other measures, White et al. administered a battery of PA tasks to measure rhyming ability, spoonerisms (i.e. errors in which the initial sounds of words are transposed, such as in no tails for toenails), non-word reading (e.g. muftig) and rapid automatic word naming. Åsberg and Dahlgren-Sandberg assessed rapid naming, sound deletion and both word and non-word spoonerisms. The results of both studies indicated that good readers with ASD performed as well as TD children on PA tasks. However, poor readers with ASD and children with dyslexia (White et al., 2006) performed worse than controls in both studies.

In summary, the research available on the PA skills of children with ASD suggests that good (or hyperlexic) readers with ASD and good readers who are TD do not differ significantly with regard to PA skills. However, unlike TD children, good reading ability is not necessarily associated with good performance on PA tasks for children with ASD. Therefore, more research on the PA skills of this population is needed in order to establish the exact role of PA in the reading abilities of children with ASD.

Language and Communication Patterns Among Bilingual Children with ASD

Only a handful of studies to date have sought to compare language development in monolingual and bilingual children with ASD. In the most comprehensive and large-scale study to date, Hambly and Fombonne (2012) recruited 75 children with ASD between the ages of 36 and 78 months from families residing in the Canadian provinces of Quebec or Ontario. Of these children, 30 were exposed to English, French or Spanish only, and 45 were exposed to two or three languages (i.e. either English or French plus a minority language; or English and French plus a minority language). The children who were exposed to two or three languages were further divided into two groups, namely simultaneous or sequential bilinguals, based on the age of exposure to the second language (i.e. before or after 12 months of age). Only children who spoke languages in which assessment measures were available in all languages spoken at home were recruited for the bilingual group.

Parents completed the MacArthur Communicative Development Inventory: Words and Sentences (MCDI; Fenson et al., 1993) in all of the languages spoken at home. In the sample, these languages included French, English, Chinese, Farsi, Hebrew, Italian, Romanian, Spanish and/or Tamil. Parents also completed a Family Background Information Questionnaire (Hambly & Fombonne, 2005) and a language environment interview that was developed specifically for the study. In addition, trained research assistants contacted the families by phone to complete the Vineland Adaptive Behavior Scales-Second Edition (VABS-II; Sparrow et al., 2005) and specific questions from the Autism Diagnostic Interview-Revised (ADI-R; LeCouteur et al., 2003). Maternal language fluency in all languages spoken in the home was also assessed during a phone interview.

Based on parent reports on the MCDI, a total conceptual vocabulary (TCV) score was calculated for the bilingual children, using the procedures described by Pearson et al. (1993). Words reported in both languages were mapped to each other so that translation-equivalent word forms were only counted once even when used in two or more languages. Then, data from the three participant groups (i.e. monolinguals, sequential bilinguals and simultaneous bilinguals) were compared using a series of one-way analyses of variance (ANOVAs). Expressive language variables included (a) the child's overall level of speech production, from the ADI-R; (b) the VABS-II expressive language subscale score; (c) the TCV score; (d) the number of words produced in the dominant language(s); and (e) the number of words produced in the minority language; the latter three variables were from the MCDI. Receptive language variables included (a) the child's overall level of language comprehension, from the ADI-R; and (b) the VABS-II receptive language subscale score. Results indicated that the monolingual and bilingual children had similar results on all measures of receptive and expressive language and reached the early language milestones at around the same age. Moreover, regardless of the type of bilingual exposure (i.e. simultaneous or sequential), no significant differences were found between the language skills of the monolingual and bilingual participants. The only significant difference was found in families in which mothers were not native speakers of the languages spoken to the children; these children had significantly lower scores on both social and language measures, suggesting that the reduced quality of the language input had a negative effect on language learning outcomes.

A study by Ohashi et al. (2012) similarly examined the language abilities of two groups of Canadian children with ASD. All of the children had received a clinical diagnosis of ASD, were between 24 and 52 months of age, had a reported spoken vocabulary of 30 or more words and had no comorbid conditions (e.g. genetic or neuromotor disorders). Of the 60 children, 20 met a set of stringent criteria for ongoing bilingual exposure at home, from the time of birth; the remaining 40 children were exposed to only one language, English, at home. The groups were matched on chronological age and non-verbal IQ scores at the time of language assessment. The researchers examined various aspects of the children's development, including (a) severity of the autism-related communication impairment, from the Autism Diagnostic Observation Scale (ADOS; Lord et al., 2002); (b) age of first words, from the ADI-R; (c) age of first phrases, from the ADI-R; (d) both receptive and expressive language raw scores on either the English or French version of the Preschool Language Scale-4 (PLS-4; Zimmerman *et al.*, 2002); and (e) the communication subscale raw score from the VABS-II. In this study, TCV was not calculated, as the PLS-4 was only administered in either French (for participants who lived in Quebec) or English.

Similarly, a recent study (Valicenti-McDermott *et al.*, 2013) utilizing a retrospective methodology compared the receptive and expressive language skills of children younger than 3 years of age. Two groups of children were compared on their receptive and expressive language skills, as well as communicative gestures: 40 monolingual English-speaking and 40 Spanish–English bilingual toddlers. Their results showed that there were no differences between the groups on cognitive abilities, autistic features and most language skills, although the bilingual children tended to vocalize and utilize gestures more often. Taken together, the findings from both studies (Ohashi *et al.*, 2012; Valicenti-McDermott *et al.*, 2013) revealed no major differences between the bilingual-exposed and monolingual-exposed groups, lending further support to the premise that bilingual exposure does not impede early language acquisition in children with ASD.

In a smaller-scale study, Petersen *et al.* (2012) examined the lexical comprehension and production skills of two groups of children with ASD – 14 bilingual Chinese–English children and 14 monolingual English-speaking children. The participants ranged from 3 to 6 years and were matched on chronological age and number and type of early intervention therapy hours they had received, as indicated by parent report. Language assessments included the MCDI (Fenson *et al.*, 1993); the Peabody Picture Vocabulary Test-III (PPVT-III; Dunn & Dunn, 1997), which measures receptive vocabulary knowledge; and the Preschool Language Scale-3 (PLS-3; Zimmerman *et al.*, 1992), which measures receptive and expressive language skills. Children in the bilingual group were also tested using the Chinese version of the PPVT (PPVT-R; Lu & Liu, 1994) as well as a Chinese version of the CDI (Tardif & Fletcher, 2008). Using the combined CDI results, a TCV score was calculated for each of the bilingual children. Two sets of multivariate analyses of covariance (MANCOVAs) with group as the independent variable and non-verbal IQ (based on selected subscales of the Mullen Scales of Early Learning; Mullen, 1995) as a covariate were performed. The results revealed that the bilingual group had larger total production vocabularies than their monolingual counterparts, but the two groups were otherwise equivalent on the remaining vocabulary and general language measures.

To our knowledge, only one study to date has examined the narrative abilities of bilingual children with ASD. Yang and Marinova-Todd (2011) examined the narrative abilities in three groups of children: 10 English–Mandarin bilingual children with ASD, 13 English monolingual children with ASD and 9 TD English–Mandarin bilingual children. Participants were asked to tell a story from a wordless picture book (*Frog, Where Are You?* by Mercer Meyer); the bilingual children produced a story both in Mandarin and in English. The narratives were analyzed according to their global structure (i.e. narrative length and the presence of obligatory story episodes and characters), local linguistic structure (i.e. use of cohesive devices, presence of grammatical errors) and the presence of evaluative devices (i.e. mental state words that express thoughts and emotions, or use of direct speech). Although the bilingual children with ASD experienced more difficulties with their narratives relative to the TD bilinguals, their performance across all narrative measures was equivalent to that of their monolingual peers with ASD. Similar to the studies on general language abilities, this study further confirms the equivalent abilities of bilingual and monolingual children with ASD in the domain of discourse skills, such as narratives.

Family Language Practices and the Impact of Imposed Monolingualism

The limited but growing research to date has shown quite consistently that bilingual children with ASD have language and communication skills equivalent to those of monolingual children with ASD. However, many bilingual families are still advised by child development professionals to speak only one language to their child. As a result, parents of children with ASD who are exposed to bilingual environments often choose to speak only one language, typically the dominant language of the society in which the family lives. In many cases, parents in these bilingual families are new immigrants; thus, the language spoken at home is not the dominant language in the society, and the parents may not be fluent in the dominant language. It is important, therefore, to determine the family language practices and attitudes toward bilingualism in those families and the effect that changing family language practices has on family dynamics, as well as on children's language and communication development.

A recent survey study examined this issue in a sample of 49 bilingual families from Canada, the United States, Greece, France, Egypt and Singapore, all of whom were associated with an autism research registry (Kay-Raining Bird *et al.*, 2012). All of the families had at least one child with ASD; 14% had two or three children with this disorder, ranging in age from 2 years 11 months to 22 years. Of the 49 respondents, 25% reported that their child with ASD was exposed to only one language on a regular basis (these included, English, French or German), 61% reported two languages and 14% reported exposure to three languages. Although 37 respondents (75%) reported that they were raising their child with ASD to be bilingual or multilingual, only three of these families reported that they were consistently encouraged by professionals to raise their child with ASD bilingually. Professional opposition to bilingual exposure came from many sources, including physicians, speech-language pathologists, psychologists, social workers and teachers. Despite professional resistance, 46% of these children reportedly had strong receptive and/or expressive language abilities in two languages, and another 22% were acquiring one language successfully in the context of bilingual exposure. Eighty-nine percent of respondents reported that they had no access to professional help or services that supported bilingual language development.

Qualitative studies

In addition, two recent qualitative studies examined the language practices and beliefs of 10 mothers who were bilingual in Mandarin and English (Yu, 2013) and 3 mothers in extended families in which English, Hindi, Arabic and at least one additional South Asian language were spoken (Jegatheesan, 2011). All mothers in both studies lived in the United States and had a child with ASD between 3 and 8 years of age. In both studies, mothers participated in detailed interviews that were conducted in one of several languages spoken by the authors. Many of the results of the two studies were remarkably similar, and revealed four main themes.

Happy and fulfilling life

All of the mothers were focused on helping their children learn the language they believed would allow them to live happy and fulfilling lives, although how they aimed to accomplish this differed across the two studies. In Yu (2013), all but one Mandarin-speaking mother believed that their children should learn to speak, understand and write English, because of its prestige and societal dominance. In contrast, all three South Asian mothers in Jegatheesan (2011) believed that their children should learn to speak both English and at least one South Asian language. They viewed English as a 'passport for participation in American society' (Jegatheesan, 2011: 191) at the same time as they highly valued their home languages (e.g. Arabic and Hindi) as hallmarks of their religious (i.e. Muslim) identity. Thus, although the mothers' goals for their children were similar across the two studies – leading a happy and fulfilling life – how they sought to accomplish this reflected differences in their cultural and religious backgrounds.

Lack of bilingual services

All of the mothers highly valued early intervention and special education services; however, they all observed that very few of these services were available to them or their children in a language other than English.

Professional opposition to bilingual exposure

Yu (2013) reported that all of the mothers in her study felt that monolingual exposure would be better for their child with ASD, and some felt strongly that bilingualism was confusing and would further delay their child's language development. In all cases, these notions about bilingualism and language development were shaped by advice from professionals such as physicians, speech-language pathologists, teachers and psychologists. The most common advice given by the professionals following a diagnosis of ASD was for the parent to start speaking only English to his or her child. In contrast, Jegatheesan (2011) reported that all three mothers in her study believed that being able to speak their native language(s) was vital for communication with non-English-speaking family members. As a result, these mothers all actively resisted professional pressure to speak only English. In this regard, one mother commented, 'He (her child) has grandparents, and they cannot speak English. So how our child can communicate with his grandmother if he knows only English? What they (professionals) are asking is unreasonable. So it is best we don't tell them anything. They don't need to know what we speak at home because it's a headache for us to make them understand. They just don't' (Jegatheesan, 2011: 196).

Challenges with English language modeling

Although all of the parents were fairly proficient in English and felt comfortable speaking it in professional settings, they reported that their ability to speak English comfortably was dependent on the context. Specifically, not all of the mothers were 'necessarily comfortable using English with their children' (Yu, 2013: 19). In Jegatheesan (2011), mothers reported enlisting the 'assistance' of community members to help their children learn English, out of concern about their own abilities in that language. For example, one of the mothers reported that, 'My English is not good, and when I speak I mix Urdu and have a strong accent. [So]…late at night we go to Walmart and let him explore because there are not many people around at that time. And I teach him to speak English to the staff and the cashier' (Jegatheesan, 2011: 192). Another mother noted that, 'I take him to fast foods (restaurants) and he orders the food himself. Sometimes in the restaurant I ask the waiter to talk to Raqib (her son) about his order, like ask him more questions about the food he orders…I make sure he [is] exposed to the American way of life' (Jegatheesan, 2011: 192).

Additional effects of imposed monolingualism

The effect of imposed monolingualism could be even more devastating for parents who are less proficient in English than the mothers in these two studies. For example, Kremer-Sadlik (2005) highlighted the fact that imposing a non-native language on a family can create social distance between family members and a child with ASD. Her report highlighted data from parent interviews and from video recordings of parent–child interactions with four children whose home language was not English. The author found that, when families followed professionals' advice to speak only English to their child, the child did not take part in family conversations, the parents addressed the child infrequently and the parents rarely used English in family conversations. Moreover, as Hambly and Fombonne (2012) noted, many parents who are advised to speak a non-native majority language to their children are not fluent themselves in that language, and thus provide models that are grammatically incorrect. Kremer-Sadlik argued that it is very important for children with ASD to speak the language of their parents and relatives, in order to be exposed to a variety of social situations at home that support social-pragmatic development, which is negatively affected by ASD. When these interactions take place in a language that the child does not understand, or when parents attempt to converse in a language in which they are not fluent, the child is deprived of important learning opportunities. Interestingly, one family in Kremer-Sadlik's study did not take professional advice and continued to speak in both languages to their child with ASD, who developed into a bilingual speaker.

This was not the case in a related study in which the authors collected information from multilingual parents of children with ASD diagnoses (Fernandez y Garcia et al., 2012). All five of the interviewed families had adopted an 'English-only' approach to communicating with their child and ceased speaking their home language following explicit recommendations from healthcare professionals and/or teachers. These families shared their experiences of trying to maintain an English-only home as well as the repercussions from this decision. The most frequent comments echoed those made by the families in Kremer-Sadlik's (2005) and Yu's (2013) studies – namely, the feeling of sadness and personal loss that resulted from having to communicate with their child in a language that was not as familiar or comfortable to them as their home language. Parents also reported speaking less with their child due to feelings of inadequacy regarding their English skills. This study, in combination with the others described in this section, highlights the unintended negative consequences that may arise from a decision to implement an English-only environment in bilingual homes. There seems to be little doubt that imposed monolingualism has the potential to significantly alter both linguistic and social development in children with ASD – two areas that are already significantly affected in this population.

ASD and Language Intervention

A search of the literature revealed only one study that specifically examined bilingual language intervention with a child with ASD. This longitudinal study followed the language development of a 3-year-old bilingual Korean–English boy who was living in the United States. The child had been diagnosed with a language delay at age 3;0 and was subsequently diagnosed with mild–moderate autism at age 3;6. He was monitored over a 24-month period by a Korean–English bilingual speech-language pathologist who also provided intervention (Seung et al., 2006). Intervention built on the connection between prelinguistic and linguistic development, including expectant waiting, imitation with animation, joint attention, gestures and pretend play. The boy's parents were trained to use intervention methods in the home in order to facilitate generalization of the boy's language use. Vocabulary building interventions were provided and, as the child made progress producing words in his primary language, English intervention was introduced at the single-word verb and noun level. Intervention also included pragmatic goals – negotiation to select a toy for an activity, transition from task to task, social greetings, social smiles, verbal requests and turn taking. Measures that were used to track the boy's progress included the MCDI: Words and Sentences (Fenson et al., 1993), PPVT-III (Dunn & Dunn, 1997), Expressive Vocabulary Test (EVT; Williams, 1997) and Reynell Developmental Language Scales (Reynell & Gruber, 1990). For the first 6 months, the child was provided with speech-language therapy in Korean only and made notable gains. After 12 months, the speech-language pathologist gradually began to integrate English into his therapy sessions until, at 18 months, therapy was provided mainly in English. After 24 months of intervention, the child had made significant gains with regard to receptive and expressive language skills in both English and Korean. In addition, significant decreases were noted with regard to problem behaviors. Although one cannot draw generalized conclusions from this single case study, it does suggest the potential benefit of bilingual speech-language intervention for this population.

Future Research Directions

Currently, a small body of evidence has compared the language and communication abilities of bilingual children with ASD and their monolingual counterparts. However, the results are fairly consistent across studies, showing no significant differences in performance between the two groups, and in some cases a tendency for the bilingual groups to do better on some of the tasks. It is also clear that there is considerable confusion among parents and professionals working with children with ASD, about the potential effect of bilingualism on their language development and communicative functioning. The results from qualitative studies strongly suggest that imposed monolingualism may be more harmful than helpful for the children's development and socialization, and that children should be offered bilingual intervention whenever possible. Additional research is needed to confirm these initial findings in order to provide essential information to both bilingual families and the practitioners who work with their children with ASD.

Clinical Implications

This review of the literature on bilingual children with ASD suggests that children from minority language families should be encouraged to continue speaking their home language, to ensure that the child is receiving high-quality social input and language input. Unfortunately, many professionals continue to recommend limiting language exposure to a single language for children with ASD and other developmental delays (Jordaan, 2008) – which, as noted previously, may have negative effects on family relationships. In addition, most language intervention with children with ASD is delivered using only a single language (Jordaan, 2008). Current research does not appear to support either of these practices. Just as the language abilities of bilingual individuals lie on a continuum, the language of intervention can also be viewed in this way (Elin Thordardottir, 2010). On one end of this continuum, language intervention can occur in only one language – often, the language spoken by a monolingual speech-language pathologist or other professional. On the other end of the continuum, language intervention can be delivered equally in both languages to which a client is exposed at home. This approach is supported by current research and is recommended by both the Canadian Association of Speech-Language Pathology and Audiology (Crago & Westernoff, 1997) and the International Association of Logopedics and Phoniatry (IALP, 2006 as cited in Elin Thordardottir, 2010). Based on these endorsements, monolingual speech-language pathologists and other early language interventionists who are not able to provide bilingual services should be encouraged to seek the assistance of interpreters in order to provide bilingual support (Jordaan, 2008). The specific strengths and weaknesses, learning environments, cultural preferences and family dynamics that affect children with ASD and their families should be taken into consideration when specific language interventions are designed.

References

Adams, M.J. (1992) *Beginning to Read: Thinking and Learning about Print*. Cambridge, MA: MIT Press.

American Psychiatric Association (2013) *Diagnostic and Statistical Manual of Mental Disorders* (5th edn). Washington, DC: Author.

Åsberg, J. and Dahlgren-Sandberg, A. (2012) Dyslexic, delayed, precocious, or normal? Word reading skills of children with autism spectrum disorders. *Journal of Research in Reading* 35, 20–31.

Baron-Cohen, S., Wheelwright, S., Lawson, J., Griffin, R., Ashwin, C., Billington, J. and Chakrabarti, B. (2005) Empathizing and systemizing in autism spectrum conditions. In F. Volkmar, R.P.A. Klin and D. Cohen (eds) *Handbook of Autism and Pervasive Developmental Disorders* (pp. 628–649). Hoboken, NJ: John Wiley & Sons.

Bradley, L. and Bryant, P.E. (1983) Categorizing sounds and learning to read: A causal connection. *Nature* 301, 419–421.

Bruner, J. and Feldman, C. (1993) Theory of mind and the problem of autism. In S. Baron-Cohen, H. Tager-Flusberg and D.J. Cohen (eds) *Understanding Other Minds: Perspectives from Autism* (pp. 223–246). Oxford: Oxford University Press.

Capps, L., Losh, M. and Thurber, C. (2000) 'The frog ate the bug and made his mouth sad': Narrative competence in children with autism. *Journal of Abnormal Child Psychology* 28, 193–204.

Centers for Disease Control and Prevention (2012) Autism spectrum disorders data and statistics. See http://www.cdc.gov/NCBDDD/autism/data.html (accessed 29 August 2013).

Crago, M. and Westernoff, F. (1997) CASLPA position paper on speech-language pathology and audiology in the multicultural, multilingual context. *Journal of Speech-Language Pathology and Audiology* 21, 223–224.

Diehl, J.J., Bennetto, L. and Young, E.C. (2006) Story recall and narrative coherence of high-functioning children with autism spectrum disorders. *Journal of Abnormal Child Psychology* 34, 87–102.

Dunn, L.M. and Dunn, L.M. (1997) *Examiner's Manual for the PPVT-III: Peabody Picture Vocabulary Test* (3rd edn). Circle Pines, MN: American Guidance Service.

Ehri, L.C. (2000) Learning to read and learning to spell: Two sides of a coin. *Topics in Language Disorders* 20, 19–36.

Elin Thordardottir (2010) Towards evidence-based practice in language intervention for bilingual children. *Journal of Communication Disorders* 43, 523–537.

Fenson, L., Dale, P.S., Reznick, J.S., Thal, D., Bates, E., Hartung, J.P., Pethick, S. and Reilly, J.S. (1993) *MacArthur Communicative Development Inventory: User's Guide and Technical Manual.* San Diego, CA: Singular Publishing Company.

Fernandez y Garcia, E., Breslau, J., Hansen, R. and Miller, E. (2012) Unintended consequences: An ethnographic narrative case series exploring language recommendations for bilingual families of children with autistic spectrum disorders. *Journal of Medical Speech-Language Pathology* 20, 10–16.

Gabig, C. (2010) Phonological awareness and word recognition in reading by children with autism. *Communication Disorders Quarterly* 31, 67–85.

Grosjean, F. (2010) *Bilingual: Life and Reality.* Cambridge, MA: Harvard University Press.

Hale, C. and Tager-Flusberg, H. (2005) Social communication in children with autism. *Autism* 9, 157–178.

Hambly, C. and Fombonne, E. (2005) *Family Background Information Questionnaire (FBIQ).* Montreal: McGill University.

Hambly, C. and Fombonne, E. (2012) The impact of bilingual environments on language development in children with autism spectrum disorders. *Journal of Autism and Developmental Disorders* 42, 1342–1352.

Heimann, M., Nelson, K.E., Tjus, T. and Gillberg, C. (1995) Increasing reading and communication skills in children with autism through an interactive multimedia computer program. *Journal of Autism and Developmental Disorders* 25, 459–480.

Hobson, R.P., García-Pérez, R.M. and Lee, A. (2010) Person-centered (deictic) expressions in autism. *Journal of Autism and Developmental Disorders* 40, 403–415.

Howlin, P., Goode, S., Hutton, J. and Rutter, M. (2004) Adult outcome for children with autism. *Journal of Child Psychology and Psychiatry* 45, 212–229.

Jegatheesan, B. (2011) Multilingual development in children with autism: Perspectives of South Asian Muslim immigrant parents on raising a child with a communicative disorder in multilingual contexts. *Bilingual Research Journal* 34, 185–200.

Jordaan, H. (2008) Clinical intervention for bilingual children: An international survey. *Folia Phoniatrica et Logopaedica* 60, 97–105.

Kay-Raining Bird, E., Lamond, E. and Holden, J. (2012) Survey of bilingualism in autism spectrum disorders. *International Journal of Language & Communication Disorders* 47, 52–64.

Kay-Raining Bird, E., Trudeau, N., Elin Thordardottir, Sutton, A. and Thorpe, A. (2005) The language abilities of bilingual children with Down syndrome. *American Journal of Speech-Language Pathology* 14, 187–199.

Kremer-Sadlik, T. (2005) To be or not to be bilingual: Autistic children from multilingual families. In J. Cohen, K.T. McAlister, K. Rolstad and J. MacSwan (eds) *Proceedings of the 4th International Symposium on Bilingualism* (pp. 1225–1234). Somerville, MA: Cascadilla Press.

Le Couteur, A., Lord, C. and Rutter, M. (2003) *Autism Diagnostic Interview – Revised.* Los Angeles, CA: Western Psychological Services.

Liberman, I.Y., Shankweiler, D. and Liberman, A.M. (1989) The alphabetic principle and learning to read. ERIC Document No. ED427291.

Lord, C., Rutter, M., DiLavore, P.C. and Risi, S. (2002) *The Autism Diagnostic Observation Scale (ADOS).* Los Angeles, CA: Western Psychological Services.

Losh, M. and Capps, L. (2003) Narrative ability in high-functioning children with autism or Asperger's syndrome. *Journal of Autism and Developmental Disorders* 33, 239–251.

Loveland, K., McEvoy, R., Tunali, B. and Kelley, M.L. (1990) Narrative story telling in autism and Down's syndrome. *British Journal of Developmental Psychology* 8, 9–23.

Loveland, K. and Tunali, B. (1993) Narrative language in autism and the theory of mind hypothesis: A wider perspective. In S. Baron-Cohen, H. Tager-Flusberg and D.J. Cohen (eds) *Understanding Other Minds: Perspectives from Autism* (pp. 247–266). Oxford: Oxford University Press.

Lu, L. and Liu, H.H. (1994) *The Peabody Picture Vocabulary Test – Revised: Taiwanese Version.* Taipei: Psychological Press.

Mirenda, P., Smith, I., Volden, J., Szatmari, P., Bryson, S., Fombonne, E., Roberts, W., Vaillancourt, T., Waddell, C., Zwaigenbaum, L., Georgiades, S., Duku, E. and Thompson, A. (2013, May) How many children with autism spectrum disorder are functionally nonverbal? In *Abstracts of the International Meeting for Autism Research* (pp. 172–173). San Sebastian: International Society for Autism Research.

Mullen, E. (1995) *Mullen Scales of Early Learning.* Circle Pines, MN: American Guidance Service.

Nagy, W. (2007) Metalinguistic awareness and the vocabulary–comprehension connection. In R.K. Wagner, A.E. Muse and K.R. Tannenbaum (eds) *Vocabulary Acquisition: Implications for Reading Comprehension* (pp. 52–77). New York: Guilford Press.

Newman, T.M., Macomber, D., Naples, A.J., Babitz, T., Volkmar, F. and Grigorenki, E.L. (2007) Hyperlexia in children with autism spectrum disorders. *Journal of Autism and Developmental Disorders* 37, 760–774.

Norbury, C.F. and Bishop, D.V.M. (2003) Narrative skills in children with communication impairments. *International Journal of Language and Communication Disorders* 38, 287–313.

Ohashi, J.K., Mirenda, P., Marinova-Todd, S., Hambly, C., Fombonne, E., Szatmari, P. and the Pathways in ASD Study Team (2012) Comparing early language development in monolingual- and bilingual-exposed young children with autism spectrum disorders. *Research in Autism Spectrum Disorders* 6, 890–897.

Paradis, J., Crago, M., Genesee, F. and Rice, M. (2003) French-English bilingual children with SLI: How do they compare with their monolingual peers? *Journal of Speech, Language, and Hearing Research* 46, 113–127.

Pearson, B., Fernandez, S. and Oller, D. (1993) Lexical development in bilingual infants and toddlers: Comparisons to monolingual norms. *Language Learning* 43, 93–120.

Perkins, M., Dobbinson, S., Boucher, J., Bol, S. and Bloom, P. (2006) Lexical knowledge and lexical use in autism. *Journal of Autism and Developmental Disorders* 36, 795–805.

Petersen, J.M., Marinova-Todd, S.H. and Mirenda, P. (2012) Brief report: An exploratory study of lexical skills in bilingual children with autism spectrum disorder. *Journal of Autism and Developmental Disorders* 42, 1499–1503.

Reynell, J.K. and Gruber, C.P. (1990) *Reynell Developmental Language Scales.* Los Angeles, CA: Western Psychological Services.

Scheele, A.F., Leseman, P.P.M. and Mayo, A.Y. (2010) The home language environment of monolingual and bilingual children and their language proficiency. *Applied Psycholinguistics* 31, 117–140.

Seung, H., Siddiql, S. and Elder, J.H. (2006) Intervention outcomes of a bilingual child with autism. *Journal of Medical Speech-Language Pathology* 14, 53–63.

Sparrow, S.S., Cicchetti, D.V. and Balla, D.A. (2005) *Vineland Adaptive Behavior Scales* (2nd edn). Circle Pines, MN: AGS Publishing.

Stanovich, K.E. (1985) Explaining the variance in reading ability in terms of psychological processes: What have we learned? *Annals of Dyslexia* 35, 67–96.

Statistics Canada (2011) Linguistic characteristics of Canadians. See http://www12.statcan.gc.ca/census-recensement/2011/as-sa/98-314-x/98-314-x2011001-eng.pdf (accessed 25 February 2013).

Tager-Flusberg, H. (1995) 'Once upon a ribbit': Stories narrated by autistic children. *British Journal of Developmental Psychology* 13, 45–59.

Tager-Flusberg, H. (2007) Evaluating the theory-of-mind hypothesis in autism. *Current Directions in Psychological Science* 16, 311–315.

Tager-Flusberg, H., Paul, R. and Lord, C. (2005) Language and communication in autism. In F. Volkmar, R. Paul, A. Klin and D. Cohen (eds) *Handbook of Autism and Pervasive Developmental Disorders* (Vol. 1; pp. 335–364). Hoboken, NJ: John Wiley & Sons.

Tardif, T. and Fletcher, P. (2008) *User's Guide and Manual for the Chinese Communicative Development Inventories (Putonghua and Cantonese).* Beijing: Peking University Medical Press.

Treiman, R. (1984) On the status of final consonant clusters in English syllables. *Journal of Verbal Learning and Verbal Behavior* 23, 343–356.

Valicenti-McDermott, M., Tarshis, N., Schouls, M., Galdston, M., Hottinger, K., Seijo, R., Shulman, L. and Shinnar, S. (2013) Language differences between monolingual English and bilingual English-Spanish young children with autism spectrum disorders. *Journal of Child Neurology* 28, 945–948.

Wagner, R., Torgeson, J. and Rashotte, C. (1999) *Comprehensive Test of Phonological Processing.* Austin, TX: Pro-Ed Inc.

White, S., Frith, U., Milne, E., Rosen, S., Swettenham, J. and Ramus, F. (2006) A double dissociation between sensorimotor impairments and reading disability: A comparison of autistic and dyslexic children. *Cognitive Neuropsychology* 23, 748–761.

Williams, K.T. (1997) *Expressive Vocabulary Test.* Circle Pines, MN: American Guidance Service.

Woodcock, R.W., McGrew, K.S. and Mather, N. (2001) *Woodcock–Johnson III Tests of Achievement*. Itasca, IL: Riverside Publishing.

Yang, S.K.T. (2011) Narrative abilities in bilingual children with autism. Unpublished masters thesis, School of Audiology and Speech Sciences, University of British Columbia, Vancouver, Canada.

Yu, B. (2013) Issues in bilingualism and heritage language maintenance: Perspectives of minority-language mothers of children with autism spectrum disorders. *American Journal of Speech-Language Pathology* 22, 10–24.

Zimmerman, I.L., Steiner, V.G. and Pond, R.E. (1992) *Preschool Language Scale* (3rd edn). San Antonio, TX: Psychological Corporation.

Zimmerman, I.L., Steiner, V.G. and Pond, R.E. (2002) *Preschool Language Scale* (4th edn). San Antonio, TX: Psychological Corporation.

3 Bilingualism and Children with Down Syndrome

Elizabeth Kay-Raining Bird

Introduction

Children with Down syndrome (DS) have cognitive and language impairments secondary to trisomy of the 21st chromosome. Language is typically more impacted than would be expected given non-verbal cognitive skills. There is considerable individual variability in the degree of impairment (Chapman & Kay-Raining Bird, 2011). In bilingual development, both languages are affected.

Bilingualism is a multifaceted concept defined here as the ability to produce, comprehend, read or write more than one language. Both child internal and child external factors affect the rate and eventual attainment of languages in bilingual settings. Among children with language and cognitive deficits, bilingual proficiency will vary as a function of the degree of impairment and the developmental level of the child. Environmental factors such as the quality and quantity of linguistic input will impact the child's development of each language in a bilingual setting.

The language experiences of bilingual children (with or without DS) vary in many ways (Baker, 2011; Kay-Raining Bird, 2006; Paradis et al., 2011). Some children are exposed to two languages from infancy, referred to as simultaneous bilingualism, or bilingual–first language learners. Other children are exposed to one language for some time before the second one is introduced (sequential bilinguals). Their languages of first and second exposure are referred to as L1 and L2, respectively. The relative frequency of exposure (input) to a child and use by the child of each language varies and often changes over time. The proficiency attained in each language varies as a function of exposure and use. Some children have relatively similar levels of proficiency in both languages (balanced bilinguals) while others have better ability in one language (the stronger or dominant language[1]) than the other (the weaker language). Some contexts nurture the development of two languages (additive bilingualism), while others have a negative impact upon bilingual development, causing plateauing or even loss of proficiency in a language (subtractive bilingualism).

Status and use of a language in the larger society affects its acquisition. Majority languages are often official languages and are valued highly,

49

evident in mass media and used by many people in a society; those languages used infrequently in the larger community have intrinsically less value in society and are termed *minority languages*. Additional variability in children's bilingual experiences is evident in the languages they use, the modality of use of the languages (i.e. signed or spoken), the typological similarity of the languages they use (e.g. same or different language families), whether they have been actively taught their languages, institutional supports for learning a language (e.g. bilingual versus immersion education options), who uses the languages and whether they are used to interact with the child directly or not and where the languages are used (e.g. school, home, community). Clearly, bilinguals are a heterogeneous population.

In this chapter, bilingualism in children with DS is explored using four hypothetical cases (see Box 3.1). While they all have DS, the cases differ in age, developmental level, bilingual proficiency and bilingual experiences.

Box 3.1 Four hypothetical bilingual children

Name	Description
Majida	Majida is a two-year-old girl with DS from the Sudan. She and her family moved to Halifax 6 months ago. Since their arrival, Majida has attended a day care where only English is spoken, while her parents work. Her family speaks only Arabic at home but both parents have some functional English skills. Majida uses gestures but not words to communicate. She is able to follow simple directions, better in Arabic than English. She gets frustrated easily when she is not successful in communicating.
Paul	Paul is a six-year-old boy of Mi'kmaq heritage with DS living on the Eskasoni First Nations reserve in Cape Breton, Nova Scotia. Paul is in the first grade of a Mi'kmaq immersion program in the reserve-operated elementary school. In this program, all core classes are taught in Mi'kmaq. Paul's parents are bilingual Mi'kmaq and English speakers but English has always been spoken more often at home. Paul is using two and three word utterances in English and knows only a few words in Mi'kmaq.
Annabel	Annabel is a 13-year-old English-speaking girl with DS. She lives in Halifax with her family who are monolingual English speakers. She attends an integrated seventh-grade class and is in the first month of a late French immersion program. In this program, all classes except English and gym are taught exclusively in French. She began the program 1 month ago and is having a hard time understanding what is going on in class. Annabel speaks English using primarily simple single-clause sentences, sometimes with grammatical morphemes omitted. She produces three words in French, which she uses functionally. Annabel reads at second-grade level and likes to tell stories. Annabel's parents are concerned and wonder whether it was a good idea for Annabel to attend a French immersion program.

Michel	Michel is a 14-year-old, seventh-grade boy with DS enrolled in an integrated English classroom in Halifax. Both French and English have been spoken in his home since Michel was born. His family knows very few other French speakers in Halifax, but Michel's extended family in southern Nova Scotia all speak French as their home language. Michel reads at fourth-grade level in English, less in French. He speaks in single and multi-clausal sentences in English but has difficulty with extended discourse. Until recently, this was also true of Michel's French skills, but Michel has begun to refuse to speak French at home and his parents are concerned that he is losing his French.

The children all live in Nova Scotia, Canada. A brief history and demographic account of Nova Scotia is provided in Box 3.2 to contextualize the cases.

Since the literature on bilingualism and DS is limited, evidence from studies of monolingual children with DS, bilingual children with typical development and bilingual children with language and/or cognitive disorders other than DS is drawn upon. When relevant, commonly held beliefs about bilingualism and children with DS or questions that are

---

Box 3.2 A description of the context: Nova Scotia, Canada

Nova Scotia is a small maritime Canadian province, located on the Atlantic Ocean. It has a population of approximately 900,000 (Statistics Canada, 2009a). The capital and largest city of Nova Scotia is Halifax. French and English are the official languages of Canada; however, in Nova Scotia, 92.1% of the population is monolingual English speaking (Statistics Canada, 2009). The original inhabitants of Nova Scotia were the Mi'kmaq. Today, 2% of the population claims Aboriginal heritage, primarily Mi'kmaq, and lives both on and off the 13 First Nations reserves in Nova Scotia (Ministry of Industry, 2008). The largest reserve in Nova Scotia is Eskasoni where the largest number of Mi'kmaq language speakers lives. European colonization began in Nova Scotia in the early 1600s, first by the French and later the British. Today, approximately 30% of the Nova Scotia population claims Scottish heritage, and Gaelic continues to be spoken by a significant minority (Gaelic Council of Nova Scotia, 2012). While French and British colonies coexisted for a time, there were frequent wars, culminating in the military domination and forcible removal of most French-speaking Acadians in the mid 1700s. While some Acadians later returned, the francophone population in Nova Scotia is only 4% of the total population (Statistics Canada, 2006). Another 4% of Nova Scotians report speaking a language other than French or English as their home language (Statistics Canada, 2009). Most recent immigrants to Nova Scotia settle in Halifax.

frequently raised by families or professionals will be addressed. The chapter ends with a discussion of the assessment of and intervention with bilingual children with DS.

Bilingualism and Down Syndrome

Language and literacy development in children with Down syndrome

A behavioral phenotype has been identified in research on monolingual children with DS. They have cognitive and language delays relative to same-age peers. Intellectual impairments vary in severity, but usually fall within the moderate to severe range. Visual cognition strengths and auditory verbal short-term memory weaknesses are well documented (Chapman & Hesketh, 2000; Jarrold et al., 2006). Verbal cognition tends to be more impaired than non-verbal cognition. The rate, but not the sequence of language development, appears to be impacted by DS; milestones are acquired in a similar order to that observed in typical children. Difficulties in language emerge early, but language learning continues to progress through adolescence. Children with DS tend to have a larger than typical gap between their receptive and expressive language skills. Consequently, young children especially could often benefit from augmentative or alternative communication (AAC) options. Receptive vocabulary is a particular strength in this population, often on par with non-verbal cognitive abilities, while morphosyntax, especially expressive morphosyntax, is a particular weakness. While many of the available studies have focused upon English development, the general phenotype holds true for other languages studied such as French, Italian, Spanish and Swedish (see Chapman & Kay-Raining Bird, 2011; Roberts et al., 2008; Rondal & Buckley, 2004 for reviews). Bilingualism does not appear to change the behavioral phenotype of a particular disorder. In French–English bilingual children with DS, a similar pattern of strengths and weaknesses in language domains was reported when examining both the stronger language (English) (Kay-Raining Bird et al., 2005) and the weaker language (French) (Feltmate & Kay-Raining Bird, 2008). Phenotypes also appear to remain stable in bilinguals with specific language impairment (SLI; Paradis et al., 2003) and autism (Hambly & Fombonne, 2011; Peterson et al., 2011). In the SLI population, for example, no differences in the type or frequency of French morphological error patterns were found in monolingual French-speaking children with SLI and French–English bilingual children with SLI. The same was found for analyses of English morphology patterns (Paradis et al., 2003).

When taught systematically, monolingual children with DS often learn to read and write (see Burgoyne, 2009; Burgoyne et al., 2012; Kay-Raining Bird & Chapman, 2011 for reviews). Some develop word recognition skills prior to school entry. Word recognition is a strength, sometimes measuring above non-verbal cognitive ability. Non-word reading (i.e. decoding), reading comprehension and phonological awareness (PA) skills tend to lag behind word recognition abilities. To date, only two case studies have reported on the reading abilities of biliterate individuals with DS. Nelson *et al.* (2008) described the reading and eye movement patterns of a 10-year-old Mexican girl with DS whose L1 was Spanish and L2 was English. This child was reported to have a moderate expressive and receptive language disorder and was reading at a first-grade level in both languages. She retold stories read in Spanish better than those read in English. Her eye movement patterns during reading were similar to those reported for typically developing beginning readers. Vallar and Papagno (1993) reported on the neuropsychological abilities of a trilingual (English, French, Italian) woman with DS who read slowly but with good intonation and accuracy in multiple languages.

Chronological age, mental age and hearing positively predict language comprehension, and language comprehension positively predicts language production in monolingual children with DS (Chapman & Kay-Raining Bird, 2011). Similarly, chronological age and mental age are positively related to ability in the stronger language in bilingual children with DS (Kay-Raining Bird *et al.*, 2005), and mental age and ability in the stronger language correlate positively with vocabulary comprehension and expressive syntax (e.g. mean length of utterance [MLU]) in the weaker language (Kay-Raining Bird *et al.*, 2005; Trudeau *et al.*, 2011). Thus, similar factors influence the language of both monolingual and bilingual children with DS and stronger language ability appears to support learning in the weaker language in bilingual children with DS. In typically developing bilingual children, positive correlations between abilities in their stronger and weaker languages are also reported (Scheele *et al.*, 2010).

The cognitive, language and literacy abilities of the children in Box 3.1 are consistent with the literature overviewed here. All four children exhibit language delays, but it is clear that the older children have better language abilities and are developmentally more mature than the younger children. The two older children exhibit literacy skills; Michel is biliterate with stronger English than French reading abilities. All children are currently exposed to two languages and are in the process of learning both languages. There is a widespread belief that bilingualism is too difficult for children with DS and will cause language delays, since these children are already challenged by language learning. A frequent response is to restrict input to a single language. These issues are examined next.

Children with Down syndrome can become bilingual

Children with DS are able to learn two languages, as demonstrated now in multiple case reports and group studies (Edgin *et al.*, 2011; Feltmate & Kay-Raining Bird, 2008; Kay-Raining Bird *et al.*, 2005; Trudeau *et al.*,

2011; Vallar & Papagno, 1993; Woll & Grove, 1996). Current evidence also shows that children with DS can become both simultaneous (Feltmate & Kay-Raining Bird, 2008; Kay-Raining Bird *et al.*, 2005; Trudeau *et al.*, 2011; Woll & Grove, 1996) and sequential (Edgin *et al.*, 2011; Feltmate & Kay-Raining Bird, 2008; Vallar & Papagno, 1993) bilinguals. However, as will be discussed later, when exposure frequency is uneven, so is acquisition of the two languages and one language becomes stronger than the other.

Simultaneous bilinguals

In typical development, simultaneous bilinguals who are exposed regularly and on an ongoing basis to two languages from birth acquire both languages of exposure, and in a similar developmental sequence as monolinguals. As well, major language milestones emerge at similar times (De Houwer, 2009; Nicoladis & Genesee, 1997; Paradis *et al.*, 2011). Michel and Paul are both simultaneous bilinguals. However, their levels of early exposure to two languages prior to school entry differed considerably, resulting in very different profiles of bilingual proficiency.

Contrary to earlier beliefs, children who experience bilingual input from birth do not confuse their languages, as demonstrated by their ability to differentiate between two languages early in development. Early differentiation can be seen at a phonological, vocabulary and pragmatic level. Babies babble differently when interacting with, for example, French and English speakers (Maneva & Genesee, 2002). Simultaneous bilingual children produce translation equivalents (TEs; words that have shared concepts in two languages, e.g. chien/dog) almost from the emergence of word productions (De Houwer, 2009; Tabors, 2008) and approximately 30% of toddlers' vocabularies are TEs (Pearson *et al.*, 1995). Two-year-old bilingual children switch languages to be pragmatically appropriate when speaking with familiar people (e.g. Nicoladis, 1998). As well, cross-linguistic influence or transfer errors are rare in the talk of simultaneous bilinguals, even at an early age (Paradis *et al.*, 2011). At one time, language mixing (switching between two languages in the same sentence, turn or conversation) was considered a sign of language confusion. More recently, however, mixing is recognized as a normal aspect of bilingual interactions (Nicoladis & Genesee, 1997; Paradis *et al.*, 2011) or a sign of a language gap that is being strategically filled by the child (Paradis *et al.*, 2011; Patterson & Pearson, 2012). Children with SLI (Gutierrez-Clellen *et al.*, 2009) and children with DS (Smith, 2010) do not mix differently or more frequently than typically developing children matched for developmental level.

Sequential bilinguals

Sequential bilingual acquisition is different and as Tabors (2008: 13) puts it, 'a much riskier business'. The likelihood that children will become proficient in both languages is more variable for sequential than for simultaneous bilinguals. Individual factors such as motivation and personality (e.g. willingness to take risks) may affect success in sequential bilingual acquisition (Hoff, 2009; Tabors, 2008). Annabel and Majida are sequential bilinguals, although Majida, by some standards would be considered simultaneous because her exposure to the L2 began before the age of three.

Importantly, knowledge of the L1 can bootstrap a child into L2 (Paradis *et al.*, 2011). One way this occurs is through the positive transfer of vocabulary knowledge via cognates, word pairs with similar phonological and/or written forms and underlying concepts, such as 'oscuro' in Spanish and 'obscure' in English (August *et al.*, 2005). PA skills, critical to learning to read an alphabetic language, also transfer from Spanish to English (e.g. Dickinson *et al.*, 2004), and morphological awareness skills, more important for reading Chinese than PA, transfer from English to Chinese (Wang *et al.*, 2006). Literacy skills seem to positively transfer even more strongly than spoken language skills (Oller & Eilers, 2002). Information that is not useful for learning an L2 also transfers cross-linguistically. Examples are speaking Spanish with an English accent or more frequent use of sentence subjects by Spanish–English bilinguals than monolingual Spanish-speaking children (Paradis, 2012). Paradis noted that transfer of this type tends to occur more often in the weaker language. While these errors can occur in simultaneous bilingual development as well, they are relatively rare and disappear early in development (Paradis *et al.*, 2011).

Rate of acquisition and proficiency in an L2 is related to whether a child is a majority language speaker learning a minority language, as is the case with Annabel, or a minority language speaker learning a majority language, as is the case with Majida (Genesee, 2004; Paradis *et al.*, 2011). With regard to majority language L1 speakers learning a minority language L2, evidence from studies of typically developing English L1 children attending French immersion programs in Canada where they acquire French as their L2 are of particular relevance (see Genesee, 2004; Paradis *et al.*, 2011 for reviews). French immersion programs in Canada begin in either kindergarten (early immersion) or after completing five or more years of schooling in English (middle or late immersion). Research shows that the English language (L1) skills of French immersion students develop on par with those of English monolingual speakers schooled only in English. In contrast, the English literacy skills of early French immersion students tend to lag behind their English-schooled peers initially, but catch up once the immersion students have completed a year of English Language Arts instruction. Importantly, early and late French immersion students acquire significantly greater functional French (minority) language skills than same-aged peers taking core French in an otherwise English-schooled environment, although French immersion students rarely achieve native-like abilities in French. Similar findings have been reported in studies of majority speakers in immersion contexts in the United States and other countries (Genesee, 2004; Paradis et al., 2011).

The situation is different for minority L1 language speakers learning a majority L2 language. Studies of bilingual programs in the United States have shown that children who are learning English as an L2 vary in their success in acquiring English language and literacy skills and academic skills. This variability, in part, depends upon the type of schooling they receive. Minority L1 speakers who are enrolled in dual language programs (where minority and majority language learners are instructed in both languages) tend to score better on all academic measures, including English literacy, than their peers in any other type of instructional program in the United States (Collier & Thomas, 2009; Genesee et al., 2005; Lindholm-Leary & Borsato, 2006; Paradis et al., 2011; Thomas & Collier, 2012). The English language skills of minority L1 children instructed in dual language programs in their minority language 90% of the time initially lag behind their peers receiving less (50%) minority language instruction; but they tend to catch up by third grade (Lindholm & Borsato, 2006; Paradis et al., 2011). Further, bilingual schooling facilitates the retention of the minority, home language (Oller & Eilers, 2002).

Bilingualism does not cause language delay

The belief that bilingualism causes language learning delays has been labeled the Bilingual Deficit Hypothesis (Oller et al., 1997) and is based on the premise that a bilingual child splits his or her resources in a limited capacity processing system between two languages, inevitably slowing growth in either (Junker & Stockman, 2002). The Bilingual Deficit Hypothesis leads to predictions that children with cognitive and/or language learning difficulties would have even greater difficulties with bilingualism because their systems are already taxed by the presence of processing disorders. Contrary to the Bilingual Deficit Hypothesis, research shows that children with communication disorders are not disadvantaged by bilingualism (Kohnert & Medina, 2009). Specifically, monolingual English-speaking and bilingual English-dominant children with DS matched on non-verbal cognition perform no differently on English measures of expressive vocabulary, receptive vocabulary and expressive morphosyntax (Feltmate & Kay-Raining Bird, 2008; Kay-Raining Bird et al., 2005) and measures of overall expressive or receptive language and cognitive skills (Edgin et al., 2011). Similar findings have been reported for children with SLI (Paradis et al., 2003) and children with autism (Hambly & Fombonne, 2011; Ohashi et al., 2012; Petersen et al., 2011).

Elin Thordardottir (2006) points out that thinking about bilingualism as a cause of language delay is a product of a monolingual mindset. Once we recognize that monolingualism and bilingualism are both normal but different developmental paths, we can expect and accept that the rate and perhaps the sequence of development may differ and that such differences do not constitute a delay. In fact, Baker (2011) cautions that referring to bilingual differences as delays perpetuates the myth of a deficit caused by bilingualism. Differences in the development of monolingual and bilingual typically developing children do exist. For example, a robust finding in the literature is that vocabulary measures are consistently lower for bilingual children than monolingual children of the same age, when only one of the bilingual child's two languages is considered. However, when both languages are considered, using either total vocabulary or total conceptual vocabulary, these differences tend to disappear (Oller *et al.*, 2007; Patterson, 1998; Pearson *et al.*, 1993). A similar finding was reported for a syntax measure taken from the MacArthur-Bates Communication Development Inventory (Fenson *et al.*, 1993). Elin Thordardottir *et al.* (2006) found that English syntactic performance was lower for French–English bilinguals than monolingual English-speaking children, but that these differences disappeared when a combined French–English syntax measure was used for the bilingual children. Such findings suggest that differences in monolingual and bilingual typical development exist, but these differences do not constitute a language delay. Of course, language and/or cognitive disorders do exist in the bilingual population. When present, both languages are affected. Supporting development in bilingual children with language and/or cognitive disorders requires separating developmental differences resulting from bilingualism from developmental differences that are symptoms of a developmental disorder. This is not an easy task. While most writers will stress the importance of separating a difference from a disorder in assessment, few have clearly delineated how developmental patterns in bilingual typically developing children and children with language impairments actually differ. One exception is Paradis (2010), who discusses these issues with regard to children with SLI.

Restrict input to a single language?

Consistent with the Bilingual Deficit Hypothesis, parents of children with DS (Elin Thordardottir, 2002; Wilken, 2003), SLI (Paradis, 2007) and autism spectrum disorder (Kay-Raining Bird *et al.*, 2011) are often counseled away from exposing their children to more than one language. Even parents of children with typical development are not immune from this advice (De Houwer, 2009), although it is offered less frequently than for children with disorders (Elin Thordardottir, 2002). As discussed above, bilingualism is possible for children with DS and does not delay their language development. Thus, the premises underlying this recommendation are false. In addition, implementing such a strategy can harm the child and the family. Children with DS often obtain substantial social benefits from becoming bilingual, as it increases their ability to interact in important life contexts and with people who are important to them. It may also increase employment and recreational opportunities for them. Therefore, bilingualism increases social inclusion and decreases social isolation for many children with DS. Asking parents to speak differently to one child than the others may extend social isolation into the home. Additionally, the chosen language may not be the preferred language of one or more family members, which can reduce both the quantity and naturalness of interactions that the child with DS experiences in the home.

There are times when reducing input to a single language *in a particular context* may be supportive of bilingualism. When a home language is not used in the larger community, it will not be perceived as valued. In this situation, a child may reject the home language in favor of the majority one, resulting in minority language loss (Paradis *et al.*, 2011). The likelihood of minority language loss increases when parents use the majority language in the home, as Michel's parents do, compared to when one or both parents speak only the minority language at home. Indeed, Michel is beginning to use French less in the home, which could reflect the beginning of French language loss. De Houwer (2007: 418) reported that 'use of just language X [the minority language] at home led to 20% more success in language X transmission than the use of language X in combination with the use of Dutch [the majority language]'.

In a survey of speech-language pathologists in 10 countries, Jordaan (2008) reported that 89% of clients' parents were advised to speak only one language to their children in the home; 74% were advised to speak only the L1 while 15% were advised to speak only the L2. The authors argued that advice to use only the L1 in the home could support retention of the home language. In contrast, advice to use only the L2 in the home will likely lead to L1 loss. The needs and informed goals of the family and child should guide decisions about language use in and out of the home.

Is there an optimal time for bilingual input?

Some authors have suggested that children with DS would benefit from developing a level of competency in one language before they are introduced to a second one (Rondal, 2000; Wilken, 2003). We know that children with DS can and do become both simultaneous and sequential bilinguals. As well, Papagno and Vallar (2001) describe a 30-year-old woman with DS who is acquiring Spanish, her fourth language. So, bilingualism in this population is not prohibited by the timing of exposure.

Consistent and intensive input in two languages from infancy on often leads to fluent bilingualism in typically developing children. The outcomes for sequential bilinguals are more variable (Tabors, 2008). The literature on L2 learning in immigrant populations shows that age makes a difference;

adults do not usually achieve the same level of L2 fluency as children over the same period of time (Hoff, 2009). Similarly, majority language speakers who enter immersion programs in kindergarten become more proficient in their L2 than children who enter immersion programs later in their schooling (Genesee, 2004). These findings are interpreted as evidence of a critical period for language learning (Johnson & Newport, 1989; Kuhl, 2011) and would suggest that earlier exposure is better for children with DS. However, L2 evidence for a critical period is confounded by the fact that the intensity and manner of L2 exposure differs in adults and children (Marinova-Todd *et al.*, 2000).

There is also considerable evidence that bilingualism facilitates the development of metalinguistic and executive functioning skills, which in turn can support L2 learning. These effects are stronger in more proficient bilinguals and after longer L2 exposure periods, respectively (Barac & Bialystok, 2012; Bialystok & Barac, 2012). Recent studies of brain plasticity suggest that even older adults have a greater capacity to acquire new information than was previously thought (Johansson, 2011). Consistent with these findings, individuals with DS continue to develop expressive language skills through adolescence on (Chapman *et al.*, 1998, 2002). Such evidence, combined with findings of positive transfer previously discussed, suggest that older children with DS can become successfully bilingual. Taken together, then, the evidence supports the notion that earlier exposure to two languages is more likely to lead to bilingual fluency. Nonetheless, older children and adults can achieve a high level of bilingual fluency under the right circumstances. Regardless of the timing of first exposure, consistent, frequent and ongoing quality exposure is needed.

Since bilingualism is often not a choice but a necessity (De Houwer, 1999), strategic timing of an L2 is a moot point for many bilingual children – they learn the languages they must learn. The question of optimal timing, then, is relevant only when bilingualism is a choice. Choice is not a simple issue and should be explored in detail with families. It involves families' beliefs and aspirations for their children. Annabel (in Box 3.1) comes from a monolingual English-speaking family and lives in a community where English is the majority language. Therefore, Annabel does not need to learn French to be a full participant in her family and community. But, Annabel and her family have chosen bilingualism. Access to immersion options is limited for people with developmental disabilities, but current evidence suggests that at-risk students can be successful in this context (Genesee, 2007). There is also an element of choice for both Michel and Paul. Most if not all of the individuals with whom they need to interact at home or in the larger community are bilingual and could communicate with Michel and Paul even if they were monolingual. However, when family and friends talk in the L2, Michel and Paul would be excluded if they did not know the L2. As well, culturally, knowing French and Mi'kmaq, respectively, is important. In both First Nations and Acadian communities in Canada, language retention is viewed as essential for cultural autonomy and health. Thus, for these children and their families, bilingualism may be critical to their sense of well-being and their identification with their communities. Bilingualism is clearly a need, not a choice, for Majida. If she does not learn Arabic, she cannot communicate fully with her parents; if she does not learn English, she cannot communicate in her day care and the larger society. For Majida, bilingualism is essential for inclusion and participation.

Language Input and Bilingualism

Input frequency

Studies have shown that input frequency in a language is positively related to performance on tests of vocabulary, reading and writing in typically developing bilingual children (De Houwer, 2007; Duursma et al., 2007; Oller & Eilers, 2002; Patterson & Pearson, 2012; Pearson et al., 1997). For example, Pearson et al. (1997) found that frequency of input accounted for between 46% and 67% of the variance on measures of proficiency in that language. Further, they reported that bilingual toddlers acquired new vocabulary in a language commensurate with the levels of exposure they received, even for exposure rates as low as 20%.

Input frequency has been studied in bilingual children with DS as well. Trudeau et al. (2011) showed that current frequency of exposure was significantly and positively correlated with vocabulary ability in the weaker, but not the stronger, language. Preliminary analyses of longitudinal measures of vocabulary and morphosyntax confirm these findings. In addition, a frequency threshold appears to exist for children with DS (but not typically developing children); children with DS who experienced less than 20% input in their weaker language showed no progress in that language over time. All children progressed in the stronger language, which was experienced at least 50% of the time in all cases (Kay-Raining Bird et al., in preparation). Input frequency has impacted the language abilities of the four children in Box 3.1. Each child has better language skills in the language experienced more frequently.

Changes in input frequency are also apparent over the lifespan of each child. For example, Michel's French language exposure went down dramatically when he entered English school. At this point, Michel is apparently in a subtractive bilingual context and is experiencing French language loss/attrition. As Majida ages and enters school, she may face a similar situation. Language loss often occurs when a child speaks a minority home language and is schooled in the majority language (Oller & Eilers, 2002).

Variation of language input

Language input varies with socio-economic status (SES) (Hart & Risley, 1995; Roseberry-McKibbin, 2008). Both the frequency and type of parent–child interactions vary with SES, which in turn affects language learning in children (Scheele et al., 2010). Higher SES families talk more to their children and use more facilitative interactions such as shared book reading, storytelling and singing with their children, who acquire language more rapidly as a result (Hart & Risley, 1995; Hoff, 2009; Scheele et al., 2010). Frequency of input and use of facilitative interactions also varies across cultures. For example, in a study of Dutch monolinguals and Turkish–Dutch and Moroccan–Dutch bilingual immigrant families in the Netherlands, the frequency that parents conversed, read books, told stories, sang songs and watched educational television shows with their children varied across the three groups and as a function of the languages spoken in each bilingual group (Scheele et al., 2010). In addition, Structural Equation Modeling showed that the role of SES differed across the three groups. SES impacted parental interactions with monolingual Dutch children in a manner consistent with previous literature, but had virtually no impact on the interactions of Turkish–Dutch parents in either language and impacted interactions of the Moroccan–Dutch parents in Dutch only (Scheele et al., 2010). This was in part due to the greater accessibility of books and educational programs in Dutch and Turkish compared to the Moroccan language. Thus, it is important to consider the specific cultural community and the languages spoken when considering both frequency and type of parent–child interactions.

Characteristics of child-directed speech to children with Down syndrome

Mothers of monolingual children with DS adjust their talk semantically and syntactically to match their child's developmental level. That is, when groups of children with DS and typical development are matched on chronological age, mothers of children with DS talk more simply to their children; when groups are matched on mental age, mothers talk with similar levels of complexity (Rondal & Docquier, 2006); and when groups are matched on syntactic ability, mothers of children with DS talk more complexly to their children with DS (Johnson-Glenberg & Chapman, 2004). Mothers of children with DS also tend to be more directive and less responsive (i.e. give commands and redirect attention more; question, comment, follow the child's lead and recast ill-formed utterances less) than mothers of typically developing children matched for developmental level (e.g. Roach et al., 1998; Venuti et al., 2012). The latter authors also report that mothers of very young children with DS talk more about their children's affect and behavior and less about the surrounding environment than mothers of typically developing children. In part, this style of interaction reflects the increased need to monitor comprehension and control the behavior of children who have a language impairment. However, responsive as opposed to directive interactions have been shown to be more facilitative of language learning in young children (e.g. Roseberry-McKibbin, 2008).

Although there are differences in mothers' interactions with children with DS, there are also similarities. Mothers of children with DS talk about familiar versus unfamiliar nouns and verbs differently, but the modifications they make are the same as those made by mothers of typically developing children matched on mental age (Cleave *et al.*, 1999; Kay-Raining Bird *et al.*, 1999). This indicates that mothers of children with DS are both sensitive to the words that their children do not know and 'teach' those words using similar strategies as mothers of typically developing children.

Assessment and Intervention

The Canadian Association of Speech-Language Pathologists and Audiologists (CASLPA), the American Speech-Language-Hearing Association (ASHA), the Royal College of Speech and Language Therapists (RCSLT) and the International Association of Logopedics and Phoniatry (IALP) have published position statements (ASHA, 1985; Crago & Westernoff, 1997; IALP, 2011) and other policy documents (ASHA 2011a, 2011b, 2004, 2005; RCSLT, 2007) that guide the assessment and treatment of children from culturally and linguistically diverse backgrounds. The policy statements of all four organizations recognize the growing diversity of caseloads and stress the need to provide respectful, evidence-based and culturally safe and competent services in either L1 or both languages.

Family- and client-centered practice

Family-centered practice (FCT) is a widely accepted approach to service delivery. The principles of FCT include recognition that the family is an integral part of the decision-making team, families have primary decision-making and care-giving responsibility for their children and assessment and treatment decisions must reflect the needs and goals of the family (Kay-Raining Bird, 2006). For a bilingual child with DS, then, families' goals and needs must be explored and discussions should focus upon how best to realize their goals.

Assess the language context

Families typically construct a deliberate pattern of language use (language policy) when communicating. Their language policy is based upon beliefs and feelings about the languages available to them and how best to manage their use (Curdt-Christiansen, 2009). For example, a family may adopt a one-parent-one-language family policy when speaking to their children at home. Family language policies vary widely, as illustrated by the children in Box 3.1. In addition, language policies change with the introduction of new events or information. Hachey *et al.* (2010) found that a diagnosis of autism, for example, often served as a 'fork' in the language policy road for families and some families changed how they communicated with their child as a result.

A variety of questionnaires have been developed to assess language context (see Baker, 2011; De Houwer, 2009; Powers, 2010; Restrepo, 1998). We developed a questionnaire to calculate current frequency of input in our lab (which can be shared on request). Direct observation in multiple contexts and with each language is also useful. Focus should be on both the quantity and the type of language input the child is receiving. Specifically, the use of strategies that facilitate language learning should be assessed (e.g. responsive style; shared book reading and storytelling activities).

Children with language impairment may be more vulnerable than typically developing children to home language loss (Kohnert & Medina, 2009). Michel is losing his French skills. This needs to be discussed with the family. If the family's goals, priorities and needs are to ensure that Michel continues to develop his French language skills, it is critical to identify ways to increase French input to Michel. This could mean modifying the family's language policy to increase the use of French in the home. More opportunities to use French outside the home could also be identified, perhaps by enrolling Michel in French recreational activities or transferring him to a French school. The pros and cons of each option should be discussed. The choice of language(s) for intervention can also support home language retention (Kohnert *et al.*, 2005). This issue will be discussed later.

Interactional patterns could also be modified to provide greater support for French language use. For example, De Houwer (2009: 138) recommends using a 'monolingual discourse strategy' in situations where a child does not respond in the language a parent uses. That is, she suggests that parents insist that the child speak the language they are using and not move on in the topic of conversation until he or she does. Michel may also have the ability to engage in direct discussions about the long-term impact of choosing not to talk in French. His personal perspectives and language goals should also be explored.

Assess both languages

Assessment of only one of a bilingual child's languages will not adequately reflect the language knowledge of the child (Patterson & Pearson, 2012; Elin Thordardottir, 2006, 2010). Therefore, both languages should be assessed, preferably by a bilingual clinician fluent in both the child's languages (e.g. Crago & Westernoff, 1997). Barriers to bilingual assessment exist, however. These include not speaking the clients' languages, a lack of valid standardized nent tools and a lack of developmental information about the clients' languages (D'Souza *et al.*, 2012). Correcting these problems will take time and will involve recruiting bilingual speakers from a large variety of language backgrounds into university programs and worksites, developing assessment tools and conducting a considerable amount of developmental and intervention research. Interestingly, monolingual clinicians are significantly more likely than bilingual clinicians to routinely assess and treat in a single language – the one they speak (D'Souza *et al.*, 2011). And many clinicians are not bilingual. A survey of speech-language pathologists across 10 countries reported that 74% of responding clinicians were monolingual and that 87% of bilingual children were being served in one language – that of the clinician (Jordaan, 2008). When bilingual therapists are not available, trained interpreters should assist clinicians (ASHA, 2004; Crago & Westernoff, 1997). Most Canadian clinicians seem to have access to interpreters, but rarely use them (D'Souza *et al.*, 2012). Similarly, clinicians reported using interpreters in only 18% of the cases surveyed by Jordaan (2008). Barriers to interpreters' use need to be investigated.

Difference versus disorder

One of the most difficult assessment tasks when working with children from diverse linguistic and cultural contexts is to distinguish a language difference from a language disorder. Standardized tests are the preferred tools for diagnosing the presence of a problem. A number of authors have discussed in detail the considerable difficulties encountered when using standardized tests for diagnosing disorders in bilingual children and others from diverse backgrounds (e.g. Roseberry-McKibbin, 2007; Wyatt, 2012). Mismatches between the characteristics of the child being assessed and those represented in the standardization sample and other cultural biases of the test are major concerns. For most children with DS, diagnosing a problem is not the primary assessment concern; a cognitive and language disorder will be present relative to same-age peers. Consequently, the assessment will focus more on determining the child's developmental abilities in each language, the relative strengths and weaknesses of various language components and how best to facilitate language growth. While standardized tests may play a role, other assessment tools such as observations, questionnaires, criterion-referenced measures and language sampling will be more useful. Nonetheless, issues of difference versus disorder remain. For instance, it is important to distinguish between patterns that reflect cross-linguistic influence from those that are evidence of a true delay when possible. An example of cross-linguistic transfer that is not evidence of language delay is the overuse of grammatical subjects when speaking Spanish. Subjects can be either overtly produced or omitted in Spanish, but they are obligatory in English. Children who are acquiring Spanish and English and are English dominant may use subjects more frequently when speaking Spanish than their monolingual Spanish-speaking peers (Paradis, 2012). *Errors* that result from cross-linguistic influence, Paradis (2012) cautions, are a normal part of bilingual development and should not be targets of intervention. The degree to which children with DS produce these errors is currently unknown.

AAC in a bilingual context

Children with DS often have expressive–receptive language gaps and can benefit from the introduction of augmentative or alternative forms of communication (AAC; Millar *et al.*, 2006). AAC provides a less transient, more visual, physically easier and more manipulable mode of communication than speech. All of these characteristics may support language learning (Kay-Raining Bird *et al.*, 2000). Children with DS are frequently introduced to sign language. In one study, 85% of children with DS in Wisconsin were introduced to sign language to support early word use (Sedey *et al.*, 1991). Other forms of AAC can be suitable for children with DS as well; selection should be based upon individual needs. Many parents fear that using sign or another form of AAC will inhibit the use of spoken language. Contrary to this belief, Millar *et al.* (2006) reported that gains in spontaneous speech followed the introduction of AAC in 79% of cases of AAC use with children with developmental disabilities that they reviewed.

Majida's frustration when trying to communicate may indicate she would benefit from the introduction of AAC. To facilitate use of speech, spoken language and AAC should be used together when communicating with Majida (i.e. total communication). For bilingual children, it seems logical that AAC should be used with both languages, although no research has been done on AAC use in bilingual children to date. That being said, the vocabulary taught in each language will likely vary. Only 30% of words in the vocabularies of bilingual typically developing toddlers are TEs (Pearson *et al.*, 1995), suggesting that what needs to be said in one language may vary from what needs to be said in the other. AAC builds upon the visual strengths of individuals with DS. Other forms of visual support, such as visual schedules, can be incorporated into intervention with Mahida and the other children in Box 3.1.

Treat one or two languages?

Gains from intervention in one language will sometimes transfer to the other language, increasing the efficiency of treatment efforts. The circumstances under which transfer occurs are not well understood (Kohnert & Medina, 2009). Patterson and Pearson (2012) reviewed the vocabulary intervention literature for typically developing children and concluded that there was little evidence for the transfer of vocabulary gains in very young children. In early development then, treating vocabulary in both languages may be best.

Parents of children with DS are routinely taught to facilitate their child's early language development. Facilitation techniques can be used by parents with all home language(s), and day-care and preschool staff can be trained also. Alternatively, a clinician may treat one language and the parents facilitate the development of the other. Caution should be exercised, however, as language facilitation strategies are based largely upon studies of middle-class parents in Western societies (e.g. Weitzman & Greenberg, 2002). van Kleeck (1994) argued that cultural differences may make certain approaches invalid and that parent training programs should be adjusted to the individual parent and culture. With bilingual children, techniques may need to be modified for each language (e.g. reading materials may not be available in Arabic; Mi'kmaq and English story structure and use differs). A third option is direct bilingual therapy. Elin Thordardottir (2010) reviewed the literature on language intervention with children with language disorders and concluded that there was no evidence that a monolingual focus in intervention resulted in better outcomes than a bilingual focus.

In contrast to younger children, preschool and school-age children transfer vocabulary gains from their stronger to the weaker language (Patterson & Pearson, 2012). Similarly, Perozzi and Sanchez (1992) reported that first graders with language impairment required fewer repetitions to learn new words when they were taught first in their L1 (stronger) language and then in their L2 than if they were taught in their L2 alone. This suggests that vocabulary instruction in developmentally more advanced children, including those with DS, might fruitfully focus first on the stronger language and transfer should be monitored. Cognates have been shown to help fifth-grade English language learners (ELLs) make accurate inferences about the meaning of English words, but these students are more likely to use a cognate strategy if they were instructed on how to do so (Dressler et al., 2011). A cognate strategy is particularly useful when it draws on the meaning of a more frequent word in one language to infer the meaning of a less frequent word in the other language (Patterson & Pearson, 2012). These strategies can be usefully taught to bilingual children with DS.

Making cross-linguistic links, as in use of a cognate strategy, requires metalinguistic skill. Typically developing bilingual children have advanced metalinguistic skills (e.g. Bialystok & Barac, 2012). Advantages become more evident as bilingual fluency increases, but even two-year-old children are more likely to override the mutual exclusivity principle when learning new words if told they are from a different language (Rhemtulla &

Nicoladis, 2003 as cited in Patterson & Pearson, 2012). Bilingual advantages have yet to be studied in bilingual children with DS. To the extent that they exist, they may ameliorate some of the language learning difficulties in this population.

Last Words

In 2009, Kohnert and Medina reported that research on bilingualism in children with communication disorders had significantly increased from previous levels between 2000 and 2008, averaging four to five published articles per year in that period. The number of studies varied across disorder type, with 72% involving children with language impairment only. The research base on bilingualism in children with developmental disabilities and DS specifically remains extremely sparse. Elin Thordardottir (2010) reviewed the literature on the efficacy of language interventions with bilingual children who have cognitive and/or language disorders. She identified only seven studies, three of which were case studies or single-subject designs. Not one published article assessed the efficacy of intervention with bilingual children with DS. This chapter examined a number of issues relevant to bilingualism in children with DS and made recommendations regarding assessment and intervention; however, in the absence of direct information, we must continue to infer from studies of other populations. It is of critical importance that the research base be expanded in the future.

Note

(1) I have chosen to use the term *stronger* instead of *dominant* throughout the chapter.

References

American Speech-Language-Hearing Association (1985) Clinical management of communicatively handicapped minority language populations. *ASHA* 26, 57–60.

American Speech-Language-Hearing Association (2004) Knowledge and skills needed by speech-language pathologists and audiologists to provide culturally and linguistically appropriate services [Knowledge and Skills]. See www.asha.org/policy (accessed 1 June 2015).

American Speech-Language-Hearing Association (2005) Cultural competence [Issues in Ethics]. See www.asha.org/policy (accessed 1 June 2015).

American Speech-Language-Hearing Association (2011a) Cultural competence in professional service delivery [Position statement]. See www.asha.org/policy (accessed 1 June 2015).

American Speech-Language-Hearing Association (2011b) Cultural competence in professional service delivery [Professional Issues Statement]. See www.asha.org/policy (accessed 1 June 2015).

August, D., Carlo, M., Dressler, C. and Snow, C. (2005) The critical role of vocabulary development for English language learners. *Learning Disabilities Research and Practice* 20, 50–57.

Baker, C. (2011) *Foundations of Bilingual Education and Bilingualism* (5th edn). Bristol: Multilingual Matters.

Barac, R. and Bialystok, E. (2012) Bilingual effects on cognitive and linguistic development: Role of language, cultural background, and education. *Child Development* 83, 413–422.

Bialystok, E. and Barac, R. (2012) Emerging bilingualism: Dissociating advantages for metalinguistic awareness and executive control. *Cognition* 122, 67–73.

Burgoyne, K. (2009) Reading interventions for children with DS. *Down Syndrome Research and Practice*, See www.down-syndrome.org/research-practice (retrieved 1 June 2015).

Burgoyne, K., Duff, F., Clarke, P., Buckley, S., Snowling, M. and Hulme, C. (2012) Efficacy of a reading and language intervention for children with DS: A randomized controlled trial. *Journal of Child Psychology and Psychiatry*, first published on-line, 1–10, http://onlinelibrary.wiley.com/doi/10.1111/j.1469-7610.2012.02557.x/pdf (accessed 7 August 2012).

Chapman, R. and Hesketh, L. (2000) Behavioral phenotype of individuals with Down syndrome. *Mental Retardation and Developmental Disability Research Reviews* 6, 84–95.

Chapman, R.S. and Kay-Raining Bird, E. (2011) Language development in childhood, adolescence, and young adulthood in persons with DS. In J. Burack, R. Hodapp, G. Iarocci and E. Zigler (eds) *The Oxford Handbook of Intellectual Disability and Development* (2nd edn; pp. 167–183). Toronto, ON: Oxford University Press.

Chapman, R.S., Hesketh, L. and Kistler, D. (2002) Predicting longitudinal change in language production and comprehension in individuals with Down syndrome: Hierarchical linear modeling. *Journal of Speech, Language, and Hearing Research* 45, 902–915.

Chapman, R.S., Seung, H.-K., Schwartz, S. and Kay-Raining Bird, E. (1998) Language skills of children and adolescents with Down syndrome: II. Production deficits. *Journal of Speech, Language, and Hearing Research* 41, 861–873.

Cleave, P.L. and Kay-Raining Bird, E. (November, 1999) Mothers' talk to children with Down syndrome: Familiar/unfamiliar verbs. Poster presented at the annual ASHA convention, San Francisco, CA.

Collier, V.P. and Thomas, W.P. (2009) *Educating English Learners for a Transformed World*. Albuquerque, NM: Dual Language Education of New Mexico, Fuente Press.

Crago, M. and Westernoff, F. (1997) CASLPA position paper on speech-language pathology and audiology in the multicultural, multilingual context. *Journal of Speech-Language Pathology and Audiology* 21, 223–224.

Curdt-Christiansen, X.L. (2009) Invisible and visible language planning: Ideological factors in the family language policy of Chinese immigrant families in Quebec. *Language Policy* 8, 351–375.

D'Souza, C., Kay-Raining Bird, E. and Deacon, H. (2012) Survey of Canadian speech-language pathology services to linguistically diverse clients. *Canadian Journal of Speech-language Pathology and Audiology* 36, 18–39.

De Houwer, A. (2007) Parental language input patterns and children's bilingual use. *Applied Psycholinguistics* 28, 411–424.

De Houwer, A. (2009) *Bilingual First Language Acquisition*. Bristol: Multilingual Matters.

Dressler, C., Carlo, M., Snow, C., August, D. and White, C. (2011) Spanish-speaking students' use of cognate knowledge to infer the meaning of English words. *Bilingualism: Language and Cognition* 14, 243–255.

Dickinson, D., McCabe, A., Clark-Chiarelli, N. and Wold, A. (2004) Cross-language transfer of phonological awareness in low income Spanish and English bilingual preschool children. *Applied Psycholinguistics* 25, 323–347.

Duursma, E., Romero-Contreras, S., Szuber, A., Proctor, P. and Snow, C.E. (2007) The role of home literacy and language environment on bilinguals' English and Spanish vocabulary development. *Applied Psycholinguistics* 28, 171–190.

Edgin, J.O., Kumar, A., Spano, G. and Nadel, L. (2011) Neuropsychological effects of second language exposure in DS. *Journal of Intellectual Disability Research* 55, 351–356.

Elin Thordardottir (2002) Parents' views on language impairment and bilingualism. Paper presented at the American Speech and Hearing Association Conference, Atlanta, GA, November.

Elin Thordardottir (2006) Language intervention from a bilingual mindset. *ASHA Leader* 6, 21.

Elin Thordardottir (2010) Towards evidence-based practice in language intervention for bilingual children. *Journal of Communication Disorders* 43, 523–537.

Elin Thordardottir, Rothenberg, A., Rivard, M.-E. and Naves, R. (2006) Bilingual assessment: Can overall proficiency be estimated from separate measurement of two languages? *Journal of Multilingual Communication Disorders* 4, 1–21.

Feltmate, K. and Kay-Raining Bird, E. (2008) Language learning in four bilingual children with DS: A detailed analysis of vocabulary and morphosyntax. *Canadian Journal of Speech-Language Pathology and Audiology* 32, 6–20.

Fenson, L., Dale, P., Reznick, S., Thal, D., Bates, E., Hartung, J., Pethick, S. and Reilly, J. (1993) *The MacArthur Communicative Development Inventory.* San Diego, CA: Singular Publishing.

Gaelic Council of Nova Scotia (2012) *Nova Scotian Gaelic.* See http://www.gaelic.ca/ (accessed 7 August 2012).

Genesee, F. (2004) What do we know about bilingual education for minority language students? In T.K. Bhatia and W. Ritchie (eds) *Handbook of Bilingualism and Multiculturalism* (pp. 547–576). Malden, MA: Blackwell Publishing.

Genesee, F. (2007) French immersion and at-risk students: A review of research findings. *Canadian Modern Language Review* 63, 655–688.

Genesee, F., Lindholm-Leary, K., Saunders, W. and Christian, D. (2005) English language learners in US schools: An overview of research findings. *Journal of Education for Students Placed at Risk* 10, 363–385.

Guiterrez-Clellen, V., Simon-Cereijido, G. and Leone, A.E. (2009) Code-switching in bilingual children with specific language impairment. *International Journal of Bilingualism* 13, 91–109.

Hachey, A., Kay-Raining Bird, E. and Hughes, J. (October, 2010) The bilingual experience of children with autism and their families: A qualitative study. The 3rd International Association for the Scientific Study of Intellectual Disabilities Europe Congress, Rome, Italy.

Hambly, C. and Fombonne, E. (2011) The impact of bilingual environments on language development in children with autism spectrum disorders. *Journal of Autism and Developmental Disorders* 42, 1342–1352.

Hart, B. and Risley, T.R. (1995) *Meaningful Differences in the Everyday Experiences of Young American Children.* Toronto, ON: Paul H. Brookes.

Hoff, E. (2009) *Language Development* (4th edn). Belmont, CA: Wadsworth Cengage Learning.

International Association of Logopedics and Phoniatrics (2011) Recommendations for working with bilingual children (updated May 2011). See http://www.linguistics.ualberta.ca/en/CHESL_Centre/~/media/linguistics/Media/CHESL/Documents/WorkingWithBilingualChildren-May2011.pdf (accessed 20 August 2015).

Jarrold, C., Purser, H. and Brock, J. (2006) Short-term memory in Down syndrome. In T.P. Alloway and S. Gathercole (eds) *Working Memory and Neurodevelopmental Disorders* (pp. 239–266). New York: Psychology Press.

Johansson, B.B. (2011) Current trends in stroke rehabilitation. A review with focus on brain plasticity. *Acta Neurologica Scandinavica* 123, 147–159.

Johnson, J. and Newport, E. (1989) Critical period effects in second language learning: The influence of maturational state on the acquisition of English as a second language. *Cognitive Psychology* 21, 60–99.

Johnson-Glenberg, M.C. and Chapman, R.S. (2004) Predictors of parent-child language during novel task play: A comparison between typically developing children and individuals with Down syndrome. *Journal of Intellectual Disability Research* 48, 225–238.

Jordaan, H. (2008) Clinical intervention for bilingual children: An international study. *Folia Phoniatrica et Logopaedica* 60, 97–105.

Junker, D.A. and Stockman, I. (2002) Expressive vocabulary of German-English bilingual toddlers. *American Journal of Speech-Language Pathology* 11, 381–394.

Kay-Raining Bird, E. (2006) The case for bilingualism in children with DS. In R. Paul (ed.) *Language Disorders From a Developmental Perspective: Essays in Honor of Robin S. Chapman* (pp. 249–275). Mahwah, NJ: Lawrence Erlbaum Associates.

Kay-Raining Bird, E. and Chapman, R.S. (2011) Literacy development in childhood, adolescence, and young adulthood in persons with DS. In J. Burack, R. Hodapp, G. Iarocci and E. Zigler (eds) *The Oxford Handbook of Intellectual Disability and Development* (2nd edn; pp. 184–199) Toronto, ON: Oxford University Press.

Kay-Raining Bird, E., Cleave, P.L. and Chapman, R.S. (July, 1999) Mother's talk about familiar and unfamiliar verbs: Does language ability make a difference? Poster presented at the International Association for the study of Child Language, San Sebastian, Spain.

Kay-Raining Bird, E., Lamond, E. and Holden, J.J. (2011) A survey of bilingualism in autism spectrum disorders. *International Journal of Language and Communication Disorders* 47, 52–64.

Kay-Raining Bird, E., Cleave, P.L., Trudeau, N., Elin Thordardottir, Sutton, A. and Thorpe, A. (2005) The language abilities of bilingual children with DS. *American Journal of Speech-Language Pathology* 14, 187–199.

Kay-Raining Bird, E., Gaskell, A., Babineau, M. and MacDonald, S. (2000) Novel word acquisition in children with Down syndrome: Does modality make a difference? *Journal of Communication Disorders* 33, 241–266.

Kay-Raining Bird, E., Trudeau, N., Cleave, P. and Sutton, A. (in preparation) A longitudinal study of bilingual ability in children with Down syndrome.

Kohnert, K. and Medina, A. (2009) Bilingual children and communication disorders: A 30-year research retrospective. *Seminars in Speech and Language* 30, 219–233.

Kohnert, K., Yim, D., Nett, K., Kan, P.F. and Duran, L. (2005) Intervention with linguistically diverse preschool children: A focus on developing home language(s). *Language, Speech and Hearing Services in the Schools* 36, 251–263.

Kuhl, P. (2011) Early language learning and literacy: Neuroscience implications for education. *Mind, Brain and Education* 5, 128–142.

Lindholm-Leary, K. and Borsato, G. (2006) Academic achievement. In F. Genesee, K. Lindholm-Leary, W. Saunders and D. Christian (eds) *Educating English Language Learners: A Synthesis of Research Evidence* (pp. 176–222). New York: Cambridge University Press.

Maneva, B. and Genesee, F. (2002) Bilingual babbling: Evidence for language differentiation in dual language acquisition. In B. Skarabela, S. Fish and A.H.J. Do (eds) *Proceedings of the 26th Annual Boston University Conference on Language Development* (pp. 383–392). Somerville, MA: Cascadilla Press.

Marinova-Todd, S., Marshall, D.B. and Snow, C. (2000) Three misconceptions about age and L2 learning. *TESOL Quarterly* 34, 9–34.

Millar, D., Light, J. and Schlosser, R.W. (2006) The impact of augmentative and alternative communication intervention on the speech production of individuals with developmental disabilities: A research review. *Journal of Speech, Language and Hearing Research* 49, 248–264.

Ministry of Industry (2008) Aboriginal Peoples in Canada in 2006: Inuit, Métis and First Nations, 2006 Census. Statistics Canada, Catalogue no. 97-558-XIE. See http://www12.statcan.ca/english/census06/analysis/aboriginal/pdf/97-558-XIE2006001.pdf (accessed 7 August 2012).

Nelson, R., Damico, J. and Smith, S. (2008) Applying eye movement miscue analysis to the reading patterns of children with language impairment. *Clinical Linguistics & Phonetics* 22, 293–303.

Nicoladis, E. (1998) First clues to the existence of two input languages: Pragmatic and lexical differentiation in a bilingual child. *Bilingualism: Language and Cognition* 1, 105–116.

Nicoladis, E. and Genesee, F. (1997) Language development in preschool bilingual children. *Journal of Speech-Language Pathology and Audiology* 21, 258–270.

Ohashi, J.K., Mirenda, P., Marinova-Todd, S., Hambly, C., Fombonne, E., Szatmari, P., Bryson, S., Roberts, W., Smith, I., Vaillancourt, T., Volden, J., Waddell, C., Zwaigenbaum, L., Georgiades, S., Duku, E., Thompson, A. and the Pathways in ASD Study Team (2012) Comparing early language development in monolingual and bilingual-exposed young children with autism spectrum disorders. *Research in Autism Spectrum Disorders* 6, 890–897.

Oller, D.K. and Eilers, R.E. (2002) Balancing interpretations regarding effects of bilingualism: Empirical and theoretical possibilities. In D.K. Oller and R.E. Eilers (eds) *Language and Literacy in Bilingual Children* (pp. 281–292). Clevedon: Multilingual Matters.

Oller, D.K., Pearson, B.Z. and Cobo-Lewis, A.B. (2007) Profile effects in early bilingual language and literacy. *Applied Psycholinguistics* 28, 191–230.

Oller, D.K., Eilers, R.E., Urbano, R. and Cobo-Lewis, A.B. (1997) Developmental precursors to speech in infants exposed to two languages. *Journal of Child Language* 24, 407–425.

Papagno, C. and Vallar, G. (2001) Understanding metaphors and idioms: A single-case neuropsychological study in a person with Down syndrome. *Journal of the International Neuropsychological Society* 7, 516–527.

Paradis, J. (2007) Bilingual children with specific language impairment. *Applied Psycholinguistics* 28, 551–564.

Paradis, J. (2010) The interface between bilingual development and specific language impairment. Keynote article for special issue with peer commentaries. *Applied Psycholinguistics* 31, 3–28.

Paradis, J. (2012) Cross-linguistic influence and code-switching. In B.A. Goldstein (ed.) *Bilingual Language Development and Disorders in Spanish-English Speakers* (pp. 73–91). Baltimore, MD: Paul H. Brookes.

Paradis, J., Crago, M., Genesee, F. and Rice, M. (2003) French-English bilingual children with SLI: How do they compare with their monolingual peers? *Journal of Speech, Language, and Hearing Research* 46, 113–127.

Paradis, J., Genesee, F. and Crago, M. (2011) *Dual Language Development and Disorders* (2nd edn). Baltimore, MD: Paul H. Brookes.

Patterson, J.L. (1998) Expressive vocabulary development and word combinations of Spanish-English bilingual toddlers. *American Journal of Speech Language Pathology* 4, 46–56.

Patterson, J.L. and Pearson, B.Z. (2012) Bilingual lexical development: Assessment and intervention. In B.A. Goldstein (ed.) *Bilingual Language Development and Disorders in Spanish-English Speakers* (pp. 113–139). Baltimore, MD: Paul H. Brookes.

Pearson, B.Z., Fernández, S.C. and Oller, D.K. (1993) Lexical development in bilingual infants and toddlers: Comparison to monolingual norms. *Language Learning* 43, 93–120.

Pearson, B.Z., Fernández, S.C., Lewedeg, V. and Oller, D.K. (1997) The relation of input factors to lexical learning in bilingual infants. *Applied Psycholinguistics* 18, 41–58.

Perozzi, J.A. and Sanchez, M.L. (1992) The effect of instruction in L1 on receptive acquisition of L2 for bilingual children with language delay. *Language, Speech and Hearing Services in Schools* 23, 348–352.

Petersen, J., Marinova-Todd, S. and Mirenda, P. (2011) Brief report: An exploratory study of lexical skills in bilingual children with autism spectrum disorder. *Journal of Autism and Developmental Disorders* 42, 1499–1503.

Powers, B.L. (2010) Bilingual Spanish-English speaking 4-year-old children: English normative data and correlations with parent reports. Doctoral dissertation, Portland State University.

Restrepo, M. (1998) Identifiers of predominantly Spanish-speaking children with language impairment. *Journal of Speech, Language, and Hearing Research* 41, 1398–1411.

Roach, M.A. Barratt, M., Miller, J.F. and Leavitt, L.A. (1998) The structure of mother-child play: Young children with Down Syndrome and typically developing children. *Developmental Psychology* 34, 77–87.

Roberts, J., Chapman, R.S. and Warren, S. (eds) (2008) *Speech and Language Development and Intervention in Down Syndrome and Fragile X Syndrome*. Baltimore, MD: Brookes Publishing.

Rondal, J.A. (2000) Bilingualism in mental retardation: Some prospective views. *Child Development and Disabilities* 26, 57–64.

Rondal, J. and Buckley, S. (eds) (2004) *Speech and Language Intervention in Down Syndrome*. London: Whurr Publishers.

Rondal, J.A. and Docquier, L. (2006) Maternal speech to children with Down syndrome: An update. *The Journal of Speech-Language Pathology and Applied Behavior Analysis* 1, 218–227.

Roseberry-McKibbin, C. (2007) *Language Disorders in Children: A Multicultural and Case Perspective*. Boston, MA: Pearson.

Roseberry-McKibbin, C. (2008) *Increasing Language Skills of Students From Low Income Backgrounds. Practical Strategies for Professionals*. San Diego, CA: Plural Publishing.

Royal College of Speech and Language Therapists (2007) Good practice for speech and language therapists working with clients from linguistic minority communities. Prepared by the RCSLT Specific Interest Group in Bilingualism. See http://www.rcslt.org/members/publications/publications2/linguistic_minorities (accessed 19 June 2014).

Scheele, A.F., Leseman, P.P.M. and Mayo, A.Y. (2010) The home language environment of monolingual and bilingual children and their language proficiency. *Applied Psycholinguistics* 31, 117–140.

Sedey, A., Rosin, P. and Miller, J. (November, 1991) The use of signs among children with Down syndrome. Poster presented at the annual convention of the American Speech-Language-Hearing Association, Atlanta, GA.

Smith, N. (2010) Code-mixing in young English-French bilinguals with Down syndrome. Undergraduate honours thesis, Dalhousie University.

Statistics Canada (2009a) Population by mother tongue and age groups, 2006 counts, for Canada, provinces and territories – 20% sample data. See http://www12.statcan.gc.ca/census-recensement/2006/dp-pd/hlt/97-555/T401-eng.cfm?Lang=E&T=401&GH=4&SC=1&S=99&O=A (accessed 2 August 2012).

Tabors, P.O. (2008) *One Child, Two Languages. A Guide for Early Childhood Educators of Children Learning English as a Second Language* (2nd edn). Baltimore, MD: Brookes Publishing.

Thomas, W.P. and Collier, V.P. (2012) *Dual Language Education for a Transformed World*. Albuquerque, NM: Dual Language Education of New Mexico, Fuente Press.

Trudeau, N., Kay-Raining Bird, E., Sutton, A. and Cleave, P. (2011) Développement lexical chez les enfants bilingues ayant le syndrome de Down. *Enfance* 2011 (3), 383–404.

Vallar, G. and Papagno, C. (1993) Preserved vocabulary acquisition in Down's syndrome: The role of phonological short-term memory. *Cortex* 29, 467–483.

van Kleeck, A. (1994) Potential cultural bias in training parents as conversational partners with their children who have delays in language development. *American Journal of Speech-Language Pathology* 3, 67–78.

Venuti, P., de Falco, S., Esposito, G., Zaninelli, M. and Borstein, M. (2012) Maternal functional speech to children: A comparison of autism spectrum disorder, Down syndrome, and typical development. *Research in Developmental Disabilities* 33, 506–517.

Wang, M., Cheng, C. and Chen, S.-W. (2006) Contribution of morphological awareness to Chinese-English biliteracy acquisition. *Journal of Educational Psychology* 98, 542–553.

Weitzman, E. and Greenberg, J. (2002) *Learning Language and Loving It: A Guide to Promoting Children's Social, Language, and Literacy Development in Early Childhood Settings* (2nd edn). Toronto, ON: The Hanen Centre.

Wilken, E. (2003) Bilingualism in children with Down syndrome in Germany. *Down Syndrome News and Update* 2 (4), 146–147.

Woll, B. and Grove, N. (1996) On language deficits and modality in children with DS: A case study of twins bilingual in BSL and English. *Journal of Deaf Studies and Deaf Education* 1, 271–278.

Wyatt, T. (2012) Assessment of multicultural and international clients with communication disorders. In D. Battle (ed.) *Communication Disorders in Multicultural and International Populations* (4th edn, pp. 243–278). St. Louis, MI: Elsevier, Mosby.

4 Communication in Children with Fetal Alcohol Spectrum Disorders: Impairment and Intervention

John C. Thorne and Truman E. Coggins

Introduction

The term *fetal alcohol spectrum disorders* (FASD) is an umbrella term used to describe the range of negative consequences that can occur due to prenatal exposure to ethyl alcohol, a spectrum of impairments that includes *fetal alcohol syndrome* (FAS). Because alcohol is consumed almost universally in human cultures, the risk for FAS or another FASD exists across socio-economic, linguistic and cultural backgrounds. This chapter will briefly explore how FASD have come to be recognized, the types of impairments found on the spectrum and how FASD are diagnosed. This will be followed by a review of the research on communication challenges found in this population as well as current thinking regarding interventions to improve outcomes for individuals with FASD. While the bulk of research on this topic has involved English-speaking populations, we have included the available research on other languages in this review.

Background

In the late 19th century, Sullivan (1899) was the first to publish a detailed examination of the developmental damage to children that can result from maternal drinking. It was not until the late 1960s, however, that researchers in France (Lemoine *et al.*, 1968) first characterized in detail the teratogenic effects of prenatal ethyl alcohol exposure (PAE), effects that were not widely recognized until the 1970s when Jones and Smith (1973) first used the term *fetal alcohol syndrome*. As a result of this important early work, FAS is now internationally recognized as a permanent birth defect syndrome resulting from PAE.

FAS is defined by the presence of growth deficiency, a unique cluster of three minor facial anomalies (i.e. small eyes, thin upper lip and smooth philtrum) and evidence of central nervous system (CNS) abnormalities, all found in the context of PAE. With best estimates indicating that FAS may be present in between 1 and 3 cases per 1000 live births, FAS is the leading known preventable cause of developmental disabilities and mental retardation worldwide (Bailey & Sokol, 2008). Because not all children with impairments in the context of PAE will end up with a diagnosis of FAS, the umbrella term *fetal alcohol spectrum disorders* is used to refer to the full range of impairments associated with PAE. FAS, therefore, represents only the most readily recognized of the FASD, largely because the distinctive FAS facial features that define it provide a specific and reliable diagnostic marker of PAE when properly assessed (Astley, 2006). Sharing a similar range and severity of CNS impairments and social costs, FASD without the facial features of FAS are many times more prevalent than FAS – perhaps approaching 1% of all children (Bailey & Sokol, 2008) – but are more difficult to diagnose because they are not accompanied by the FAS facial phenotype. Without that objective biological marker, exposure risk remains unknown for many children, a particular problem for children in foster or adoptive placements where the biological mother is often unavailable or unwilling to provide exposure information. As a result, much of the research in the field has been driven by an attempt to identify other biological, behavioral or cognitive markers of damage caused by PAE that are as specific to exposure as the face of FAS – so far without clear success.

In multilingual and multicultural populations, the presence of PAE is an important risk factor that can complicate the task of determining difference versus disorder when children present with communication challenges. When FAS or another FASD is present in these children, the challenges inherent in negotiating multiple sociocultural and linguistic contexts may be exacerbated by underlying neurodevelopmental impairments. The possibility that PAE has caused neurodevelopmental impairments should be kept in mind as interventions are considered and implemented for any child, no matter his or her background, and clinicians should always take steps to gather the information they need to understand the level of exposure risk that is present. This is best done in the context of an interdisciplinary assessment that carefully examines both the body structures and body functions that can be impaired by PAE (Astley, 2004).

Impairment in FASD

The extent and nature of the damage caused by PAE is, of course, related to the dose and timing of exposure, so the range of impairments seen in individuals with PAE is highly variable. The CNS is the most vulnerable body system to PAE. Throughout development, a variety of developmental processes, cell types and regions in the brain can be damaged by that exposure (e.g. synaptogenesis, neuronal migration and differentiation, myelination; see Guerri, 2002). As expected, these disruptions in development can lead to structural and neurochemical abnormalities throughout the CNS. Frontal lobes and the caudate nucleus of the basal ganglia appear to be particularly vulnerable to damage (Astley, Aylward et al., 2009).

As might be expected, group differences in performance on intelligence tests between children with PAE and their unexposed peers are well documented. IQ scores reported for children with FASD, however, cover the range from profoundly handicapped to above average intelligence. For example, Streissguth et al. (1996) examined the intellectual abilities of 473 individuals with documented PAE. More than 90% of children with FASD had an IQ broadly within the average range. Indeed, even among children with FAS, approximately 75% have IQ scores above 70 (Astley & Clarren, 2001; Riley & McGee, 2005). But IQ does not tell the full story. Many children with FASD, including those who have IQ scores in the average range, are found to have deficits across a variety of functional and cognitive domains. Commonly reported differences have included attention, reaction time, visual spatial learning, fine/gross motor control and balance, verbal learning, executive function, working memory, mathematical reasoning, non-verbal inductive reasoning, information processing and language (see Astley, Olson et al., 2009; Kodituwakku, 2007; Mattson et al., 2011 for reviews).

Not surprisingly, given that structures that support executive functioning seem particularly vulnerable to PAE (e.g. caudate nucleus, frontal lobes), impairments of the executive function are seen more often in children with FASD than in their peers – with inattention being, perhaps, the most common concern in children with FASD. In addition, deficits in planning, set shifting, problem solving, social skills and adaptive functioning are also commonly reported, as are clinically significant problems maintaining appropriate behaviors (Astley, Olson et al., 2009; Kodituwakku, 2007; Riley & McGee, 2005; Schonfeld et al., 2006; Vaurio et al., 2011).

Fine motor, gross motor and visual-motor deficits are also associated with PAE (Mattson et al., 2011; Riley & McGee, 2005). Tone abnormalities, tremulousness, oral motor (suck-swallow) difficulties and delayed motor milestones are found in early childhood, while impaired balance, reduced fine motor control, visual spatial problems, as well as motor immaturities and other 'neurologic soft signs' are reported in older children. These findings are consistent with reports of clumsiness and speed/accuracy trade-offs in children with FASD (Jirikowic et al., 2008; Riley & McGee, 2005).

Behaviors suggesting both over- and under-responsivity to stimuli consistent with poor sensory modulation have been described among clinic-referred children with FASD (Franklin *et al.*, 2008; Jirikowic *et al.*, 2008). These kinds of sensory processing problems may underlie motor and postural deficits and contribute to poor behavioral regulation in these individuals.

Among clinical samples of individuals affected by PAE there is also a high rate of comorbid mental health problems (O'Connor & Paley, 2006; Streissguth & O'Malley, 2000). Even at low levels, PAE has been associated with an increased risk for mental health problems, particularly in young females (Sayal *et al.*, 2007). In addition, research suggests that PAE may be an independent risk factor for the development of alcohol abuse disorders in adulthood (see e.g. Alati *et al.*, 2006; O'Malley, 2007).

Whenever PAE is found in the context of other risk factors, it may exacerbate challenges for the developing child and increase the risk for secondary disabilities later in life (Streissguth *et al.*, 2004). This is true whether those additional risk factors are adverse prenatal and postnatal exposures with a known biological risk associated (e.g. polydrug exposure, abuse and/or neglect), or when there are sociocultural risk factors such as poverty or a minority language/cultural status that may represent an environmental barrier to the individual meeting his or her full potential in certain social contexts.

Diagnosis in FASD

Whenever PAE is suspected, an FASD diagnosis can be considered. The degree of impairment found in body structures and functions that define FAS is used to define diagnostic categories that fall under the umbrella of FASD. The four factors that go into a diagnosis are: (1) prenatal and postnatal growth, (2) the FAS facial phenotype, (3) CNS integrity and (4) evidence for and degree of PAE.

The FASD 4-digit diagnostic code is the most comprehensive, systematic and widely used method internationally for assessing and diagnosing FASD (3rd edition, Astley [2004]; free guidelines, measurement tools/software available at www.fasdpn.org). The other major diagnostic systems, the *Canadian Guidelines for FASD Diagnosis* (Chudley *et al.*, 2005) and the *Guidelines for Identifying FAS* from the Centers for Disease Control (CDC; Bertrand *et al.*, 2005), incorporate methods/measurement tools from the 4-digit code, but use modified diagnostic criteria.

In the 4-digit code, FAS is diagnosed when an individual exhibits (1) *growth deficiency* (height and/or weight ≤10th percentile); (2) *FAS facial phenotype* including small eyes (palpebral fissure length more than 2 SD below the mean), a smooth philtrum and a thin upper lip meaning Ranks 4 or 5 for each on the *University of Washington Lip-Philtrum Guide* (Astley, 2004); and (3) *significant CNS abnormality* (2 SD from the mean in three or more domains of brain function, or direct structural/neurological evidence such as microcephaly or seizures). The expression of this constellation of features *at these values* has high specificity for PAE, and as such can serve as a proxy indicator of PAE when exposure is unknown (see Astley, 2006). If alcohol exposure is confirmed, but these criteria are not met, another FASD diagnosis can be given. In the 4-digit code, these FASD diagnoses do not imply a causal role between exposure and the identified abnormalities in the CNS. Instead, they simply describe the degree and type of impairment and document PAE as an important risk factor present.

Communication in Individuals with FASD

The majority of research into communication disorders in FASD is based on English-speaking children; however, similar results are found regardless of language in the available research. While not all children with an FASD will have communication disorders, current evidence suggests they may be among the most common impairments associated with FASD. For instance, in a survey of a large clinic-referred FASD population presented by Astley (2010), 299 out of 1270 children with a significant CNS impairment were reported as having significant impairment in the domain of language (i.e. performance 2 SD from the mean). At 24% of the population, this rate of language impairment was higher than any other single functional domain surveyed with the exception of attention deficit hyperactivity disorder (ADHD) (425 children or 33%). While, to date, no detailed and systematic attempt has been made to characterize the direct level of risk for language disorder that PAE poses, it is clear that, at least in children for whom there is sufficient concern to trigger a clinical assessment, the domain of language functioning is one of the most commonly found to be impacted in children with an FASD.

Language and communication disorders have been documented for children with FASD in all areas from hearing and auditory/phonological processing to morphosyntax, semantics, verbal memory, discourse cohesion, functional communication, as well as pragmatics and social communication (see e.g. Aragón *et al.*, 2008; Chasnoff *et al.*, 2010; Church & Kaltenbach, 1997; Cone-Wesson, 2005; Streissguth *et al.*, 1994; Wyper & Rasmussen, 2011). Children with FASD are frequently described as having particular difficulty with the processing of complex information (see e.g. Kodituwakku, 2007) and responding to dynamically changing social situations (Coggins *et al.*, 2003), so early development may not be a reliable indicator of success as communication demands increase in complexity through the school years. Indeed, Coggins *et al.* (2007), when looking at a subset of 393 school-aged children from the same clinical population examined by Astley (2010), found severe communicative disorders in at least one domain of language in 38% of children with an FASD. This figure rose to 60% when measures of narrative discourse were included in the assessment. When mild disorders (−1.25 to −2.00 SD) were included in the analysis, 68% of this sample demonstrated an impairment of some aspect of language.

Despite these findings, however, the research on the effect of PAE on speech and language development provides an inconsistent picture. For instance, as might be expected in a highly heterogeneous group, case studies indicate a wide range of impairments and severities, ranging from absence of speech to mild articulation disorders (Mattson *et al.*, 2011). Retrospective group studies have found impairments related to PAE ranging from pragmatics to word comprehension and receptive language functioning, naming ability, mixed expressive and receptive language disorders, verbal memory and functional communication disorders, and disorders of vocabulary, sentence imitation and grammatical comprehension (see e.g. Abkarian, 1992; Chasnoff *et al.*, 2010; Wyper & Rasmussen, 2011). In a long-term prospective study, 14-year-old children with PAE exhibited deficits in phonological skills needed for pseudoword reading (Streissguth *et al.*, 1994). Although most studies of speech, language and communication characteristics associated with PAE have been conducted with English-speaking children, population studies with children in Italy have also shown specific impairments in language comprehension and academic achievement (Aragón *et al.*, 2008).

Recent research indicates early language delays in multilingual children (Afrikaans and Xhosa speaking) in South Africa with high levels of PAE (Davies *et al.*, 2011). This is consistent with a series of earlier prospective studies that found early language impairment to be associated with PAE up to 3 years of age (Fried & Watkinson, 1988; Gusella & Fried, 1984). However, this earlier research, which looked at children with lower levels of PAE, did not see similar delays upon follow-up at 5 and 6 years of age using measures of vocabulary and basic morphosyntax (Fried *et al.*, 1992). And, indeed, another study that also looked at children with lower levels of PAE (Greene *et al.*, 1990) found no impairments in expressive or receptive language in 1-, 2- and 3-year-old children using basic measures such as mean length of utterance (MLU).

Taken together, these findings suggest greater risk of language disorder with greater PAE, and a preliminary indication that vocabulary and some earlier-developing aspects of language may be relatively robust in the face of PAE. Indeed, it may be later-developing, more complex aspects of language that are most vulnerable to PAE. Evidence for this line of thinking is found in research that focuses on integrative language functioning needed to produce cohesive and coherent discourse. For instance, Coggins *et al.* (2003) found that school-aged children with FASD struggle to balance social cognitive and linguistic demands during contextually integrated discourse including narrative discourse (Coggins *et al.*, 2007), and Timler *et al.* (2005) found that these children may not consistently consider the perspective of the listener during interaction. Detailed analysis of how school-aged children use definite and indefinite noun phrases to *introduce* new information and *refer to* known information during a narrative generation task indicates that, as a group, children with FASD make more frequent errors than their typically developing peers. So, for instance, a child with FASD is more likely than a typically developing peer to *introduce* a character into a story using the form 'The boy', a referential form which indicates that the BOY is already part of the shared common ground of knowledge between the speaker and listener (i.e. the storyteller has used a form that *refers to* known information, rather than one that *introduces* new information on the first mention of the information). These types of errors create an additional processing load on the listener by, for instance, initiating a futile search in memory for the antecedent occurrence in the discourse of the entity referred to by the referential form. The risk that a child with an FASD will make a substantial number of these errors increases based on the severity of the CNS abnormality and FASD diagnostic category (Thorne, 2010).

As yet, it is unclear whether difficulties with later-developing aspects of discourse seen in children with FASD are rooted in an underlying difficulty with social perspective taking, or come about due to reduced cognitive control abilities that make it difficult for these children to monitor and adjust to the rapid changes to the context that occur during discourse. What is clear is that more complex aspects of communicative discourse need to be addressed in both assessment and intervention for this population.

In summary, the language and communication outcomes associated with PAE appear to be highly variable both across individuals and developmental stages. Some children may have language abilities relatively spared early on, only to face significant challenges as language demands increase. Others will face significant challenges across all developmental stages. And some children's language and communication abilities will be spared as they face challenges in other domains of functioning. What is clear, however, is that PAE is an important risk factor to consider whenever language and communication are assessed. For children from multilingual and multicultural backgrounds, of course, the presence of neurodevelopmental impairment in the cognitive systems that support both effective language learning and successful implementation of communicative behavior will make the challenge of navigating multiple social contexts that much more challenging. Clinicians and caregivers who provide support for these individuals will need to keep the complex profile of challenges that may be present due to PAE in mind as they design and implement interventions.

Intervention

So, as we've seen, PAE exerts a broad range of harmful effects on the developing brain. In fact, Kodituwakka and Kodituwakku (2011: 205) have aptly noted that 'neurocognitive deficits and behavioral-emotional disturbances are ubiquitous in this clinical group'. Since the risk for FASD cuts across all social, cultural and economic boundaries, these wide-ranging deficits and disturbances place an even greater responsibility on teachers and clinicians who work with children from multilingual and/or multicultural environments.

Until recently, the bulk of the treatment approaches for FASD was based on personal testimonials, clinical judgments or professional endorsements (e.g. Kleinfeld & Wescott, 1993). While not theory driven or empirically validated, these early approaches yielded two basic truths. First, the challenges faced by children with FASD are brain based and affect how they perceive and process information. Second, getting a desired behavior from a child with a brain-based impairment often means changing the environment rather than changing the child. Thus, increasing structure, creating routines and/or using visual supports have become widely accepted means of addressing problematic behaviors.

In the following sections, we examine two intervention literatures that have emerged for instructing and treating children with FASD. We first focus on selected educational interventions that address the special needs of children with FASD during daily classroom instruction. We then turn our attention to several evidence-based, clinical interventions that focus more directly on remediating the behavioral and/or social problems in children with FASD. While the observations and findings have largely been derived from experiences with children from middle-class families in the United States, we believe that the findings and implications are directly relevant for multilingual and multicultural populations.

Educational interventions

Even though alcohol is a toxic agent that can damage brain cells, organization and structures, children with FASD often come to the attention of an educational system because of behavioral challenges, not because their mothers consumed alcohol during pregnancy. Thus, teachers run the risk of interpreting a child's non-compliant and/or challenging classroom behaviors as annoying, resisting or refusing rather than a manifestation of a neurologically based disability. Adding to this enigma, the measured IQ of children with FASD often falls broadly within the average range of functioning, compounding the risk that these vulnerable children go unrecognized and/or are misdiagnosed. This baffling state may be even more acute when cultural or linguistic differences mask subtle neurocognitive impairments and are interpreted as the reason for differences in performance. Even though there is widespread agreement that children with FASD benefit from specialized curricula, these youngsters often do not receive important accommodations in their classrooms or the functional supports they need (Kalberg & Buckley, 2007).

Two 'best practice' curricula have been developed as potentially effective methods for children with FASD. Both intervention methods are built on environmental modifications and functional supports to assist the child in reaching optimal educational outcomes.

The first curriculum, *Teaching Students with Fetal Alcohol Spectrum Disorder: Building Strengths, Creating Hope* (Clarren, 2004), is part of the programming for students with special needs series by the Alberta Learning Resource Center (Special Programs Branch) in Alberta, Canada. *Teaching Students with FAS* is a curriculum to assist educators in 'thinking about and understanding the complex learning and behavioral issues associated with FASD' (Clarren, 2004: 15). The curriculum is built around the belief that identifying individual strengths and needs is the starting point for children who have CNS damage associated with PAE.

Teaching Students with FASD provides key accommodations to support learning and performance. These environmental supports structure the learning environment in a way that allows the child to compensate for impairments in attention, memory and self-regulation that may be standing in the way of learning new behaviors and skills.

The second specialized curriculum was developed by the National Organization on Fetal Alcohol Syndrome – South Dakota (NOFAS-SD). The *Fetal Alcohol Spectrum Disorders Educational Strategies: Working with Students with a Fetal Alcohol Spectrum Disorder in the Education System* curriculum resource guide was published in 2009. The curriculum is a collaborative, team approach model that draws on all available expertise in the school district and surrounding community to assist classroom teachers in meeting the complex needs of children with FASD.

According to NOFAS-SD, there are 'five keys' necessary for successful outcomes when working with the unusual learning patterns of youngsters exposed to alcohol. These fundamental features are structure, consistency, variety, brevity and persistence. Educators and caregivers must provide external structure (e.g. reducing visual and auditory distractions or providing visual cues) wherever possible as students lack internal structure. Responses and daily routines need to be predictable to assist children in learning about their environment. Because children with FASD have genuine difficulty in focusing and sustaining their attention, explanations and descriptions must be simple, short and presented in a variety of ways. Finally, educators must be tenacious in their approach to teaching by refusing to yield and continuously repeating, rephrasing and revising.

Like *Teaching Students with FASD*, the NOFAS-SD resource guide is intended for educators and professionals who provide support services. And like *Teaching Students with FASD*, the NOFAS-SD material is a collection of plans and techniques from experienced parents and seasoned professionals. The guide details environmental strategies (e.g. visual cues, teaching routines), communication strategies (e.g. having students repeat information, peer tutors), executive function strategies (e.g. self-monitoring) and social skills strategies (e.g. reducing stress, creating a positive classroom environment).

In sum, changing the environment rather than changing the child is an effective way of getting a desired behavior from an individual with brain-based difficulties. Teachers and parents have used their experiences to develop a trove of creative ideas and practical accommodations that structure and reinforce daily learning activities. Their collected knowledge for working with individuals with FASD can be readily adapted for a multicultural context.

Evidenced-based clinical interventions

There are a growing number of evidence-based interventions demonstrating that targeted treatments are effective in minimizing many of the negative social and behavioral outcomes associated with FASD. One promising intervention also shows the positive impact of dealing with the clinically concerning behaviors of these children by focusing on family systems in order to reduce daily stressors that often accompany raising children with alcohol-related, neurocognitive impairments. Since language impairments often co-occur with behavioral problems (Coggins *et al.*, 2007; Guralnick, 1999; McGee *et al.*, 2009; Redmond & Rice, 1998; Thorne & Coggins, 2008) and since good language and social communication help children 'travel a more positive life path' (Carmichael Olson & Montague, 2011: 69), these selected interventions provide speech-language pathologists and other support professionals with solid starting points for improving specific cognitive or adaptive skills in children with FASD.

Cognitive control intervention

As detailed above, children with FASD often have compromised executive functions and higher-order processes that guide, monitor or direct their interactions. Cognitive control therapy (CCT) is built on a developmental–interaction model where a set of cognitive mechanisms or controls develop in concert with changes in a child's personality and demands of the environment (Santostefano, 1985). CCT is a 'progressive skill building intervention' (Kalberg & Buckley, 2007: 283) designed for children and adolescents with cognitive dysfunctions. The goal is to help children reflect on what they know in order to facilitate learning.

The essence of CCT is the successful interplay between internal processes and the external environment. From the CCT perspective, children with short attention spans, difficulty organizing and sticking with tasks and/or coping with the demands of a changing environment, are seen as individuals with dysfunctional cognitive controls. Adnams and colleagues (reported in Riley *et al.*, 2003) explored CCT treatment in a selected sample of five school-age children with FAS (mean age 8;4 years) from a multilingual community in South Africa who were living with substance-abusing caregivers in adverse environments. The five children received CCT intervention 1 hour each week for 10 months from experienced therapists. The primary goal of this research was to assess whether this skill-building intervention would improve children's understanding of their learning difficulties and behavioral challenges.

The results from this feasibility study revealed improvements in behavior for the CCT group but no meaningful differences in cognitive or academic skills when compared to the controls. To be fair, the primary goal of a feasibility study is not to establish statistical significance but rather to determine the clinical viability of an untested intervention and whether further investigation is warranted. On this point, the authors maintain that 'qualitative improvements were noted by the therapists in the children's self-sufficiency, motivation, cooperation, self-confidence and emotionality' (Riley *et al.*, 2003: 366). While this approach is not yet fully validated, Kalberg and Buckley (2007: 283) maintain that CCT intervention 'is showing promising results'.

Working memory intervention

A deficit in working memory is a frequently reported impairment among children with FASD. Working memory is a hypothesized 'mental workspace' (Loomes *et al.*, 2007) to store and process relevant information. An individual uses working memory to recognize how current events relate to previous experiences, which according to Watson and Westby (2003: 196), 'allows for hindsight, forethought, and a sense of time'. Boudreau and Costanza-Smith (2011) provide the following examples of everyday activities predicated on working memory: following multiple-step directions that build on each other, mentally completing a math equation with two digits or larger numbers, writing a series of recently heard sentences and following the actions of multiple characters throughout a story.

Loomes and colleagues (2007) examined the effect of rehearsal training on working memory in children with PAE. Rehearsal is a strategy that has been effective in a variety of clinical populations (e.g. ADHD, autism, intellectual deficits) to keep from losing or forgetting information. All of the children in this study ($n = 33$) fell along the FASD continuum. The Loomes research team told their experimental subjects they would teach them a special way of remembering information and instructed them to use whispered rehearsal of the test stimuli. The control subjects received no rehearsal instructions. The results suggest that brief rehearsal training can improve performance on a working memory task (i.e. storing and processing a series of single-digit numbers).

While the initial findings from Loomes and colleagues suggest that rehearsal training may mitigate working memory difficulties in FASD, the clinical significance remains unknown. The researchers did not provide a detailed description of their experimental subjects so we don't have a clear picture of the cognitive and behavioral profiles of the children whose working memory improved with this brief intervention. Moreover, these findings have yet to be replicated in other children with FASD, and certainly have not been investigated in multilingual or multicultural contexts. Since replication is a critical component in the validation of a successful intervention, the efficacy of this intervention should be viewed with caution.

Social skills intervention

Peer interactions provide an essential context for learning and developing information about the social uses of language specific to a shared cultural context. When these interactions take place in multilingual and multicultural contexts, the learning task can be challenging for even the most socially skilled individuals. Given the exceptionally high proportion of children with FASD who have social problems that increase with age, promoting social problem solving is viewed by many as a pivotal intervention goal. O'Conner and colleagues (2006) have adapted Frankel and Myatt's (2003) *Children's Friendship Training* (CFT) program to improve the social functioning of children with FASD who have experienced multiple social interaction failures.

The CFT addresses the specific components that contribute to satisfying and successful social interactions. The goal of this intervention is to assist children in creating and maintaining friendships. Frankel and Myatt (2003) contend that quality friendships, between two individuals who consider themselves as equals, are arguably the single most salient measure for learning social skills and feeling good about oneself.

To examine the effects of child friendship training, O'Connor and colleagues (2006) recruited 100 children with PAE histories and their families to participate in their longitudinal treatment study. The children ranged in age from 6;0 to 12;0 years and were assessed for features of FASD by a physician using the 4-digit code (Astley, 2004). Using this diagnostic guide, 11% of children received a diagnosis of FAS, 43% a diagnosis of partial FAS and 46% a diagnosis of static encephalopathy, alcohol exposed.

Children were assigned to one of two conditions: a child friendship treatment condition (n = 51) or a delayed treatment control condition (n = 49). The friendship treatment group completed the 12-week CFT program. At the same time, each child's respective parents attended concurrent sessions on issues related to FASD and the social skills that their children were learning. The CFT treatment utilized environmental accommodations to train socially valid behaviors (e.g. having a conversation, resolving conflicts and entering a peer group) while decreasing challenging and intrusive behaviors. Children in the CFT treatment group also completed a follow-up assessment three months after the final treatment session.

The findings revealed clear evidence that social skills could be improved in children with FASD. Not only did the results reveal that children's knowledge of appropriate social skills improved during treatment, but in addition this improvement was retained three months thereafter. Importantly, parents also reported a significant decrease in their children's problematic behaviors.

Social communication intervention

Children with PAE have documented difficulties providing sufficient information to their partners during conversational and narrative discourse (e.g. Coggins *et al.*, 1998; Hamilton, 1981; Thorne *et al.*, 2007). These limitations appear to be the result of an array of subtle, yet meaningful compromises in language, social cognition and higher-order executive functions (Coggins *et al.*, 2007). Maladaptive social experiences, which often co-occur with substance abuse, also negatively impact the social language behaviors that children must develop to predict and explain people's behavior (Cicchetti, 2004; Cicchetti *et al.*, 2003). Thus, children with PAE are subject to multiple risk factors that limit the kind of practical knowledge they need to use in socially demanding situations. Again, these challenges are exacerbated when the increased demands of a multicultural social context are part of the child's environment.

Timler and colleagues (2005) designed a multidimensional treatment to teach children with PAE the skills they need to be competent communicators in social situations. The Social Communication Intervention (SCI) program takes into account both the behaviors and skills that clinicians need to teach as well as the environmental support that children need to be competent communicators.

The SCI treatment focuses on the linguistic skills that support theory of mind and the social cognitive skills that purport to teach children what to do and say when confronted with social dilemmas. The SCI blends three intervention components in teaching these interrelated skills to school-age youngsters during individual and group sessions. The components include: (1) role-playing techniques to assist children in assuming the perspectives of others; (2) a checklist to guide children through a routine for resolving social dilemmas; and (3) the direct modeling of socially appropriate responses by a clinician.

The preliminary research supporting the effectiveness of the SCI is encouraging. Timler and colleagues (2005) used a single-case experimental design to examine the effectiveness of SCI with a 9;8-year-old girl who had a documented PAE and an array of neurocognitive and social-emotional deficits. The intervention was conducted over six weeks, with two weeks of individual treatment (i.e. two, one-hour sessions per week) and four weeks of group treatment (i.e. three, two-hour sessions per week with two school-age peers). Treatment data revealed that the intervention was effective in increasing the number of strategies the participant used for obtaining social goals and promoting mental state verb production. While further study is warranted, the feasibility of this intervention is promising for clinicians who have caseloads that include youngsters with social communication difficulties.

Caregiver-family intervention

Challenging behaviors can be particularly nettlesome for parents and family members, and culture-specific attitudes about agency and personal responsibility are an important factor shaping how families react to those behaviors. Carmichael Olson and colleagues (2007, 2011) have designed a caregiver-focused intervention for families experiencing considerable stress raising children with FASD who exhibit 'clinically concerning behavior problems' (Carmichael Olson & Montague, 2011: 82). In contrast to behavioral interventions that focus directly on children's challenging behaviors, Carmichael Olson maintains that the most efficacious way of abating non-compliant or competitive behaviors is by changing parental attitudes and behaviors through positive supports.

Families moving forward (FMF) is a positive parenting intervention that addresses concerning or disruptive behaviors in children from 4;0 to 12;0 years with FASD. Positive parenting interventions teach skills, practices and methods for dealing with challenging behaviors. This family systems intervention targets highly stressed parents and/or caregivers who have children with low adaptive functioning and high levels of problematic behaviors. The FMF program is a consultation intervention that teaches parents how to implement environmental accommodations using evidence-based parenting training strategies, motivational interviewing and coaching techniques.

The FMF intervention is delivered individually to families by an experienced clinician who has specialized training with the FMF model. The FMF intervention has three primary aims: (1) to help parents reframe their child's neurological impairment; (2) to help parents devise environmental accommodations; and (3) to create action plans to reduce self-selected behavioral problems.

Randomized control trial outcome data have been gathered and summarized (Carmichael Olson & Montague, 2011). The initial efficacy study involved 52 families who were raising children with FASD and who presented with problematic behaviors. The families were divided into two groups – one group received the FMF intervention while the second group received 'the community standard of care' (Carmichael Olson & Montague, 2011: 83). Families were reported to be diverse in terms of ethnic background, social class, income level and type of family structure (adoptive, birth, foster; grandparents, single parents, two-parent families). Relative to the controls, the FMF group 'reported significantly greater family needs met, a greater sense of parenting efficacy, more parental self-care and decreased child disruptive behavior' (Carmichael Olson & Montague, 2011: 83).

Efficacy data supporting the family-oriented FMF intervention model is currently underway. While the intervention holds promise, the initial data in support of the intervention have only appeared in summary form (see Carmichael Olson & Montague, 2011) rather than in a peer-reviewed, data-based scientific journal. Thus, there are questions regarding the effectiveness, efficiency and effects of the intervention that remain unanswered. More information regarding this inventive treatment is available at http://depts.washington.edu/fmffasd.

In sum, the educational programs and evidence-based clinical interventions presented here provide state-of-the art information that can be used to maximize the impact of intervention, and hold exciting possibilities for children with FASD from diverse cultural and/or linguistic backgrounds. A foundational tenet of both intervention approaches is that the difficulties children with FASD exhibit in learning and interacting are the result of brain-based compromises that present lifelong challenges. Thus, those who work with children on the FASD spectrum must 'reframe' their understanding of and approach to children's behavioral shortcomings to reflect an attitude of 'can't do' rather than a mindset of 'won't do' (Carmichael Olson & Montague, 2011; Clarren, 2004). Clarren (2004) has noted that professionals and parents report a significant shift in their perceptions once they accept that children with FASD have a neurologically based (i.e. brain-based) disability.

Conclusion

Individuals with FASD present complicated neurodevelopmental profiles where co-occurring conditions are not the exception, but the rule. These complicated profiles are manifest across social, cultural and economic lines and frequently disrupt important cooperative learning experiences. Perhaps more than any other clinical population, children with FASD live in a state of double jeopardy due to the fact that maternal drinking frequently co-occurs with multiple life stressors that also have the potential for adverse neurocognitive and behavioral outcomes (Coggins et al., 2007).

Co-occurring risks in children with FASD contribute to a myriad of co-occurring deficits. The continuum of outcomes associated with fetal alcohol exposure has made differential diagnosis a challenging proposition, and one that is most competently accomplished in the context of an interdisciplinary team assessment. An accurate team diagnosis should be based on verifiable facts (Astley, 2011). The 4-digit diagnostic code is built on this thesis and uses quantitative measurement scales with specific case definitions to increase diagnostic accuracy. A number of empirical studies have demonstrated the utility of the 4-digit diagnostic code to measure the spectrum of disabilities under the umbrella of FASD (Astley, 2011; Thorne et al., 2007; Timler & Olswang, 2001; Timler et al., 2005).

Earlier we noted that even though language disorders are among the most frequently reported impairments in FASD, a distinctive clinical profile has yet to emerge. However, the lack of evidence to support a prevalent profile may be an artifact of gathering language performance data in contrived contexts using standardized instruments. Interestingly, when language is examined using more dynamic and interactive assessment paradigms, under real-time conditions that resemble naturalistic environments (e.g. conversations and narratives), performance is more compromised than would be predicted from standardized tests. This finding suggests that the language performance of children with FASD may be particularly influenced by environmental variables. Following this argument, one might expect a child to have more difficulty using language in real-world social situations that demand higher levels of inference, processing and integrative language. In a multicultural context, navigating interactions with individuals who do not share your cultural or linguistic background is a prime example of a social situation that places significant demands on the child's capacities.

Children with FASD present a range of complex difficulties in many areas of functioning. To be sure, these children can and do learn, but often in non-conventional ways. Increasingly, educational policies in North America, Western Europe and Australia favor the inclusion of children with FASD into regular classrooms. The ultimate goal of educating students with PAE is to determine the most effective combination of strategies, techniques and modifications to promote appropriate expectations and levels of support.

Common to all children with an FASD are cognitive and behavioral deficits resulting from CNS damage. Evidence-based clinical interventions have addressed specific domain deficits (e.g. social skills; language and communication), general processing deficits (e.g. cognitive control, working memory) and systems deficits (positive parenting). Collectively, these empirically supported studies provide positive evidence that treatments are effective in (1) teaching children many of the multivariate skills they need to function in everyday social interactions; (2) teaching clinicians about environmental supports that can assist children in compensating for the neurobiological and environmental risks that impede learning; and (3) teaching parents positive support strategies that can reduce challenging behaviors in their alcohol-affected children. Adapting these programs and interventions for children from diverse multilingual and/or multicultural backgrounds should have a positive and penetrating impact on the relationships among the family who are raising them, the educators and professionals who serve them and the community organizations that support them.

References

Abkarian, G. (1992) Communication effects of prenatal alcohol exposure. *Journal of Communication Disorders*, 25, 221–240.

Alati, R., Al Mamun, A., Williams, G., O'Callaghan, M., Najman, J. and Bor, W. (2006) In utero alcohol exposure and prediction of alcohol disorders in early adulthood. *Archive of General Psychiatry* 63. See http://archpsyc.jamanetwork.com/ (accessed 31 May 2012).

Aragón, A., Coriale, G., Fiorentino, D., Kalberg, W., Buckley, D., Gossage, J., Ceccanti, M, Mitchell, E. and May, P. (2008) Neuropsychological characteristics of Italian children with fetal alcohol spectrum disorders. *Alcoholism: Clinical and Experimental Research* 32 (11), 1909–1191.

Astley, S. (2004) *Diagnostic Guide for Fetal Alcohol Spectrum Disorders: The Four-Digit Diagnostic Code* (3rd edn). Seattle, WA: FAS Diagnostic and Prevention Network, University of Washington. See http://fasdpn.org (accessed 28 May 2014).

Astley, S. (2006) Comparison of the 4-digit diagnostic code and the Hoyme diagnostic guidelines for fetal alcohol spectrum disorders. *Pediatrics* 118 (4), 1532–1545.

Astley, S. (2010) Profile of the first 1,400 patients receiving diagnostic evaluations for fetal alcohol spectrum disorder at the Washington State Fetal Alcohol Syndrome Diagnostic & Prevention Network. *Canadian Journal of Clinical Pharmacology* 17 (1) Winter, e132–e164.

Astley, S. (2011) Diagnosing fetal alcohol spectrum disorders (FASD). In S. Abubato (ed.) *Prenatal Alcohol Use and FASD: A Model Standard of Diagnosis, Assessment and Multimodal Treatment* (pp. 3–28). Oak Park, IL: Bentham Science.

Astley, S. and Clarren, S. (2000) Diagnosing the full spectrum of fetal alcohol exposed individuals: Introducing the 4-digit diagnostic code. *Alcohol & Alcoholism* 35, 400–410.

Astley, S. and Clarren, S. (2001) Measuring the facial phenotype of individuals with prenatal alcohol exposure: Correlations with brain dysfunction. *Alcohol & Alcoholism* 36 (2), 147–159.

Astley, S., Aylward, E., Olson, H.C., Kerns, K., Brooks, A., Coggins, T.E., Davies, J., Dorn, S., Gendler, B., Jirikowic, T., Kraegel, P., Maravilla, K. and Richards, T. (2009) Magnetic resonance imaging outcomes from a comprehensive magnetic resonance study of children with fetal alcohol spectrum disorders. *Alcoholism: Clinical & Experimental Research* 33 (10), 1–19.

Astley, S., Olson, H., Kerns, K., Brooks, A., Aylward, E., Coggins, T.E., Davies, J., Dorn, S., Gendler, B., Jirikowic, T., Kraegel, P., Maravilla, K. and Richards, T. (2009) Neuropsychological and behavioral outcomes from a comprehensive magnetic resonance study of children with fetal alcohol spectrum disorders. *Canadian Journal of Clinical Pharmacology* 16 (1), e178–e201.

Bailey, B. and Sokol, R. (2008) Pregnancy and alcohol use: Evidence and recommendations for prenatal care. *Clinical Obstetrics and Gynecology* 51 (2), 436–444.

Bertrand, J., Floyd, L. and Weber, M. (2005) Guidelines for identifying and referring persons with fetal alcohol syndrome. *Morbidity and Mortality Weekly Report: Recommendations and Reports* 54 (RR-11), 1–14.

Boudreau, D. and Costanza-Smith, A. (2011) Assessment and treatment of working memory deficits in school-age children: The role of the speech-language pathologist. *Language, Speech, and Hearing Services in Schools* 42, 152–166.

Carmichael Olson, H. and Montague, R. (2011) An innovative look at early intervention for children affected by prenatal alcohol exposure. In S. Abudato and D. Cohen (eds) *Prenatal Alcohol Use and FASD: Diagnosis, Assessment and New Directions in Research and Multimodal Treatment* (pp. 64–107). Oak Park, IL: Bentham Science.

Carmichael Olson, H., Jirikowic, T., Kartin, D. and Astley, S. (2007) Responding to the challenge of early intervention for fetal alcohol spectrum disorders. *Infants and Young Children*, 20, 172–189.

Chasnoff, I., Wells, A., Telford, E., Schmidt, C. and Messer, G. (2010) Neurodevelopmental functioning in children with FAS, pFAS, and ARND. *Journal of Developmental & Behavioral Pediatrics* 31 (3), 192–201.

Chudley, A., Conry, J., Cook, J., Loock, C., Rosales, T. and LeBlanc, N. (2005) Fetal alcohol spectrum disorder: Canadian guidelines for diagnosis. *Canadian Medical Association Journal* 172 (5 Suppl), S1–21.

Church, M. and Kaltenbach, J. (1997) Hearing, speech, language, and vestibular disorders in the fetal alcohol syndrome: A literature review. *Alcoholism, Clinical and Experimental Research* 21 (3), 495–512.

Cicchetti, D. (2004) An odyssey of discovery: Lessons learned through three decades of research on child maltreatment. *American Psychologist* 58, 731–741.

Cicchetti, D., Rogosch, F., Maughan, A., Toth, S. and Bruce, J. (2003) False belief understanding in maltreated children. *Development and Psychopathology* 15 (4), 1067–1091.

Clarren, S. (2004) Teaching strategies for students with fetal alcohol spectrum disorder: Alberta learning. See https://education.alberta.ca/media/377037/fasd.pdf (accessed 24 August 2015).

Coggins, T.E., Friet, T. and Morgan, T. (1998) Analyzing narrative productions in older school-age children and adolescents with fetal alcohol syndrome: An experimental tool for clinical applications. *Clinical Linguistics & Phonetics* 12, 221–236.

Coggins, T.E., Timler, G.R. and Olswang, L.B. (2007) A state of double jeopardy: Impact of prenatal alcohol exposure and adverse environments on the social communicative abilities of school-age children with fetal alcohol spectrum disorder. *Language, Speech, and Hearing Services in Schools* 38 (2), 117–127.

Coggins, T.E., Olswang, L.B., Carmichael Olson, H. and Timler, G.R. (2003) On becoming socially competent communicators: The challenge for children with fetal alcohol exposure. *International Review of Research in Mental Retardation* 27, 121–150.

Cone-Wesson, B. (2005) Prenatal alcohol and cocaine exposure: Influences on cognition, speech, language, and hearing. *Journal of Communication Disorders* 38 (4), 279–302.

Davies, L., Dunn, M., Chersich, M., Urban, M., Chetty, C., Olivier, L. and Viljoen, D. (2011) Developmental delay of infants and young children with and without fetal alcohol spectrum disorder in the Northern Cape Province, South Africa. *African Journal of Psychiatry* 14, 298–305.

Frankel, F. and Myatt, R. (2003) *Children's Friendship Training*. New York: Brunner-Routledge.

Franklin, L., Deitz, J., Jirikowic, T. and Astley, S. (2008) Children with fetal alcohol spectrum disorders: Problem behaviors and sensory processing. *The American Journal of Occupational Therapy* 62 (3), 265–273.

Fried, P. and Watkinson, B. (1988) 12- and 24-month neurobehavioural follow-up of children prenatally exposed to marihuana, cigarettes and alcohol. *Neurotoxicology and Teratology* 10 (4), 305–313.

Fried, P., O'Connell, C. and Watkinson, B. (1992) 60- and 72-month follow-up of children prenatally exposed to marijuana, cigarettes, and alcohol: Cognitive and language assessment. *Journal of Developmental and Behavioral Pediatrics* 13 (6), 383–391.

Greene, T., Ernhart, C., Martier, S., Sokol, R. and Ager, J. Jr. (1990) Prenatal alcohol exposure and language development. *Alcoholism: Clinical and Experimental Research*, 14 (6), 937–945.

Guerri, C. (2002) Mechanisms involved in central nervous system dysfunctions induced by prenatal ethanol exposure. *Neurotoxicity Research* 4 (4), 327–335.

Guralnick, M. (1999) Family and child influences on the peer-related social competence of young children with developmental delays. *Mental Retardation and Developmental Disabilities* 5, 21–29.

Gusella, J. and Fried, P. (1984) Effects of maternal social drinking and smoking on offspring at 13 months. *Neurobehavioral Toxicology and Teratology* 6 (1), 13–17.

Hamilton, M. (1981) Linguistic abilities of children with fetal alcohol syndrome. Unpublished doctoral dissertation, University of Washington.

Jirikowic, T., Carmichael-Olson, H. and Kartin, D. (2008) Sensory processing, school performance, and adaptive behavior among young school-aged children with FASD. *Physical and Occupational Therapy in Pediatrics* 28 (2), 117–136.

Jones, K. and Smith, D. (1973) Recognition of the fetal alcohol syndrome in early infancy. *The Lancet* 302 (7836), 999–1001.

Kalberg, W. and Buckley, D. (2007) FASD: What types of intervention and rehabilitation are useful? *Neuroscience & Biobehavioral Reviews* 31 (2), 278–285.

Kleinfeld, J. and Wescot, S. (eds) (1993) *Fantastic Antone Succeeds! Experiences in Educating Children with Fetal Alcohol Syndrome.* Anchorage: University of Alaska Press.

Kodituwakku, P. (2007) Defining the behavioral phenotype in children with fetal alcohol spectrum disorders: A review. *Neuroscience & Biobehavioral Reviews* 31 (2), 192–201.

Kodituwakku, P. and Kodituwakku, E. (2011) From research to practice: An integrative framework for the development of interventions for children with fetal alcohol spectrum disorders. *Neuropsychology Review* 21 (2), 204–223.

Lemoine, P., Harousseau, H., Borteryu, J. and Menuet, J. (1968) Les enfants de parents alcooliques: Anomalies observées à propos de 127 cas (Children of alcoholic parents: Abnormalities observed in 127 cases). *Ouest Medicine* 21, 165–175.

Loomes, C., Rasmussen, C., Pei, C., Manji, S. and Andrew, G. (2007) The effect of rehearsal training on working memory span of children with fetal alcohol spectrum disorder. *Research in Developmental Disabilities* 29, 113–124.

Mattson, S., Crocker, N. and Nguyen, T. (2011) Fetal alcohol spectrum disorders: Neuropsychological and behavioral features. *Neuropsychology Review* 21 (2), 81–101.

McGee, C., Bjorquist, O., Riley, E. and Mattson, S. (2009) Impaired language performance in young children with heavy prenatal alcohol exposure. *Neurotoxicology and Teratology* 31, 71–75.

National Organization on Fetal Alcohol Syndrome – South Dakota (2009) *Fetal Alcohol Spectrum Disorders Educational Strategies: Working with Students with a Fetal Alcohol Spectrum Disorder in the Education System.* Center for Disabilities, Sanford School of Medicine of the University of South Dakota. See http://www.usd.edu/medical-school/center-for-disabilities/fetal-alcohol-spectrum-disorders-education-strategies-handbook.cfm (accessed 28 May 2014).

O'Connor, M. and Paley, B. (2006) The relationship of prenatal alcohol exposure and the postnatal environment to child depressive symptoms. *Journal of Pediatric Psychology* 31 (1), 50–64.

O'Connor, M., Frankel, F., Paley, B., Schonfeld, A., Carpenter, E., Laugeson, E. and Marquardt, R. (2006) A controlled social skills training for children with fetal alcohol spectrum disorders. *Journal of Consulting & Clinical Psychology* 74 (4), 639–648.

O'Malley, K. (2007) *ADHD and Fetal Alcohol Spectrum Disorders (FASD)*. New York: Nova Science.

Redmond, S. and Rice, M. (1998) The socioemotional behaviors of children with SLI: Social adaptation or social deviance? *Journal of Speech Language Hearing Research* 41, 688–700.

Riley, E. and McGee, C. (2005) Fetal alcohol spectrum disorders: An overview with emphasis on changes in brain and behavior. *Experimental Biology and Medicine (Maywood, N.J.)* 230 (6), 357–365.

Riley, E., Mattson, S., Li, K., Jacobson, W., Coles, C., Kodituwakku, P., Adams, C. and Korkman, M. (2003) Neurobehavioral consequences of prenatal alcohol exposure: An international perspective. *Alcoholism: Clinical and Experimental Research* 27, 362–373.

Santostefano, S. (1985) *Cognitive Control Therapy with Children and Adolescents*. New York: Pergamon Press.

Sayal, K., Heron, J., Golding, J. and Emond, A. (2007) Prenatal alcohol exposure and gender differences in childhood mental health problems: A longitudinal population-based study. *Pediatrics* 119 (2), e426–434.

Schonfeld, A., Paley, B., Frankel, F. and O'Connor, J. (2006) Executive functioning predicts social skills following prenatal alcohol exposure. *Child Neuropsychology* 12 (6), 439–452.

Streissguth, A. and O'Malley, K. (2000) Neuropsychiatric implications and long-term consequences of fetal alcohol spectrum disorders. *Seminars in Clinical Neuropsychiatry* 5 (3), 177–190.

Streissguth, A., Barr, H., Kogan, J. and Bookstein, F. (1996) *Understanding the Occurrence of Secondary Disabilities in Clients with Fetal Alcohol Syndrome (FAS) and Fetal Alcohol Effects (FAE), Final Report to the Centers for Disease Control and Prevention* (CDC), August. Seattle: University of Washington, Fetal Alcohol & Drug Unit, Tech. Rep. No. 96-06.

Streissguth, A., Barr, H., Olson, H.C., Sampson, P., Bookstein, F. and Burgess, D. (1994) Drinking during pregnancy decreases word attack and arithmetic scores on standardized tests: Adolescent data from a population-based prospective study. *Alcoholism: Clinical and Experimental Research* 18 (2), 248–254.

Streissguth, A., Bookstein, F., Barr, H., Sampson, P.D., O'Malley, K. and Young, J. (2004) Risk factors for adverse life outcomes in fetal alcohol syndrome and fetal alcohol effects. *Journal of Developmental and Behavioral Pediatrics* 25 (4), 228–238.

Sullivan, W.C. (1899) A note on the influence of maternal inebriety on the offspring. *Journal of Mental Science* 45, 489–503.

Thorne, J.C. (2010) Tallying reference errors in narratives: Integrative language function, impairment, and fetal alcohol spectrum disorders. Doctoral dissertation, University of Washington. See http://hdl.handle.net/1773/16321 (accessed 28 May 2014).

Thorne, J.C. and Coggins, T.E. (2008) A diagnostically promising technique for tallying nominal reference errors in the narratives of school-aged children with fetal alcohol spectrum disorders (FASD). *International Journal of Language & Communication Disorders* 43 (5), 570–594.

Thorne, J.C., Coggins, T.E., Carmichael Olson, H. and Astley, S. (2007) Exploring the utility of narrative analysis in diagnostic decision making: Picture-bound reference, elaboration, and fetal alcohol spectrum disorders. *Journal of Speech, Language, and Hearing Research* 50 (2), 459–474.

Timler, G.R. and Olswang, L.B. (2001) Variable structure/variable performance: Caregiver and teacher perspectives of a school-age child with fetal alcohol syndrome. *Journal of Positive Behavior Interventions* 3, 48–56.

Timler, G.R., Olswang, L.B. and Coggins, T.E. (2005) 'Do I know what I need to do?' A social communication intervention for children with complex clinical profiles. *Language, Speech, and Hearing Services in Schools* 36 (1), 73–85.

Vaurio, L., Riley, E. and Mattson, S. (2011) Neuropsychological comparison of children with heavy prenatal alcohol exposure and an IQ-matched comparison group. *Journal of the International Neuropsychological Society* 17, 463–473.

Watson, S. and Westby, C. (2003) Strategies for addressing the executive function impairments of students prenatally exposed to alcohol and other drugs. *Communication Disorders Quarterly* 24, 194–204.

Wyper, K. and Rasmussen, C. (2011) Language impairments in children with fetal alcohol spectrum disorder. *Journal of Population Therapeutics and Clinical Pharmacology* 18 (2), e364–e376; June 21.

5 Multilingual Perspectives on Language in Children with Williams Syndrome

Vesna Stojanovik

General Description of Williams Syndrome

Williams syndrome (WS) is a rare genetic disorder first identified in 1961 by Williams and his colleagues in New Zealand (Williams *et al.*, 1961). It is typically found in 1 in 15,000–20,000 live births (Karmiloff-Smith, 2012), although a study in Norway has reported incidence of 1 in 7,500 (Stromme *et al.*, 2002). It occurs due to a deletion of approximately 25 genes on chromosome 7. WS is characterized by physical abnormalities, high blood pressure and renal problems, increased blood calcium levels, failure to thrive in infancy, abnormal sensitivity to certain types of sounds (hyperacusis), a characteristic face morphology known as 'elfin' face and mild to moderate learning difficulties.

On the level of brain organization, WS is characterized by a reduced brain volume, particularly in the parietal regions (Eckert *et al.*, 2006) and in the corpus callosum (Schmitt *et al.*, 2001). The brain volume of WS brains reaches about 80% of the brain volume in neurotypical individuals (Chiang *et al.*, 2007) and increased cortical thickness has been reported (Thompson *et al.*, 2005). When the reduced brain volume is considered, the frontal lobes, superior temporal gyrus, amygdala, fusiform gyrus and cerebellum in the brains of adults with WS are relatively preserved whereas the parietal and occipital lobes, the thalamus, the basal ganglia and the midbrain are smaller in volume (Karmiloff-Smith, 2012). It has also been found that the amygdala and the cerebellum are larger than the rest of the WS brain; in fact, a large cerebellum has been shown to be present in early childhood in WS (Jones *et al.*, 2002).

Of particular interest to linguists, developmental psychologists/ psycholinguists, speech and language pathologists (SLPs) and neuroscientists is the fact that the WS neurocognitive profile is uneven. Individuals with WS have mild to moderate learning difficulties, with profound impairments in planning, problem solving and spatial cognition compared to relative strengths in social cognition, linguistic abilities, face processing and auditory rote memory (Mervis, 1999). It should be stressed, however, that these are *relative* strengths and weaknesses, which may not hold for *all* individuals with WS, and they have not gone unchallenged. A very small proportion of individuals with WS have severe learning difficulties and very little or no language, and also a small proportion have average IQs. Individuals with WS also have a unique personality profile characterized by gregariousness, overfriendliness and anxiety (Klein-Tasman & Mervis, 2003).

From the 1980s onward, studies on WS have made a substantial contribution toward the *nature–nurture* question. The very fact that individuals with WS have been shown to have a profile of relative strengths and weaknesses has lent itself to being the subject of theoretical debate with regard to the independence of language, in particular, from general cognitive abilities. This debate has mainly focused around issues such as whether WS offers evidence for innate modularity, i.e. the neural specialization of certain cognitive functions in ontogeny (according to Fodor [1983]), or whether it shows that neural specializations for certain cognitive functions occur as a result of the interaction between the brain, genes and the environment (Karmiloff-Smith, 1998).

This chapter is organized as follows: first a summary of research to date with regard to language, communication/social interaction patterns and literacy in English-speaking children with WS will be presented; this will be followed by a more detailed review of studies on language, communication/social interaction patterns and literacy of children with WS speaking languages other than English; the chapter will end with future research suggestions and clinical implications for assessment and intervention.

A Summary of Language, Communication/Social Interaction Patterns and Literacy in English-Speaking Children with Williams Syndrome

Early research into language, communication/interaction patterns and literacy in WS focused almost exclusively on English. It was not until the early 1990s that the first studies on language and communication/ interaction patterns in children with WS speaking languages other than English started to appear. Research into literacy in WS is fairly sparse, with only a handful of studies published so far. Research into literacy only started to develop in the 1980s, with the majority of studies being conducted on English-speaking individuals and only three studies based on languages other English.

Early studies on language in WS

The early studies on WS were typically carried out as part of multidimensional studies, which would normally include the assessment of behavioral, medical, physiological, cognitive and linguistic aspects of the WS profile, providing a general description of the WS phenotype (Stojanovik, 2014). Although rather broad and general in nature, they tended to emphasize the linguistic strengths of this atypical population. For example, one of the earliest studies by von Arnim and Engel (1964) characterized the profiles of four individuals with WS, aged 5–15 years, whose IQs ranged from 43 to 56 and who had physical growth problems, poor motor coordination, outgoing personalities, recurrent signs of anxiety and an unusual command of language. 'Their loquacity combined with friendliness and a great ability to make interpersonal contacts makes them appear brighter and more intelligent than in fact they are' (von Arnim & Engel, 1964: 375). Just over a decade later, Jones and Smith (1975: 719) described the personality of individuals with WS as 'friendly, loquacious, and cocktail party manner'. They presented data including 14 children and adults with WS ranging between 3 months and 23 years of age with full-scale IQ scores of between 41 and 80, with a mean of 56. A later study by Bennett et al. (1978) which included seven children with WS, aged between 4;6 and 8;5, using the McCarthy (1972) Scales of Children's Abilities, reported better performance on measures of verbal ability than on fine and gross motor skills measures.

In the 1980s, the research base on the WS neurocognitive profile started to grow fairly rapidly; however, studies still mainly used standardized test batteries as the method to investigate linguistic and other cognitive abilities in individuals with WS. Interestingly, despite the fact that earlier studies pointed toward linguistic strengths in individuals with WS, most of these studies did not find superior verbal functioning compared to other cognitive abilities or motor skills (Arnold et al., 1985; Crisco et al., 1988; Kataria et al., 1984). Some of these studies also recognized the individual variation within the syndrome by providing data on individual participants. For example, Pagon et al. (1987), who administered the Wechsler Intelligence Scale for Children (WISC; Wechsler, 1974) to a group of nine individuals with WS aged between 10 and 20, reported that seven individuals in the group scored above floor (floor = 45) on the verbal scale, and had verbal IQs of between 47 and 85. Five of these individuals also scored above floor on the performance IQ scale and their performance IQs were between 45 and 69. The differences between the verbal and non-verbal performance were non-significant. However, one individual with a high verbal IQ score showed an obvious verbal advantage. Four of the nine individuals with WS fell within the 'severely mentally retarded range' (Pagon et al., 1987: 90) with regard to their general functioning. In contrast, significant differences between verbal and performance IQ were reported in a series of papers by Udwin and colleagues (Udwin *et al.*, 1986, 1987; Udwin & Yule, 1990, 1991). These four papers are based on data from a large group of 44 individuals with WS (referred to as infantile hypercalcaemia, which was a former label for WS) aged between 6;0 and 15;9 years who were administered the WISC. There was individual variation in that a number of participants scored below floor on the verbal and performance scales, but the verbal IQs for the remaining participants ranged between 45 and 109 (mean = 62.4), while the performance IQs ranged between 45 and 73 (mean = 55.9). These scores point to a marginal verbal advantage, although both verbal and non-verbal scores are within 2 standard deviations below the mean so any verbal advantage is relative.

Research from the late 1980s to 2015

Throughout the 1990s, there were still a few studies being published which used a standardized IQ test battery as their main method to investigate language and non-verbal abilities in individuals with WS, such as Dall'Oglio and Milani (1995) and Greer *et al.* (1997); however, experimental studies also started to appear. For example, Bellugi *et al.* (1988) who used a number of different language tasks in a study of three teenagers with WS argued that individuals with WS show a dissociation between their verbal and non-verbal skills, with verbal abilities being above non-verbal. In a series of studies that followed in the late 1980s and early 1990s, Bellugi and her colleagues showed that adolescents and adults with WS have relatively good morphosyntactic and lexical-semantic abilities when assessed on tasks that specifically tap these abilities, particularly when compared to individuals with Down syndrome (DS) of similar chronological and mental ages (MAs), arguing that WS provides evidence for the independence of language from other cognitive abilities (Bellugi *et al.*, 1989, 1992, 1994). A criticism of these studies, however, is that only the data of a small number of subjects have actually been published. As Bellugi *et al.* (1994: 25) state: 'over 100 WS subjects have been tested by the LCN (Laboratory for Cognitive Neuroscience), to date. The results presented here focus primarily on a core group of 10 adolescents'. Given what we now know about the heterogeneity within the WS population (Porter & Coltheart, 2005; Stojanovik *et al.*, 2006), the 10 selected individuals are unlikely to be representative of the WS population.

Clahsen and Almazan (1998) studied a number of different syntactic phenomena using specific tasks for each phenomenon. They investigated passive sentences via a sentence-picture matching task, anaphoric and reflexive pronouns via a sentence-picture judgment task and regular and irregular past-tense formation via two elicited production tasks. They reported that the ability of individuals with WS to comprehend reversible passives, regular past-tense morphology and reflexive anaphors compared to children with specific language impairment (SLI) is intact. Furthermore, in the regular and irregular past-tense formation tasks, the children with WS were able to apply the *–ed* affixation rule to existing regular verbs (e.g. *scowl*) and to novel verbs with stems that do not rhyme with any existing irregular verbs (e.g. *spuff*). However, they were not very successful in supplying irregular affixation to existing irregular verbs (e.g. *swim*) and novel verbs with stems that rhyme with existing irregular verbs (e.g. *crive*). The authors conclude that disorders such as WS and SLI provide evidence for a theoretical distinction between a computational system, which deals with rule learning (e.g. -ed past-tense marking), and an associative memory system for language, which is concerned with the learning of individual lexical items, such as irregular verbs.

In the last decade or so, the majority of studies investigating language abilities in WS have employed experimental tasks and/or have elicited spontaneous speech data with standardized language measures only being used (when used) to provide baseline assessment, or for the purposes of matching individuals with WS to other participant groups (e.g. Clahsen *et al.*, 2004; Joffe & Varlocosta, 2007; Stojanovik *et al.*, 2004; Thomas *et al.*, 2001; Zukowski, 2004). These have shown a rather mixed picture of findings, with some arguing for superior linguistic skills over non-verbal skills (Clahsen *et al.*, 2004; Clahsen & Almazan, 1998; Zukowski, 2004) and others showing that linguistic skills are not superior and are on a par with general cognitive abilities (Stojanovik *et al.*, 2004; Thomas *et al.*, 2001). Interestingly, Joffe and Varlocosta (2007) reported that individuals with WS performed worse than MA-matched controls on comprehension and production of wh- questions and comprehension of passive sentences. This study therefore suggests that linguistic abilities are not always a relative strength, and furthermore, that linguistic abilities can be a relative weakness compared to general cognitive abilities in this population. Perovic and Wexler (2007) suggested that some aspects of complex grammar, and especially those which may be acquired late by typically developing (TD) children, may be unattainable for children with WS. They studied two complex syntactic constructions, i.e. binding and raising, in two groups of children with WS (a younger group of 6–12 year olds and a group of 12–16 year olds), compared to TD controls matched on non-verbal MA, verbal MA and grammar. They found that the younger children with WS were poorer than the older children with WS on their interpretation of personal pronouns in binding constructions (e.g. Mowgli said that Baloo bear was tickling him), but their performance was in line with the two groups of younger TD controls. However, both groups of children with WS performed poorly on raising constructions (e.g. It seems that Paul will marry Jane).

Studies that have investigated morphosyntactic abilities in older individuals (adolescents and adults) with WS also show that they perform below their vocabulary age and chronological age (CA) peers with regard to their grammatical abilities. For example, in a sentence imitation task, which required the participants (aged between 8 and 30) to repeat relative clauses, adolescents and adults with WS performed at a level equivalent to 5-year-old children (Grant *et al.*, 2002).

Particularly useful in enlightening the disagreement in findings with regard to whether linguistic abilities are interdependent with general cognitive abilities is a large-scale study by Mervis *et al.* (2004). The study provides data from participants with WS spanning a wide age-range (5–47) on a number of different standardized language and non-verbal measures. The correlations between language and visuospatial construction skills suggest that these two cognitive skills are not independent of each other. An additional analysis indicated that verbal working memory may be mediating the relationship between receptive vocabulary and visuospatial construction. This suggests that verbal working memory may be more important for language acquisition (especially vocabulary and syntax) for individuals with WS than for TD individuals.

The above discussion focused either on morphosyntactic abilities in WS or on verbal skills in general as measured by a standardized IQ test battery. A conclusion that could be drawn from that discussion is that verbal abilities are not superior to non-verbal abilities in most cases, although there is some degree of individual variation and there are a small number of studies that show a marginal verbal advantage in WS. It should be pointed out, however, that what is taken as 'verbal advantage' in WS may be subject to debate. For example, showing that individuals with WS have better language abilities than those with known severe language difficulties, such as individuals with DS (who often have better non-verbal than verbal abilities), is not very strong evidence for the existence of a verbal advantage in WS. The evidence would be stronger if studies could show that language abilities exceed the general non-verbal level of functioning and this has not been shown so far, at least where morphosyntactic skills are concerned.

There is some evidence from studies investigating receptive vocabulary skills in WS which may be more relevant for the question of verbal advantage. In particular, when adolescents and adults with WS are compared to other populations with learning difficulties, such as individuals with DS, they usually show very good receptive vocabularies. They often score better than what would be expected for their MA on standardized measures of receptive vocabulary such as the British Picture Vocabulary Scales or its US equivalent, the Peabody Picture Vocabulary Test (PPVT; Bellugi *et al.*, 1988; Clahsen *et al.*, 2004). Such findings suggest that if there is verbal superiority in WS, it is with regard to receptive vocabulary. However, this may not be specific to WS, because children with DS often have receptive vocabulary as their relative strength (Glenn & Cunningham, 2005). In addition, a review paper by Mervis and Beccera (2007) reports the results of PPVT scores for a very large cohort of 238 children and adolescents with WS aged between 4 and 17. The mean standard score achieved was 79.85 (with a range of 40–118). Importantly, the majority of children (78%) achieved a score of at least 70 but only a small percentage (8%) scored at least 100 (Mervis & Beccera, 2007). This suggests that although receptive vocabulary can be a relative strength when compared to other language and non-verbal abilities in WS, it is often below the level expected when compared to children in the general population who are of a similar CA.

Language acquisition in infancy

Until quite recently, research into language in WS tended to focus on children above the age of 4, with not much being known with regard to language acquisition in early infancy. In the last couple of decades, however, there have been a number of studies. In general, language acquisition is delayed in WS (Mervis & Klein-Tasman, 2000; Mervis & John, 2012). Mervis and colleagues have conducted the majority of studies on early language development in WS and, in particular, they have conducted a few longitudinal studies of English-speaking individuals with WS. For example, in a longitudinal study, Mervis et al. (2003) followed the early vocabulary development of 13 children with WS using the MacArthur–Bates Communicative Development Inventory (CDI; Fenson et al., 1993). All of the participants were below the fifth percentile when they achieved the 10 expressive word stage; and all but one remained below fifth percentile when they achieved the 50–100 expressive word stage. The median for achieving a 100-word expressive vocabulary was 37 months (range: 26–68 months) whereas TD children achieve a 100-word expressive vocabulary typically at around 18 months (Fenson et al., 2007).

Few studies have addressed the grammatical abilities of young children with WS. These have reported that grammatical development is delayed in WS. In a longitudinal study including 22 young children with WS, Mervis et al. (2003) reported that only 18% of the children in the sample (that is four children) were producing at least one two-word combination at 30 months. Correlational analyses showed that grammatical ability was strongly related to expressive vocabulary.

Although both expressive vocabulary and grammatical ability are delayed, the relationship between these two skills is similar to what is found in TD children (Mervis et al., 2004). Also just like TD children, the early vocabularies of children with WS contain the child basic-level categories (Mervis, 1999). However, unlike TD children and those with DS, children with WS do not show referential pointing prior to the onset of referential language (Mervis et al., 2004). Also, toddlers with WS have been reported to engage less in triadic joint attention than MA-matched TD children with smaller expressive vocabularies (Mervis & John, 2012). This may have implications for their early language acquisition in that they may have more limited opportunities to acquire new vocabulary as efficiently as TD children and hence may explain the initial delay seen in WS with regard to language acquisition.

Social communication/interaction in WS

Communication/social interaction abilities were first investigated in the 1990s. The first descriptions of the communication skills of adolescents with WS characterized them as being 'highly social' (Reilly *et al.*, 1990: 373) and having 'remarkable social understanding' (Reilly *et al.*, 1990: 389). Later on, Jones *et al.* (2000) described individuals with WS as hypersocial. This was based on findings from a series of tasks in which Jones and colleagues (2000) found that individuals with WS included more inferences about the affective states and motivations of story characters than did TD children or children with DS. In addition, individuals with WS provided a greater number of descriptions of affective states and evaluative comments during an interview task and were more likely to ask the interviewer personal questions. Rice *et al.* (2005) interpreted this highly social personality as meaning that social communication is not a weakness in children with WS.

However, there are also different reports which suggest difficulties with social interaction and communication skills. Using the Children's Communication Checklist (CCC) (Bishop, 1998), Laws and Bishop (2003) compared caregiver or teacher reports of the pragmatic abilities of children and young adults with WS to those of individuals with DS and those with SLI. They reported significant levels of pragmatic language impairment and difficulties with social relationships in the WS group. The WS group was also described as using considerably more stereotyped conversation than either the DS or SLI groups. It should be noted, however, that when compared to children with autism, who are known to have difficulties with social communication, children with WS perform significantly better on the pragmatic scales on the CCC-2 (Bishop, 2003) and also on the Social Relations Scale (Philofsky *et al.*, 2007).

Stojanovik (2006) used a semi-structured conversation task to investigate the social interaction skills of individuals with WS. The children with WS had difficulties with exchange structure and with responding appropriately to interlocutors' requests for information and clarification. They also had significant difficulties with interpreting meaning and providing enough information for their conversational partner, often providing too little information. This suggests that social interaction abilities in children with WS may not be a relative strength as originally reported. However, as mentioned earlier, there is individual variation. A case study by Tarling *et al.* (2006) reports on the remarkable conversational success of a 12-year-old child with WS who, despite being quite dysfluent, having the linguistic abilities of a 5-year-old and a non-verbal IQ of about 50, managed to repair a number of possible conversation breakdowns by having exceptional sensitivity to the emotional state of his conversational partner, as well as being aware when his interlocutor was having difficulties understanding what he was trying to say.

Figurative language

Successful communication skills also involve interpreting other people's intended meaning, which is not always the literal meaning of what was said. This requires an understanding of figurative language. A few studies have investigated how individuals with WS understand figurative language, in particular idiomatic expressions. Idiom comprehension starts to develop from early childhood and continues to improve into adolescence and through adulthood. Studies by Annaz *et al.* (2009) and Sullivan *et al.* (2003) show that the understanding of figurative language is an area of weakness for children with WS and they would certainly have difficulties in communication contexts when figurative language is used. In a study which included older children and young adults with WS as well as CA- and IQ-matched adolescents with Prader–Willi syndrome and adolescents with non-specific intellectual disability, Sullivan *et al.* (2003) reported that individuals with WS had difficulty distinguishing between lies and ironic jokes, consistently interpreting ironic jokes as lies. However, their performance was similar to the two groups of individuals with learning difficulties, suggesting that this difficulty may not be syndrome specific.

Recent research on the development of the comprehension of metaphor and metonymy in 6- to 10-year-old children with WS reported by Annaz *et al.* (2009) showed that while for TD children, there is a linear relation between increasing CA and understanding of lexicalized metaphor and metonymy, this does not hold for children with WS, although there was a significant relation with the level of vocabulary comprehension. Furthermore, metaphor comprehension was worse than expected for the level of receptive vocabulary for the WS group compared to metonymy comprehension which was in line with their receptive vocabulary level. Both metaphors and metonyms are figurative expressions which are thought to be fundamental aspects of conceptual thinking (Lakoff & Johnson, 1980). They both refer to a different concept to the one that is stated literally but they are different in that metonomy relies on contiguity within one conceptual domain while metaphors involve relationships across conceptual domains (Annaz *et al.*, 2009). For example, when we use metonomy and say: 'There is a new face in the office', we mean a new person rather than an actual face (Annaz *et al.*, 2009). Face and person are within the same conceptual domain which is 'animate being'. Metaphor, on the other hand, relies on the resemblance between two different concepts. For example, when we say: 'The ship ploughs the sea', we mean that the ship moves through the water just like a plough through soil (Hudson, 2000). The authors interpret this by suggesting that comprehension of metaphors and metonymy might be handled by two separate mechanisms. Namely, metonyms may be part of vocabulary and treated as synonyms in WS; they fall more squarely within the language domain. Metaphor comprehension, on the other hand, spans cognition and language, and hence engages additional cognitive mechanisms.

Prosody

Successful communication is also dependent on the person's ability to interpret not only *what* people say (the actual words) but *how* people say words, phrases and utterances. It is also very important for people to be able to express and understand different emotional states (e.g. happiness, sadness, like and dislike) as well being able to express and understand which words are the most important in an utterance. All of these phenomena are conveyed by the term *prosody*. Prosody is also used to disambiguate potentially ambiguous utterances.

One of the first studies to investigate the cognitive profile of individuals with WS noted that adolescents with WS had expressive prosody which was over-rich in affect intonation (Reilly *et al.*, 1990). After this report, research into prosody in WS was somewhat dormant for the following 15 years until the publication of the study by Catterall *et al.* (2006), which assessed the production and expression of prosody in two adolescents with WS using a battery of tasks (i.e. producing and understanding prosody for the purposes of disambiguation of potentially ambiguous utterances, signaling the most important word in an utterance, signaling questions versus declaratives, conveying affective states such as likes and dislikes). Both adolescents with WS displayed impaired expressive and receptive prosodic abilities and had pervasive difficulties, compared to CA controls, in all aspects of the understanding and production of prosody. A year later, Stojanovik *et al.* (2007) compared prosody among 14 children with WS, ages 6 through 13, to language comprehension matches and CA matches. They found that three linguistic aspects of prosody (i.e. producing and understanding prosody for the purposes of disambiguation of potentially ambiguous utterances, producing and understanding prosody to signal the most important word in an utterance and understanding prosody to signal questions versus declarative intonation) were as expected for the level of language comprehension in WS; furthermore, the ability to express questions versus declaratives via intonation was at a CA appropriate level. With regard to affective intonation, one affect function of prosody (understanding and expressing likes versus dislikes) was assessed and it was found that this is as expected for CA in WS (Stojanovik *et al.*, 2007).

However, in a spontaneous speech task, in which children with WS were asked to generate a story from a wordless picture book, they were reported to use a much wider pitch range than either language age- or CA-matched controls (Setter *et al.*, 2007). This study also reported that the children with WS were judged by phonetically naïve listeners as being twice as emotionally involved as TD children, either matched on receptive language or CA. Using developmental trajectory analysis, Stojanovik (2010) showed that when MA is taken into account, children with WS do not show either a delay in onset or a slowed rate of development in any aspect of linguistic prosody apart from a delayed onset in using prosody to regulate conversational behavior (questioning versus declarative intonation). However, the evidence suggests that children with WS do manage to catch up with their CA peers in their ability to use prosody to regulate conversation (as Stojanovik *et al.* [2007] reported). The developmental trajectory analysis also showed that, relative to CA, children and adolescents with WS have a delayed onset of ability to use prosody to signal the most important word in an utterance. In addition, they also show a delayed rate of development in the ability to perceive and produce prosody to disambiguate phrases and the ability to use prosody to perceive the most prominent word in an utterance (Stojanovik, 2010).

Literacy in WS

As mentioned earlier, in comparison to the wealth of research into language and communication abilities in individuals with WS, research into their literacy abilities has been very modest in volume with only eight published studies in the past three decades (Griffiths, 2012). Although children with WS do have literacy difficulties, there have only been a handful of studies investigating literacy skills in the WS population. The general picture is that literacy abilities are variable within the adult WS population with some individuals never being able to read at all, whereas others are able to decode and comprehend what they have read at a level equivalent to a student entering university (Mervis, 2009). This variability is also seen within children with WS, with some being able to decode and comprehend at an age-appropriate level whereas others are unable to read at all.

The earliest study to report on the level of reading ability in individuals with WS was Pagon *et al.* (1987). Reading was assessed using the Peabody Individual Achievement Test (Dunn & Markwardt, 1970) which includes decoding and comprehension. The standardized scores for the nine children and adolescents with WS ranged from 41 to 99. When translated into school-level reading achievement, the children appear to have reading abilities equivalent to between first and ninth grade. A series of studies by Udwin and colleagues followed in which reading was assessed as part of a multidimensional battery of tests in a large group of 44 children and adolescents with WS aged between 6 and 16. Reading variability was obvious. In Udwin *et al.* (1987), half of the sample (22 children) gained at least a basal score on the Reading Composite, measured using a battery that assesses decoding and reading comprehension. Among these 22 children and adolescents with WS, the mean reading accuracy age level was 7 years 10 months (range between 6 years 2 months and 11 years 4 months) and the reading comprehension age level was 7 years 9 months (age range 6 years 3 months to 12 years). In a follow-up study, which included 23 of the original 44 participants (this time the mean age was 21 years), Udwin and colleagues (1996) reported that 14 participants achieved a basal level on the Neale Analysis of Reading (Neale, 1966), whereas 17 achieved a basal level on the Wechsler Objective Reading Dimensions Test (WORD) (Rust *et al.*, 1993). This study again suggests that not all individuals with WS are able to read and for some this persists into adulthood.

The obvious question to ask is why some participants with WS are unable to read. A partial answer to this question is provided in a study by Howlin *et al.* (1998), which included some of the participants from the earlier Udwin *et al.* studies. The study found that reading abilities were related to IQ: those participants who had an IQ of below 50 were unable to read, whereas a large proportion (78%) of the participants with an IQ of between 50 and 69 were able to read. All participants with an IQ above 70 were able to read.

The studies above report findings on reading assessments which form part of larger standardized IQ batteries. None of the studies cited above used TD control groups nor did they address the link between component reading skills (such as phonological awareness or language comprehension) and level of reading ability. Some recent studies have addressed these issues. For example, Laing *et al.* (2001) reported that a group of individuals with WS (which included both children and adults) had slightly lower performance on a phoneme deletion task compared to a group of reading-age-matched controls; although the WS group also had lower mean performance on all other phonological awareness tasks, this difference was not reliable. The individuals with WS also found it harder to read non-words than real words.

Language, Communication/Social Interaction Patterns and Literacy Among Children with Williams Syndrome Who Speak Languages Other than English

There have been studies on individuals with WS speaking a number of different languages, including Romance (French, Italian, Spanish, Portuguese), Germanic (German), Greek, Uralic (Hungarian) and Semitic

(Hebrew). There have also been a few published cross-linguistic studies which compare individuals with WS with different native languages on specific linguistic phenomena. Research on literacy in children with WS speaking languages other than English is more limited and currently only includes studies on Spanish, Italian and Hebrew. This part of the chapter will provide a summary of a number of studies conducted with individuals with WS speaking languages other than English and a critical review of the implications of the findings for our understanding of the WS phenotype.

Although research into language and communication/interaction skills in children with WS speaking languages other than English is relatively recent, this type of research is essential for two main reasons: firstly, to establish which patterns may be syndrome specific and which may be language specific; secondly, to evaluate the significance of the theoretical advances made by studying the syndrome based on English. With regard to the latter, different studies have shown that WS provides evidence for the neural specialization of cognitive functions from birth (innate modularity), or that WS offers evidence of how the subtle changes in the brain structure and function interact with genes and the environment to produce the specific phenotype (neuroconstructivist view) (Stojanovik, 2011).

Morphosyntax

As mentioned earlier, a study on English-speaking children with WS has argued that individuals with WS have relatively good morphological abilities relative to their non-verbal MA, and in particular, a preserved computational system for grammatical rules and an impaired associative memory system (Clahsen & Almazan, 1998). However, English is a language which only has a few inflectional morphemes. In order to argue that children with WS truly have good morphological skills and a spared computational system for grammar, we need data from morphologically rich languages. In this respect, studies on languages other than English have been invaluable. For example, Kraus and Penke (2002) showed a similar pattern for German-speaking children with WS with regard to noun plurals and participles in that the participants with WS had better performance on the regular as opposed to the irregular forms. For participles, this was evident only when frequent and infrequent participles were considered separately. While a large percentage of errors (84%) with irregular participles in the control children were due to overregularization of infrequent verbs, in children with WS there was a different pattern. Forty percent of errors with irregular participles were due to overregularization of frequent verbs and not infrequent verbs. For nouns, this was evident in the correctness scores for regular and irregular inflection. There were no differences between the children with WS and controls with regard to regular plural forms, but the children with WS supplied significantly fewer irregular plural forms than controls. This study only had two participants, and due to this small sample size, the findings should be interpreted cautiously.

A study of 14 Hungarian-speaking children with WS focusing on plurals and accusatives has also shown that children with WS perform better on regular than irregular forms (Pleh *et al.*, 2003). The control group also found irregulars harder, but the proportion of errors on these was much higher for the WS group. In addition, short-term memory measures were also administered and it was reported that the children with WS who had lower memory spans, made more errors on the irregular forms. Interestingly, in the TD group, memory span was not related to errors on irregular forms.

Unlike the previous two studies mentioned on German and Hungarian, a study on Hebrew-speaking adolescents with WS by Levy and Hermon (2003) did not report strong morphological skills. Hebrew is a Semitic language; roots are formed by consonants and morphology is indicated by various prefixes, suffixes and infixes. Irregular forms are rare in Hebrew and they were not investigated in this study, hence all the morphological markers examined were regular. The study by Levy and Hermon (2003) assessed 10 adolescents with WS (between 12 and 17 years of age) and two control groups: a younger MA-matched group (CA 5 years) and an older group (CA 11 years). These two MA-matched groups spanned the MA range of the WS group. The study found that individuals with WS were good at extracting the basic consonantal root structure of Hebrew words. However, this finding was expected because very young TD Hebrew-speaking children are able to do this (Levy, 1988). In addition, on all the other morphological paradigms studied, individuals with WS performed similarly to MA-matched controls (younger ones who were CA 5).

The conclusion from the regular–irregular debate is not definitive. Studies involving Germanic and Uralic languages suggest that individuals with WS have much better performance with regular than irregular morphology, which would support the argument that generating rules is a strength in individuals with WS. The data from Hebrew cannot be used to either support or refute this distinction because irregular forms are rare in Hebrew and the study cited did not investigate them. The data from regular morphology suggest that Hebrew-speaking individuals with WS are not better than expected for their non-verbal MA; hence, it is not clear whether generating rules truly is a relative strength in individuals with WS. The reason may be that Hebrew's very different way of morphological marking makes it particularly difficult for individuals with WS to master. Data from other Semitic languages or from Chinese for example, in which the regular–irregular distinction does not apply in its original form, would be a great test for this theoretical assumption.

Studies on other aspects of grammar have also been conducted and these have shown that language abilities in WS are more in line with their general non-verbal abilities rather than being a specific strength. For example, Volterra *et al.* (1996) studied the lexical and morphosyntactic abilities of 17 Italian-speaking children and adolescents with WS. They reported that while lexical comprehension was similar to what was found in the MA-matched controls, the grammatical abilities of the children with WS were lower than expected for their MA. This study revealed a number of interesting findings with regard to morphological errors which would have been difficult to detect in children with WS speaking a language like English with a sparse morphological system. For example, the children with WS produced errors which are rarely or never reported in TD Italian children. These included: errors with gender agreement, substitutions of prepositions, word order errors and verb conjugations. However, the authors stress the remarkable individual variation within the WS population.

Findings from French on grammatical gender assignment also point to the fact that language abilities in WS may be impaired (Karmiloff-Smith *et al.*, 1997). A gender concord paradigm was used to assess gender agreement and gender assignment. Participants were asked to provide the critical gender agreement information carried out by the article and the adjective either for real words or for nonsense words. It was reported that although both groups (the WS and the MA-matched controls) produced more errors with nonsense words than with the real words, the groups did not differ in the number of errors they made on real words but they did differ on the number of errors made on the nonsense words. However, when nonsense words were presented with a numeral, which does not provide any clue as to the gender of the noun (e.g. *deux*/two, as in *deux faldines*), and when participants had to rely only on the word ending to infer the gender of the noun, the children with WS performed at chance, and lower than young normal controls. The authors interpreted this finding as suggesting that individuals with WS performed poorly on grammatical gender agreement and assignment, and they suggest that individuals with WS may follow a different path and may resemble second language learning. However, Monnery *et al.* (2002) challenged the interpretation of these results, arguing that individuals with WS did not have difficulty with gender agreement, which relies on syntactic rules, but that they had difficulties with lexical retrieval.

A study by Bernicot *et al.* (2003) reported on the lexical, structural (morphological and syntactic) and pragmatic abilities of seven French-speaking children with WS aged between 6 and 19 in a story generation task. They reported that children with WS performed similarly to a CA-matched group with regard to lexical and morphological measures. The lexical measure was a lexical diversity measure which was based on dividing the number of different words by the total number of words (similar to a type-token ratio). The morphological measure was the number of morphological errors produced by the participants. The results of the lexical diversity measure reported in this study was similar to what has also been reported for English-speaking individuals with WS (Stojanovik & van Ewijk, 2008), which used a very similar methodology (i.e. a narrative generation task) and calculated lexical diversity using two measures. In addition, the fact that there was not a difference between the number of morphological errors between the WS and the control group in the Bernicot *et al.* study is similar to what was also found by Stojanovik *et al.* (2004). It seems that children with WS do not make many morphological errors in spontaneous speech and these kinds of tasks are not sensitive in identifying the morphological difficulties these children have.

Social communication/interaction

The understanding of idiomatic expressions has been studied in French-speaking children and adolescents with WS (Lacroix *et al.*, 2010a). The analyses of the data showed that although children with WS had a slower rate of development regarding the comprehension of idiomatic expressions, their understanding of idioms increased with increasing CA. Due to their slower rate of development, the study concluded that individuals with WS may never reach typical proficiency with regard to idiom comprehension. Given that idiomatic expressions fall within the domain of figurative language, this study supports the findings for English that figurative language is an area of difficulty in WS.

Narratives

There have been a few cross-linguistic studies involving investigations of narratives and prosody. Narratives have been investigated in Italian-, French- and English-speaking children with WS (Reilly *et al.*, 2005) in a single study. It reported that Italian-speaking children with WS used the highest number of social evaluation devices in their stories and more than the English- and French-speaking children with WS; however, the English-speaking children with WS used more than the French-speaking children. An interesting finding was that although the three groups of children with WS differed between them with regard to the number of evaluative devices, they all used more evaluation in the stories than their respective control groups. These authors propose that this extensive use of social evaluation across three different cultures suggests that this may be a 'marker' of the WS phenotype, but they also argue that the intensity of the WS social behavior is 'influenced by the individual culture's display rules and social conventions for expressing sociability' (Reilly *et al.*, 2005: 312).

Prosody

An English–French cross-linguistic comparison investigated the use of pitch range in children with WS in a spontaneous speech task (Lacroix *et al.*, 2010b). The investigation included 8 French children with WS and 2 control groups (one matched for MA and one for CA) and 13 English-speaking children with WS and 2 control groups as above. The English and the French children with WS had similar CAs (mean age for the English group = 9 years 6 months and mean age for the French group = 10 years 8 months). The study found that the English-speaking children with WS had a narrower pitch range in semitones compared to their French counterparts; however, both WS groups had a significantly higher pitch range than both control groups, suggesting that a wide pitch range may be syndrome specific, but is certainly also influenced by the specific cultural context of the child.

Production and comprehension of prosody was also investigated in an English–Spanish study, using the same test battery: Profiling Elements of Prosody for Speech and Communication (PEPS-C) (Peppé *et al.*, 2003) for English and its Spanish adaptation (Martínez-Castilla & Peppé, 2008). The study compared Spanish and English children with WS who were matched for chronological and non-verbal MA. The findings of the study suggest that the profiles of the children with WS speaking two different languages seem to mirror, to a great extent, the patterns observed in TD children (Martinez *et al.*, 2012). Aspects of prosody which are acquired later in TD children are more difficult for children with WS in both languages.

Literacy

Three published studies have investigated literacy abilities in children with WS speaking languages other than English. Two studies were published in 2004: Levy and Anteby (for Hebrew) and Menghini *et al.* (for Italian). Levy and Anteby (2004) studied word reading and reading-related skills in 17 adolescents and young adults with WS. They reported that 6 out of the 17 participants could not read non-words at all, and 4 participants were unable to read words and non-words. Rapid automatized naming (RAN) did not correlate with reading ability; however, word reading correlated with IQ and performance on phonological awareness tasks. In particular, phoneme deletion and expressive vocabulary were correlated with single-word reading, and single-word reading and phoneme identification correlated with the reading of non-words. Learning to read Hebrew, which has a very opaque orthography, is likely to be more challenging than learning a Roman alphabet which is more transparent. Hebrew involves integrating visuospatial information along several axes because the vowels are marked below and above the consonants. Italian, on the other hand, has a very shallow orthography and hence it is easier to master (Wydell & Butterworth, 1999).

Menghini *et al.* (2004) investigated the reading abilities of 16 Italian-speaking individuals with WS, including children (mean age 17 years 7 months; range 10;9–30;2). They found that the WS group was significantly lower than the MA-matched control group (mean age 7 years 7 months) on syllable deletion and rhyme detection. Syllable deletion was significantly correlated with both word and non-word reading. Single-word reading was reported to be as expected for the MA group but the WS group was poorer at reading non-words than real words. Also, the WS group was lower on reading comprehension than the control group.

Gayarzibal and Cuetos (2008) investigated the reading abilities of 12 Spanish-speaking children with WS aged between 8 and 15 years. Unlike the Menghini study, the children with WS did not have difficulty with reading non-words; however, they were weaker than the controls on reading real words. This is unexpected and suggests serious reading difficulties because Spanish has a transparent orthography. The WS group performed at the same level as the MA-matched group on syllable deletion and non-word repetition, but lower than the control group on rhyming. There were no correlations between phonological processing measures and reading ability. Gayarzibal and Cuetos suggest that the differences between their study and the Menghini *et al.* study may lie in the fact that the participants in the Menghini *et al.* study were mainly adults and may have therefore developed compensatory strategies for word reading. Another reason they suggest could be the method of instruction for the Spanish individuals with WS, which may have relied on a 'look and say' strategy rather than phonics.

Summary and Future Research Implications

The literature review above suggests that children and adolescents with WS do not have language abilities that are above what would be expected for their non-verbal MA. There are areas of strengths and weaknesses in their linguistic profile; for example, strengths in receptive vocabulary and possibly regular morphology (at least for some languages and for some morphemes). In spite of early reports of friendliness and loquaciousness, there is also a range of social communication difficulties reported. These include difficulties with appropriateness of conversations, interpreting figurative language and forming social relationships. Wide pitch range appears to be characteristic of the WS profile and this finding has received cross-linguistic support.

There is still a small body of research on early language acquisition in WS, in particular with regard to grammatical development. Also, there is hardly any research on how the different language profiles we find in this population may reflect the different size of the chromosomal deletion.

With regard to research including languages other than English, the findings so far across different languages seem to be fairly consistent in delineating the strengths and weaknesses in this population. Thus, there is a general agreement that vocabulary is relatively stronger than grammar in all languages studied, although it should be noted that this pattern is not unique for individuals with WS. This pattern is also quite commonly found in the DS population (Chapman *et al.*, 1991). Phonological awareness skills seem to be generally as expected for MA with some specific weaknesses which may either be language specific or dependent on the age of the population studied. It is fair to say though that despite the few studies on WS on languages other than English, the body of research is still in its infancy and data from different languages and language families are needed in order to elucidate the possible 'syndrome-specific' language and communication skills.

There has been limited research into the role of wider oral language skills (including vocabulary, syntax, semantics) and visuo-perceptual deficits for reading and spelling in children with WS. Also there need to be longitudinal studies which trace the development of general language skills and reading in order to establish the causality between reading and general language development (Griffiths, 2012) as it has already been shown that children who are at a familial risk of dyslexia (Snowling *et al.*, 2007) show a positive correlation between reading outcomes and oral language skills.

Clinical Implications

Assessment

The review above highlighted that there are huge individual differences in WS as there are in other atypical populations as well as in the typical population; and although we talk about a WS profile, characterizing exactly what this profile is, is not an easy task. Although the general picture seems to be that receptive concrete vocabulary is a relative strength as well as regular morphology (at least for some type of structures and for some languages), all other aspects of the WS language profile show either a delay or impairment. Hence, assessment should be as comprehensive as possible and it should include all aspects of language (from phonological awareness, through expressive and receptive vocabulary, expressive and receptive grammatical abilities including complex syntactic structures as well as pragmatic aspects of language). The research studies reviewed above also showed that the way that different skills are assessed can impact the results obtained. For example, spontaneous speech tasks do not seem to be as sensitive to morphological difficulties as elicited tasks. Therefore, one should ideally combine both types of assessment (spontaneous speech and elicited tasks). On the other hand, sometimes, social communication skills (especially when they may be a particular strength) are best assessed via spontaneous speech tasks; hence, assessment should be as comprehensive as possible if intervention is to be well designed.

Intervention

Language and communication

To date, there have been no intervention studies on language and communication in WS; hence, there is the urgent need for building an evidence base. The lack of referential pointing in WS prior to the onset of referential language is important for intervention (Mervis *et al.*, 2004). Usually, the onset of referential pointing is taken as a sign that the child is ready for vocabulary acquisition. However, this is not the case for children with WS and they may be ready for speech and language intervention targeting vocabulary development before the onset of referential pointing. In addition, some children with WS may benefit from intervention which targets comprehension and production of referential gestures in order to improve their non-verbal abilities (Mervis *et al.*, 2004). It should also be noted that intervention studies do not take the 'one fits all' approach as this is unlikely to be effective for this heterogeneous group. Currently, there is lack of evidence with regard to the type, frequency or indeed the effectiveness of speech and language therapy in children with WS, yet there are so many areas of language in WS that could potentially benefit from intervention. Semel and Rosner (2003) provide excellent suggestions on various intervention strategies and techniques that would be appropriate for this population, such as structured therapy, mediational strategies and naturalistic approaches.

Literacy

Although WS has been recognized for half a century and although the few research studies to date that have investigated literacy in this population suggest difficulties, there has as yet not been an intervention study. There has only been one study described in Mervis (2009) which is based on a conference presentation by Becerra *et al.* (2008) and discusses the impact of a reading intervention method on the reading abilities of a large group of 44 older children and adolescents with WS. Of these 44 children, 20 were exposed to whole word (sight) reading and 24 to the phonics method. The study reports that most of the children who had been exposed to the phonics method could read at or above their general cognitive level. Most of the children who were exposed to the whole word reading method, read below their general cognitive level. Eight children in the sample could not read at all and they had all been exposed to the whole word method. This study suggests, therefore, that children with WS perhaps benefit more from being exposed to the phonics as opposed to the whole word method, which is not surprising given that the phonics method of instruction has been found to be more effective than the whole word method in TD children (Ehri, 2004) as well as children with learning difficulties, such as those with DS (Cupples & Iakono, 2002). To conclude, experimental and quasi-experimental studies that will investigate the effectiveness of different reading approaches for individuals with WS are a priority of research in this area. As Griffiths (2012: 329) points out: 'there is an urgent need for an evidence base to inform practitioners of effective reading intervention in WS'.

Overall Summary

This chapter produced an overview of language, communication and literacy abilities in individuals with WS across languages. Current knowledge suggests that individuals with WS have difficulties in the three domains reviewed and the evidence for this comes not only from English-speaking individuals, but also from those speaking other languages. There is an imbalance between research into language and communication skills, which is much more common, and literacy skills, which have been studied to a lesser extent. There are hardly any language, communication or intervention studies in WS and this is a gap that future research will need to fill.

References

Annaz, D., van Herwegen, J., Thomas, M., Fishman, R., Karmiloff-Smith, A. and Runblad, G. (2009) Comprehension of metaphor and metonymy in children with Williams syndrome. *International Journal of Language and Communication Disorders* 44, 962–1078.

Arnold, R., Yule, W. and Martin, N. (1985) The psychological characteristics of infantile hypercalcaemia: A preliminary investigation. *Developmental Medicine and Child Neurology* 27, 49–59.

Becerra, A.M., John, A.E., Peregrine, E. and Mervis, C.B. (2008) Reading abilities of 9–17-year-olds with Williams syndrome: Impact of reading method. Paper presented at the Symposium on Research in Child Language Disorders, Madison, WI, June.

Bellugi, U., Poizner, H. and Klima, E. (1989) Language modality and the brain. *Trends in Neurosciences* 12, 380–388.

Bellugi, U., Wong, P. and Jernigan, T.L. (1994) Williams syndrome: An unusual neuropsychological profile. In S.H. Broman and J. Grafman (eds) *Atypical Cognitive Deficits in Developmental Disorders: Implications for Brain Function* (pp. 23–56). Hillsdale, NJ: Lawrence Erlbaum Associates.

Bellugi, U., Marks, S., Bihrle, A. and Sabo, H. (1988) Dissociations between language and cognitive functions in Williams Syndrome. In D. Bishop and K. Mogford (eds) *Language Development in Exceptional Circumstances* (pp. 177–189). Edinburgh: Churchill Livingstone.

Bellugi, U., Bihrle, A., Neville, H., Jernigan, T. and Doherty, S. (1992) Language, cognition, and brain organization in a neurodevelopmental disorder. In M. Gunnar and C. Nelson (eds) *Developmental Behavioural Neuroscience* (pp. 201–232). Hillsdale, NJ: Lawrence Erlbaum.

Bennett, F.C., La Veck, B. and Sells, C.J. (1978) The Williams elfin facies syndrome: The psychological profile as an aid in syndrome identification. *Pediatrics* 61, 303–306.

Bernicot, J., Lacroix, A. and Reilly, J. (2003) La narration chez les enfants atteints du syndrome de Williams: Aspects structuraux et pragmatiques. *Enfance* 3, 265–281.

Bishop, D.M. (1998) *Children's Communication Checklist*. London: The Psychological Corporation.

Bishop, D.V.M. (2003) *Children's Communication Checklist 2*. London: The Psychological Corporation.

Catterall, C., Howard, S., Stojanovik, V., Szczerbinski, M. and Wells, B. (2006) Investigating prosodic ability in Williams syndrome. *Clinical Linguistics and Phonetics* 20, 531–538.

Chapman, R.S., Schwartz, S.E. and Kay-Raining Bird, E. (1991) Language skills of children and adolescents with Down syndrome: I. Comprehension. *Journal of Speech, Language and Hearing Research* 34, 1106–1120.

Chiang, M.-C., Reiss, A.L., Lee, A., Bellugi, U., Galaburda, A., Korenberg, J., Mills, D.L., Toga, A.W. and Thompson, P.M. (2007) 3D pattern of brain abnormalities in Williams syndrome visualised using tensor-based morphometry. *NeuroImage* 36, 1096–1109.

Clahsen, H. and Almazan, M. (1998) Syntax and morphology in Williams syndrome. *Cognition* 68, 167–198.

Clahsen, H., Ring, M. and Temple, C. (2004) Lexical and morphological skills in English-speaking children with Williams syndrome. In S. Bartke and J. Siegmüller (eds) *Williams Syndrome Across Languages* (pp. 221–244). Amsterdam: Benjamins.

Crisco, J.J., Dobbs, J.M. and Mulhern, R.K. (1988) Cognitive processing of children with Williams syndrome. *Developmental Medicine and Child Neurology* 30, 650–656.

Cupples, L. and Iacono, T. (2002) The efficacy of 'whole word' versus 'analytic' reading instruction for children with Down syndrome. *Reading and Writing: An Interdisciplinary Journal* 15, 549–574.

Dall'Oglio, A.M. and Milani, L. (1995) Analysis of the cognitive development in Italian children with Williams syndrome. *Genetic Counselling* 6, 175–176.

Dunn, L.M. and Markwardt, F.C. (1970) *Peabody Individual Achievement Test*. Circle Pines, MI: American Guidance Service.

Eckert, M.A., Galaburda, A.M., Mills, D.L., Bellugi, U., Korenberg, J.R. and Reiss, A.L. (2006) The neurology of Williams syndrome: Cascading influences of visual system impairment? *Cellular and Molecular Life Sciences* 63, 1867–1875.

Ehri, L.C. (2004) Teaching phonemic awareness and phonics: An explanation of the National Reading Panel meta-analyses. In P. McCardle and V. Chhabra (eds) *The Voice of Evidence in Reading Research* (pp. 153–186). Baltimore, MD: Brookes.

Fenson, L., Dale, P.S., Reznick, J.S., Thal, D., Bates, E., Hartung, J.P., Pethick, S. and Reilly, J.S. (1993) *MacArthur Communicative Development Inventories: User's Guide and Technical Manual*. San Diego, CA: Singular Publishing Group.

Fenson, L., Marchman, V.A., Thal, D., Dale, P.S., Reznick, J.S. and Bates, E. (2007) *MacArthur Communicative Development Inventories: User's Guide and Technical Manual* (2nd edn). Baltimore, MD: Brookes.

Fodor, J. (1983) *The Modularity of Mind*. Cambridge, MA: MIT Press.

Garayzabal, H.E. and Cuetos, V.F. (2008) Aprendizaje de la lectura en los niños con síndrome de Williams. *Psicothema* 20, 672–677.

Glenn, S. and Cunningham, C. (2005) Performance of young people with Down syndrome on the Leiter-R and British Picture Vocabulary Scales. *Journal of Intellectual Disability Research* 49, 239–244.

Grant, J., Valian, V. and Karmiloff-Smith, A. (2002) A study of relative clauses in Williams syndrome. *Journal of Child Language* 29, 430–416.

Greer, M.K., Brown, F.R., Shashidhar, G., Choudry, S.H. and Klein, A.J. (1997) Cognitive, adaptive, and behavioural characteristics of Williams syndrome. *American Journal of Medical Genetics (Neuropsychiatric Genetics)* 74, 521–525.

Griffiths, Y. (2012) Literacy. In E. Farran and A. Karmiloff-Smith (eds) *Neurodevelopmental Disorders Across the Lifespan* (pp. 313–335). Oxford: Oxford University Press.

Howlin, P., Davies, M. and Udwin, O. (1998) Syndrome specific characteristics in Williams syndrome: To what extent do early behavioural patterns persist into adult life. *Journal of Applied Research in Intellectual Disabilities* 11, 207–226.

Hudson, G. (2000) *Essential Introductory Linguistics*. Oxford: Blackwell.

Joffe, V. and Varlocosta, S. (2007) Patterns of syntactic development in children with Williams syndrome and Down's syndrome: Evidence from passives and wh-questions. *Clinical Linguistics and Phonetics* 21, 705–727.

Jones, K.L. and Smith, D.W. (1975) The Williams elfin facies syndrome: A new perspective. *Journal of Paediatrics* 86, 718–723.

Jones, W., Bellugi, U., Lai, Z., Chiles, M., Reilly, J., Lincoln, A. and Adolphs, R. (2000) Hypersociability in Williams syndrome. *Journal of Cognitive Neuroscience* 12 (S1), 30–46.

Jones, W., Hesselink, J.R., Courchesne, E., Duncan, T., Matsuda, K. and Bellugi, U. (2002) Cerebellar abnormalities in infants and toddlers with Williams syndrome. *Developmental Medicine and Child Neurology* 44, 688–694.

Karmiloff-Smith, A. (1998) Development itself is the key to understanding developmental disorders. *Trends in Cognitive Sciences* 2, 389–398.

Karmiloff-Smith, A. (2012) Brain: The neuroconstructivist approach. In E.K. Farran and A. Karmiloff-Smith (eds) *Neurodevelopmental Disorders Across the Lifespan: A Neuroconstructivist Approach* (pp. 37–58). Oxford: Oxford University Press.

Karmiloff-Smith, A., Grant, J., Berthoud, I., Davies, M., Howlin, P. and Udwin, O. (1997) How intact is 'intact'? *Child Development* 68, 274–290.

Kataria, S., Goldstein, D.J. and Kushnik, T. (1984) Developmental delays in Williams ('elfin facies') syndrome. *Applied Research in Mental Retardation* 5, 419–423.

Klein-Tasman, B.P. and Mervis, C.B. (2003) Distinctive personality characteristics of 8-, 9-, and 10-year olds with Williams syndrome. *Developmental Neuropsychology* 23, 269–290.

Kraus, M. and Penke, M. (2002) Inflectional morphology in German Williams syndrome. *Brain and Cognition* 48, 410–413.

Lacroix, A., Aguert, M., Dardier, V., Stojanovik, V. and Laval, V. (2010a) Idiom comprehension in French-speaking children and adolescents with Williams syndrome. *Research in Developmental Disabilities* 31, 608–616.

Lacroix, A., Stojanovik, V., Dardier, V. and Laval, V. (2010b) Prosodie et syndrome de Williams: Une étude inter-culturelle. *Enfance* 3, 287–300.

Laing, E., Hulme, C., Grant, J. and Karmiloff-Smith, A. (2001) Learning to read in Williams syndrome: Looking beneath the surface of atypical reading development. *Journal of Child Psychology and Psychiatry* 42, 729–739.

Lakoff, G. and Johnson, M. (1980) *Metaphors We Live By*. London: University of Chicago Press.

Laws, G. and Bishop, D. (2003) A comparison of language abilities in adolescents with Down syndrome and children with specific language impairment. *Journal of Speech, Language and Hearing Research* 46, 1324–1339.

Levy, Y. (1988) On the early learning of formal grammatical systems: Evidence from studies of the acquisition of gender and countability. *Journal of Child Language* 15, 179–187.

Levy, Y. and Hermon, S. (2003) Morphological abilities of Hebrew-speaking adolescents. *Developmental Neuropsychology* 23, 61–85.

Levy, Y. and Antebi, V. (2004) Word reading and reading-related skills in Hebrew-speaking adolescents with Williams syndrome. *Neurocase* 10, 444–451.

Martínez-Castilla, P. and Peppé, S. (2008) Developing a test of prosodic ability for speakers of Iberian Spanish. *Speech Communication* 50, 900–915.

Martinez-Castilla, P., Stojanovik, V., Setter, J. and Sotillo, M. (2012) Prosodic abilities in English and Spanish children with Williams syndrome: A cross-linguistic study. *Applied Psycholinguistics* 33, 1–22.

McCarthy, D. (1972) *McCarthy Scales of Children's Abilities*. New York: Psychological Corporation.

Menghini, D., Verucci, L. and Vicari, S. (2004) Reading and phonological awareness in Williams syndrome. *Neuropsychology* 18, 29–37.

Mervis, C.B. (1999) The Williams syndrome cognitive profile: Strengths, weaknesses, and interrelations among auditory short-term memory, language and visuo-spatial constructive cognition. In E. Winograd, R. Fivush and W. Hirst (eds) *Ecological Approaches to Cognition: Essays in Honour of Ulric Neisser* (pp. 193–227). Mahwah, NJ: Lawrence Erlbaum.

Mervis, C. (2009) Language and literacy development of children with Williams syndrome. *Topics in Language Disorders* 29, 149–169.

Mervis, C.B. and Klein-Tasman, B.P. (2000) Williams syndrome: Cognition, personality, and adaptive behaviour. *Mental Retardation and Developmental Disabilities Research Reviews* 6, 148–158.

Mervis, C.B. and Beccera, A.M. (2007) Language and communicative development in Williams syndrome. *Mental Retardation and Developmental Disabilities Research Reviews* 13, 3–15.

Mervis, C.B. and John, A.E. (2012) Precursors to language and early language. In E. Farran and A. Karmiloff-Smith (eds) *Neurodevelopmental Disorders Across the Lifespan: A Neuroconstructivist Approach* (pp. 187–204). Oxford: Oxford University Press.

Mervis, C.B., Robinson, B.F., Rowe, M.L., Beccera, A.L. and Klein-Tasman, B.P. (2003) Language abilities of individuals who have Williams syndrome. In L. Abbeduto (ed.) *International Review of Research in Mental Retardation 27* (pp. 35–81). Orlando, FL: Academic Press.

Mervis, C.B., Robinson, B.F., Rowe, M.L., Becerra, A.M. and Klein-Tasman, B.P. (2004) Relations between language and cognition in Williams syndrome. In S. Bartke and J. Siegmuller (eds) *Williams Syndrome Across Languages* (pp. 63–92). Amsterdam: Benjamins.

Monnery, S., Seigneuric, A., Zagar, D. and Robinchon, F. (2002) A linguistic dissociation in Williams syndrome: Good at gender agreement but poor at lexical retrieval. *Reading and Writing: An Interdisciplinary Journal* 15, 589–612.

Neale, M.D. (1966) *Neale Analysis of Reading Ability*. London: MacMillan.

Pagon, R., Bennet, F., La Veck, B., Stewart, K. and Johnson, J. (1987) Williams syndrome: Features in late childhood and adolescence. *Paediatrics* 80, 85–91.

Peppé, S., McCann, J. and Gibbon, F. (2003) *Profiling Elements of Prosodic Systems – Children (PEPS-C)*. Edinburgh: Queen Margaret University College.

Perovic, A. and Wexler, K. (2007) Complex grammar in Williams syndrome. *Clinical Linguistics and Phonetics* 21, 729–745.

Philofsky, A., Fidler, D.J. and Nepburn, S. (2007) Pragmatic language profiles of school-age children with autism spectrum disorders and Williams syndrome. *American Journal of Speech-Language Pathology* 16, 368–380.

Pleh, C., Likacs, A. and Racsmany, M. (2003) Morphological patterns in Hungarian children with Williams syndrome and the rule debates. *Brain and Language* 86, 377–383.

Porter, M.A. and Coltheart, M. (2005) Cognitive heterogeneity in Williams syndrome. *Developmental Neuropsychology* 27, 275–306.

Reilly, J., Klima, E.S. and Bellugi, U. (1990) Once more with feeling: Affect and language in atypical populations. *Development and Psychopathology* 2, 367–391.

Reilly, J., Bernicot, J., Vicari, S., Lacroix, A. and Bellugi, U. (2005) Narratives in children with Williams syndrome: A cross-linguistic perspective. *Perspectives on Language and Language Development* 303–312. [Springer Digital Version.] doi:10.1007/1-4020-7911-7_22

Rice, M.L., Warren, S.F. and Betz, S.K. (2005) Language symptoms of developmental language disorders: An overview of autism, Down syndrome, fragile X, specific language impairment, and Williams syndrome. *Applied Psycholinguistics* 26, 7–27.

Rust, J., Golombok, S. and Trickey, J. (1993) *Wechsler Objective Reading Dimensions* (WORD). Sidcup: The Psychological Corporation.

Schmitt, J.E., Eliez, S., Warsofsky, I.S., Bellugi, U. and Reiss, A. (2001) Corpus callosum morphology of Williams syndrome: Relation to genetics and behaviour. *Developmental Medicine and Child Neurology* 43, 155–159.

Semel, E. and Rosner, S.R. (2003) *Understanding Williams Syndrome: Behavioural Patterns and Interventions*. London: Lawrence Erlbaum Associates.

Setter, J., Stojanovik, V., van Ewijk, L. and Moreland, M. (2007) Affective prosody in children with Williams syndrome. *Clinical Linguistics and Phonetics* 21, 659–672.

Snowling, M.J., Mutter, V. and Carroll, J.M. (2007) Children at family risk of dyslexia: A follow-up in adolescence. *Journal of Child Psychology and Psychiatry* 48, 609–618.

Stojanovik, V. (2006) Social interaction deficits in children with Williams syndrome. *Journal of Neurolinguistics* 19, 157–173.

Stojanovik, V. (2010) Understanding and production of prosody in children with Williams syndrome: A developmental trajectory approach. *Journal of Neurolinguistics* 23, 112–126.

Stojanovik, V. (2011) Later language. In E.K. Farran and A. Karmiloff-Smith (eds) *Neurodevelopmental Disorders Across the Lifespan: A Neuroconstructivist Approach* (pp. 204–221). Oxford: Oxford University Press.

Stojanovik, V. (2014) Language in genetic disorders and cognitive modularity. In L. Cummings (ed.) *The Cambridge Handbook of Communication Disorders* (pp. 541–558). Cambridge: Cambridge University Press.

Stojanovik, V and van Ewijk, L. (2008) Do children with Williams syndrome have unusual vocabularies? *Journal of Neurolinguistics* 21, 18–34.

Stojanovik, V., Perkins, M. and Howard, S. (2004) Williams syndrome and specific language impairment do not support claims for developmental double dissociations and innate modularity. *Journal of Neurolinguistics* 17, 403–424.

Stojanovik, V., Perkins, M. and Howard, S. (2006) Linguistic heterogeneity in Williams syndrome. *Clinical Linguistics and Phonetics* 20, 547–552.

Stojanovik, V., Setter, J. and van Ewijk, L. (2007) Intonation abilities in children with Williams syndrome: A preliminary investigation. *Journal of Speech, Language and Hearing Research* 50, 1606–1617.

Stromme, P., Bjornstad, P.G. and Ramstad, K. (2002) Prevalence estimation of Williams syndrome. *Journal of Child Neurology* 17, 269–271.

Sullivan, K., Winner, E. and Tager-Flusberg, H. (2003) Can adolescents with Williams syndrome tell the difference between lies and jokes? *Developmental Neuropsychology* 23, 85–103.

Tarling, K., Perkins, M. and Stojanovik, V. (2006) Conversational success in Williams syndrome: Communication in the face of cognitive and linguistic limitations. *Clinical Linguistics and Phonetics* 20, 583–590.

Thomas, M.S.C., Grant, J., Barham, Z., Gsodl, M., Laing, E., Lakusta, L., Tyler, L.K., Grice, S., Paterson, S. and Karmiloff-Smith, A. (2001) Past tense formation in Williams syndrome. *Language and Cognitive Processes* 16, 143–176.

Thompson, P.M., Lee, A.D., Dutton, R.A., Geaga, J.A., Hayashi, K.M., Eckert, M.A., Bellugi, U., Galaburda, A.M., Korenberg, J.R., Mills, D.L., Toga, A.W. and Reiss, A.L. (2005) Abnormal cortical complexity and thickness profiles mapped in Williams syndrome. *The Journal of Neuroscience* 25, 4146–4158.

Udwin, O. and Yule, W. (1990) Expressive language of children with Williams syndrome. *American Journal of Medical Genetics Supplement* 6, 108–114.

Udwin, O. and Yule, W. (1991) A cognitive and behavioural phenotype in Williams syndrome. *Journal of Clinical and Experimental Neuropsychology* 13, 232–244.

Udwin, O., Davies, M. and Howlin, P. (1996) A longitudinal study of cognitive abilities and educational attainment in Williams syndrome. *Developmental Medicine and Child Neurology* 38, 1020–1029.

Udwin, O., Yule, W. and Martin, N. (1986) Age at diagnosis and abilities in idiopathic hypercalcaemia. *Archives of Disease in Childhood* 61, 1164–1167.

Udwin, O., Yule, W. and Martin, N. (1987) Cognitive abilities and behavioural characteristics of children with idiopathic infantile hypercalcaemia. *Child Psychology and Psychiatry* 28, 297–308.

Volterra, V., Capirci, O., Pezzini, G., Sabbadini, L. and Vicari, S. (1996) Linguistic abilities in Italian children with Williams syndrome. *Cortex* 32, 663–677.

von Arnim, G. and Engel, P. (1964) Mental retardation related to hypercalcaemia. *Developmental Medicine and Child Neurology* 6, 366–377.

Wechsler, D. (1974) *Intelligence Scale for Children – Revised*. New York: Psychological Corporation.

Williams, J.C., Barratt-Boyes, B.G. and Lowe, J.B. (1961) Supravalvular aortic stenosis. *Circulation* 24, 1311–1318.

Wydell, T.N. and Butterworth, B. (1999) A case study of an English-Japanese bilingual with monolingual dyslexia. *Cognition* 70, 273–305.

Zukowski, A. (2004) Investigating knowledge of complex syntax: Insights from experimental studies of Williams syndrome. In M. Rice and S. Warren (eds) *Developmental Language Disorders: From Phenotypes to Etiologies* (pp. 99–119). Mahwah, NJ: Lawrence Erlbaum Associates.

Part 2

Language Disorders in Specific Languages

6 Language Disorders in Cantonese-Speaking Children

Carol K.S. To

The purpose of this chapter is to provide readers with information on cultural and linguistic features of Cantonese and how different types of language disorders are manifested in the language. The clinical implications of these linguistic and cultural characteristics are discussed with practical suggestions for speech-language pathologists (SLPs) at the end of the chapter.

Cantonese or the Yue dialect belongs to one of the seven dialect groups of Modern Chinese, which also include Mandarin (Putonghua), Wu, Xiang, Gan, Kejia and Min. Speakers of these dialects are mutually unintelligible and the overlap of vocabulary and syntactic structures varies among dialects. Cantonese is spoken by 55.6 million people in southern China, as well as in Chinese communities in many countries such as Australia, Canada and the United States (Lewis, 2009). Cantonese is the major language spoken by the Chinese population in Hong Kong (Census and Statistics Department, 2012), which is one of the most densely populated cities in the world, situated in the southern corner of Mainland China. Within a land area of 1104 km², the total population exceeded 7 million in 2011 (Census and Statistics Department, 2012). Hong Kong was a British colony between the years 1842 and 1997 and English has been the official language since the colonization period. After the handover to Mainland China in 1997, the national language of China, Mandarin (also called Putonghua for the oral form), became another official language in Hong Kong. However, Cantonese remains the dominant oral language in Hong Kong.

Chinese Culture

Chinese cultures differ from Western cultures in many ways. Although Chinese cultures have been remarkably influenced by the West in recent times, certain cultural values are inherent and still maintained among many Chinese nowadays. The ethical, social, political and educational values of Chinese society have been shaped by Confucianism, the most influential philosophy in Chinese culture for nearly 2000 years.

Family structure and child-rearing practices

One of the most prominent concepts of Confucianism is family and the hierarchy within the family. Chinese families value responsibility for family members and harmony (Ng & Ingram, 1989). When younger generations grow up, they have the responsibility to take care of the older generations. For example, if older people are sick, the younger generation has a sense of responsibility to look after them and support them physically and financially. Multiple generations of families often live in the same household. With this arrangement, grandparents can be taken care of and can look after their grandchildren. This family structure directly impacts Chinese parents' child-rearing practice and interaction style.

Many traditional Chinese parents focus on developing their children's obedience, proper conduct and moral values, while paying less attention to children's development of independence, assertiveness and creativity as in the Western parenting styles (Ho, 1986). Chinese children are therefore found to be more aware of behavioral rules than their Western peers and are comfortable with following rules (Moneta, 2004). A way to maintain harmony is to respect older family members and avoid direct conflicts. Younger members of the family may defer to older members for advice (Ng & Ingram, 1989). Children are taught to control and suppress their emotions, in particular negative emotions. They might be less ready to express and discuss what they feel with their parents when compared to their English-speaking counterparts.

The traditional Chinese parenting style is reflected in the way that parents interact with their children, including the content and context of parental talk to children (van Kleeck, 1994). In their survey, Johnston and Wong (2002) revealed that (Canadian) Chinese mothers were less likely to treat their children as potentially equal conversational partners than Canadian mothers of Western European descent were. It was also reported that Chinese mothers did not read stories to their children. In addition, play and having fun were not considered to be part of children's learning by the Chinese mothers. Instead, direct teaching via structured activities was the dominant teaching mode for the Chinese parents.

Humility and modesty are important virtues valued by Confucians. Chinese parents believe that praising too much may have a negative impact on their children since children may become too arrogant about their current achievements and such an attitude would inhibit future progress. Therefore, Chinese parents usually provide limited amounts of praise to their children (Leung, 2002). This is in contrast to most Western cultures in which adults are more likely to reward effort and provide encouragement so as to foster children's self-esteem.

Education

Education is very important in Chinese cultures. In Confucianism, one's education level is closely related to social status and occupation. Chinese believe that people who are highly educated are more likely to be the leaders of society. Leaders are characterized by their intelligence, scholarly works, good standard of ethics and moral character. This concept has been deeply rooted in the Chinese cultures and is still prominent. Chinese parents expect their children to work hard and wish them to do well at school. Obtaining good grades therefore becomes Chinese children's mission.

Chinese teachers are relatively directive when teaching (Lynch & Hanson, 1998) and are highly regarded by both children and their parents. Students are expected to learn through observation and attentive listening. Therefore, asking questions that challenge teachers' assumptions is not encouraged and may be considered impolite and unacceptable. In other words, silence is more appreciated in Chinese classrooms. In contrast, students in Western cultures learn by exploration and asking many questions. The difference between Chinese and Western students' style of learning are noticeable in American classrooms. Cheng (1989) reported that (American-)Asian students were often quiet in class and seldom volunteered to participate in class activities when compared to their American peers. Teachers from the dominant American culture may misinterpret the behaviors of Asian students as being passive and inattentive (Cheng, 1989).

Interpersonal interaction

Chinese cultures signal and interpret politeness slightly differently from Western cultures. Using family names and titles to address people is more polite than using first names (Cheng, 2012). Chinese speakers tend to be more indirect, reserved and implicit. Chinese also tend not to make direct comments or give their own opinions. Even when they express their ideas, Chinese speakers are more implicit, less extreme and tend to use modal words such as 'could' or 'may' to soften their tone. These behaviors may also be a way to avoid direct confrontation and retain harmony in the interaction. Chinese speakers also differ in non-verbal communication when compared to English speakers. Chinese may avoid making direct and prolonged eye contact, in particular for younger generations to elders or for juniors to authority. Smiling is a sign of agreement and approval in Western culture. But smiling in Chinese culture sometimes signals embarrassment or a polite apology.

It should be noted that contemporary Chinese cultures have a wide range of diversity. Through globalization, some Chinese families may have adopted Western culture and may be moving away from the traditional

Confucian values. Moreover, certain sociopolitical factors may weaken the Confucian influence. For example, Cheng (2012) pointed out that the one-child-per-family policy in Mainland China may be linked to changes in family dynamics and a more permissive parenting style. Although Hong Kong does not have the one-child policy, the size of the nuclear family is small and similar changes in children's behaviors and parenting style can be observed in Cantonese families. However, certain Confucian concepts are still deeply rooted in the Chinese culture. For instance, the importance of family and the value of education are consistent across generations (Huang & Gove, 2012).

Linguistic Characteristics of Cantonese

Phonology

The syllable structures of Cantonese include V, VC, CV, CVC and syllabic consonants. In contemporary Cantonese, there are 17 initial consonants, namely, /p, pʰ, t, tʰ, k ,kʰ, ts, tsʰ, f, s, h, w, j, l, m, n, ŋ/. Among these consonants, /ŋ/ is disappearing at the syllable-initial position. Final consonants include /p, t, k, m, n, ŋ/. The eight Cantonese vowels include /i, u, y, a, œ, ɛ, ɔ, ɐ/. The 11 diphthongs are /iu, ou, au, ɐu, ui, ai, ɐi, ei, ɔi, œy, ɛu/.

Like other Chinese languages, Cantonese is a tone language that makes use of pitch differences to mark lexical meaning. There are six contrastive tones in Cantonese differing in tone heights and tone contours, namely, high-level tone (Tone 1), high-rising tone (Tone 2), mid-level tone (Tone 3), low-falling tone (Tone 4), low-rising tone (Tone 5) and low-level tone (Tone 6). In addition to these level and contour tones, there are three shorter variants ending with a final stop. These variants include high-stopped tone (Tone 7), mid-stopped tone (Tone 8) and low-stopped tone (Tone 9). To illustrate, taking the syllable /si/ as an example, Tone 1 絲 /si1/ means 'silk', Tone 2 史 /si2/ means 'history', Tone 3 試 /si3/ means 'to try', Tone 4 時 /si4/ means 'time', Tone 5 市 /si5/ means 'market' and Tone 6 是 /si6/ means 'yes'/'is'. In addition, Cantonese is more syllable-timed than English, meaning that each Cantonese syllable receives approximately an equal amount of stress while English syllables receive varying amounts of stress depending on the speaker's emphasis and the word class. For example, in the English sentence, 'They re**cord** a new **re**cord', the first record is a verb and the second is a noun differing in the stress pattern. Such a functional use of stress contrast is absent in Cantonese.

Word classes

The general properties of the main word classes of nouns, pronouns, verbs, adjectives, adverbs and conjunctions in Cantonese and other

Chinese dialects, including Mandarin, are generally similar to English. However, the proportional use of the main word classes in English and Chinese is reported to be different. Unlike English, verbs but not nouns were found to be the most common word class in the conversation of young Chinese toddlers at 22 months of age (Tardif, 1996). In order to investigate this verb-bias pattern in Chinese children, Tardif *et al.* (1997) compared the proportion of different word classes in adult-to-child speech and in children's speech in English, Italian and Mandarin Chinese. Unlike the English- and Italian-speaking children, the Mandarin-speaking children used more verbs than nouns, consistent with previous studies. Tardif *et al.* (1997) suggested that differences in the adult input between Mandarin and the other two languages may account for the language-specific patterns in children's distribution of word classes. Adult input in Mandarin was characterized by more types and tokens of verbs than nouns, while a reverse pattern was observed in English and Italian. Moreover, Mandarin adults tended to emphasize verbs by placing them in utterance final position and there were very few morphological markings on verbs in Mandarin. Given these verb-dominant patterns in adult-to-child speech, Mandarin-speaking children may also exhibit similar patterns (Tardif *et al.*, 1997).

Morphosyntax

Cantonese differs from English in many ways in the domain of morphosyntax. Like English, the canonical word order of Cantonese is subject-verb-object (SVO). However, there is more flexibility in word ordering in Cantonese than English. For example, object-subject-verb (OSV) is also a productive structure in Chinese. There is no tense marking, no case, gender or animacy markings on pronouns, as well as no plural inflection in Cantonese. On the other hand, Cantonese makes use of lexical devices such as temporal adverbs, aspect markers, nominal classifiers and particles to achieve similar functions.

Aspect markers

Cantonese like other Chinese dialects has a sparse verb morphological system. Verb-tense markings and agreement marking in verbs are absent in Cantonese. Temporal information is mainly conveyed by aspect marking on verbs or using explicit lexical devices of temporal adverbials. Aspect is different from tense. Tense concerns when an event occurs within a time frame, i.e. whether the event took place in the past or it takes place in the present or it will happen in the future. Aspect concerns the status of an action or an event, including completeness, continuousness, duration, habituality and progressiveness, regardless of when the event happens. For example, the perfective aspect does not relate to the past tense as it may refer to an event in the future (see Table 6.1). Aspect markers in Cantonese are attached to the verb as a suffix and are sometimes regarded as a kind of verb particle (Matthews & Yip, 1994). Unlike tense markings in English, aspect markers are not grammatically obligatory. This means that a grammatically correct sentence can have no aspect marker. There are six commonly used aspect markers in Cantonese (Matthews & Yip, 1994).

Pronouns

Pronoun markings in Cantonese are also limited and there are no gender, case or animacy markings. There is one first-person pronoun 我 /ɔ5/ and one second-person pronoun 你 /lei5/ used in both subject and object positions – 'I' and 'me' – in Cantonese are both represented by 我 /ɔ5/ and 'you' is represented by 你 /lei5/. There is only one third-person pronoun in Cantonese, 佢 /kʰœy5/, referring to 'he', 'him', 'she', 'her' and 'it'. The suffixes 哋 /tei6/ and 嘅 /kɛ3/ are used to indicate plural and possessive, respectively. For example, 'we' is represented by /ɔ5 tei6/ and 'his' is represented by /kʰœy5 kɛ3/. Without the cues from gender, case

Table 6.1 Aspect markers in Cantonese

Marker	Aspect	Usage	Example
咗 /tsɔ2/	Perfective	To emphasize the completion of an event	我做咗功課先去玩. (I will play after I have finished the assignment.)
過 /kʷɔ3/	Experiential	To emphasize an event is an experience and has happened at least once.	佢去過澳洲 (He has been to Australia.)
住 /tsy6/	Continuous/durative	To emphasize continuous activity without a change of state	佢聽住歌踩單車 (He is listening to music when cycling.)
吓 /ha5/	Delimitative	To emphasize an event of brief duration	聽歌放鬆吓 (Listen to some music to relax for a while.)
緊 /kɐn2/	Progressive	To emphasize an ongoing activity, similar to the progressive –ing form	佢食緊早餐 (He is having breakfast.)
開 /hɔi1/	Habitual	To emphasize an habitual activity over a period of time	我搭開巴士 (I usually take the bus.)

Source: Adapted from Matthews and Yip (1994).

and animacy markings, Chinese listeners appear to rely more on inference rather than pronouns in resolving discourse reference (LaPolla, 1990).

Classifiers

Cantonese, like other Chinese dialects, has an elaborate array of classifiers that categorize entities according to their properties, particularly shape and function. Classifiers in Cantonese are unique to nouns. Classifiers are always an obligatory grammatical element when referring to common nouns with numerals and when the common objects are definite referents (e.g. '一 /jɐt7/ (one) 隻 /tsɛk8/ (classifier) 貓 /mau1/ (cat)'). The classification system is somewhat cognitively based, reflecting inherent conceptual structures (Tai, 1994). There are about 60 classifiers in Cantonese (Matthews & Yip, 1994), which can be subcategorized into mensural (quantity) classifiers and sortal (kind/type) classifiers (Lyons, 1977). The main function of mensural classifiers is to measure nouns in terms of *quantity*, similar to the word class of quantifiers in English. This type of classifier includes container-based classifiers, e.g. '一 /jɐt7/ (one) 樽 /tsœn1/ (bottle) 酒 /tsɐu2/ (wine)', standard measurements, e.g. '一 /jɐt7/ (one) 磅 /pɔŋ6/ (pound) 提子 /tʰɐi4tsi2/ (grapes)' and collective classifiers, e.g. '一 /jɐt7/ (one) 群 /kʷɐn4/ (group) 動物 /tuŋ6mɐt9/ (animal)'. Sortal classifiers on nouns specify the *kind/quality* of the referents, particularly the perceived features of objects (e.g. flatness, length and size). For example, classifiers like 條 /tʰiu4/ and 枝 /tsi1/ are used to encode long objects (e.g. snakes and pens); 塊 /fai3/ and 張 /tsœŋ1/ flat objects (e.g. boards and paper); 粒 /lɐp7/ tiny objects (e.g. beads); and 幢 /tuŋ6/ stacked up or high-up objects (e.g. buildings, piles of books).

Sentence-final particles

There is a large inventory of sentence-final particles (SFPs) in Cantonese with approximately 30–90 types in everyday speech (Kwok, 1984; Leung, 1992). They are very common in daily Cantonese speech even though some of them are grammatically optional. Luke (1990) estimated that SFPs were found in continuous talk on average every 1.5 seconds and regarded SFPs as the hallmark of Cantonese. There is no known direct grammatical counterpart like SFPs in English. SFPs occur individually or in clusters of two or three in sentence-final position (Leung, 1992). An important role of SFPs is to convey the moods, attitudes, feelings and emotions of a speaker (Matthews & Yip, 1994). SFPs are also responsible for modality, focus and conditional reasoning of utterances (Lee & Law, 2001). Hence, the same utterance with different SFPs could be interpreted differently. For example, the meaning of the utterance, *'He will go'*, changes with the use of different SFPs:

(1) /kʰœy5 wui5 hœy3 k̲ʷa̲3/ (He might go SFP.) [Interpretation: He might go.] /kʷa3/ is often used to express a prediction with uncertainty.

(2) /kʰœy5 wui5 hœy3 p̠ɔ̠3/ (He will go SFP.) [Interpretation: (I am emphasizing that) he will go as well.] /pɔ3/ is often used to emphasize some information to the listener.

(3) /kʰœy5 wui5 hœy3 w̠ɔ̠5/ (He will go SFP.) [Interpretation: (His mother says) he will go.] /wɔ5/ is often used to report what someone has said.

Intonation is another means of expressing some of the functions served by SFPs. Intonation is realized by changing pitch contour and the acoustic correlate of pitch is the fundamental frequency (F0). Cantonese is a tone language in which the lexical tones are realized by changing pitch contour and F0. A change in pitch height or contour of a Cantonese syllable may potentially alter the meaning. Chan (1996) proposed that the tonal system in Cantonese may restrict the use of sentential intonation in conveying higher-level pragmatic implications. However, more recently, researchers have claimed that intonation at the sentence level coexists with lexical tones in Cantonese and is used to convey different intentions. The lexical tones are carried on the overall intonation contour of an utterance (e.g. Chan, 2001). Chao (1968: 39) put forward the analogy of 'small ripples riding on larger waves' to describe the relationship between lexical tone at the syllable level and intonation at the utterance level in Chinese. However, there is limited empirical evidence on the production and perception of Cantonese intonation in relation to different pragmatic functions and their relationship remains unclear.

Written language and orthography

Like some other Chinese dialects, Cantonese is basically an oral language. The corresponding form of written language being used is Modern Standard Chinese (MSC), which is shared by all Chinese speakers. Recently, Cantonese speakers in Hong Kong developed a variety of written Cantonese, which usually appears in informal genres such as comic books, magazines, newspapers and personal correspondence. In formal registers, such as textbooks, formal documents and novels, MSC is still the traditional form. Cantonese corresponds less closely to MSC than Putonghua. They differ in terms of vocabulary and syntactic structures. About one-third of Cantonese words are dialectal and do not have a written form (Li *et al.*, 1995). Syntactically, both Cantonese and Putonghua have the canonical SVO structure. However, there are some differences in other syntactic structures, such as comparative constructions, adverb–verb order in some contexts and direct/indirect object order.

There are generally four ways that languages can be expressed in visible form: pictographic, logographic (also called ideographic), syllabic and alphabetic (Harris & Coltheart, 1986). These four principles are grouped into two systems, 'Pictographic and logographic are "word-writing" systems, in which individual characters generally stand for whole words. In contrast, syllabic and alphabetic systems are "sound-writing" systems, in which individual characters generally stand for individual sounds within a word' (Harris & Coltheart, 1986: 10). The main feature of a logographic system such as Chinese is that characters do not represent the individual sounds.

About 95% of Chinese characters are compounds consisting of more than one component unit (Cheng, 1987), while others are characters which cannot be broken down into smaller productive units (e.g. 水 'water'). A majority of the Chinese characters (about 80%) belong to the category of phonetic–semantic compounds composed of a semantic component carrying information about the meaning of the character, and a phonetic component carrying full or partial information about the pronunciation of the whole character (Zhu, 1987 as cited in Hoosain, 1991). It was estimated that there are about 800 pronounceable phonetic components in Chinese (Hoosain, 1991). For example, as shown in Table 6.2, the Chinese character for 'pond' is 塘 /tʰɔŋ4/. The two component characters are 土 /tʰou2/, a semantic component that means 'soil' and 唐, a phonetic component pronounced as /tʰɔŋ4/. The meaning of the component 唐 is 'Chinese' which is not directly related to the meaning of the character and only provides information on the pronunciation of the whole character 塘. Among the compound characters that are in modern and frequent use, only around 18.5% of them share an identical pronunciation with the phonetic component (Zhu, 1987 as cited in Hoosain, 1991). Due to sound change resulting in variation in pronunciation over the years, a majority of phonetic–semantic compounds may only share partial pronunciation as the phonetic component, such as sharing the same rhyme, or may have a totally different pronunciation (Leong, 1986). Therefore, one may not be able to reliably predict the exact pronunciation of novel characters using the strategy of pronouncing the phonetic components. Moreover, the phonetic component is not always

Table 6.2 Examples of different phonetic–semantic compounds

Target	Components		Contribution to the whole character
塘 /tʰɔŋ4/ 'pond'	土	/tʰou2/ 'soil'	Semantic
	唐	/tʰɔŋ4/ 'Chinese'	Phonetic
忠 /tsʊŋ1/ 'loyal'	中	/tsʊŋ1/ 'central'	Phonetic and semantic
	心	/sɐm1/ 'heart'	Semantic
鏈 /lin2/ 'chain'	金	/kɐm1/ 'gold'	Semantic
	連	/lin4/ 'connect'	Phonetic and semantic
念 /lim6/ 'think'	今	/kɐm1/ 'now'	Phonetic but changed substantially
	心	/sɐm1/ 'heart'	Semantic

totally independent of the meaning. Some 'phonetic' components also encode partial meaning of the character. The relatively low consistency in the role of phonetic and semantic components may help explain why acquisition of Chinese character reading is complicated and different from that in alphabetic languages.

The shape of all Chinese characters is like a square. All components of each compound character are assembled within the square configuration and the arrangement follows the orientations of top-down (e.g. 香 /hœŋ1/ 'fragrant'), left to right (e.g. 好 /hou2/ 'good') and outside to inside (e.g. 悶 /mʊn6/ 'bored'). Each component in compound characters can be further broken down into even smaller units called strokes. There are approximately eight basic strokes involving one movement of the writing instrument (e.g. 丶, 一, 丨, 丿).

There are two conventions of Chinese characters, traditional and simplified scripts. For example, the characters for 'love' in the traditional and simplified scripts are 愛 and 爱, respectively. Hong Kong and Taiwan use the traditional script while most parts of Mainland China and Singapore use the simplified script. Normally, children in Hong Kong are required to learn to read and write the traditional script at school. Sometimes, children in Hong Kong may learn the simplified script spontaneously through exposure to books, the internet and advertisements since the correspondence between the traditional and simplified scripts is quite high. Another major difference between character learning in Hong Kong and Mainland China is the use of the Pinyin system for pronunciation of Putonghua in the mainland. Pinyin is an alphabetic script, which indicates the pronunciation of each character and can be regarded as a Romanization system of Putonghua. The Pinyin system is taught to children in the mainland during school entry so that they can use the knowledge from the script to learn the pronunciation of new characters. In early-grade textbooks, Pinyin is often printed above the characters. In contrast, there is no equivalent alphabetic system for coding pronunciation in Cantonese.

Developmental Language Disorders in Cantonese

Due to the cultural and linguistic differences between Cantonese and English speakers, Cantonese has provided a very fruitful ground for researchers to examine the manifestations of various language disorders through exploring cross-linguistic similarities and differences in children with language disorders. At the same time, linguistic and cultural differences may pose challenges to English-speaking clinicians when working with Cantonese-speaking children and their families. The following section reviews studies of Cantonese-speaking children with language disorders. The information aims to inform clinicians about the language development and disorders of children learning Cantonese as their first language (L1).

A large body of work on childhood communication disorders has been done in Cantonese over the past two decades, in particular for children with specific language impairment (SLI) and dyslexia. Studies on children with autism spectrum disorders (ASD) are emerging.

Specific language impairment

Among the various language domains, morphosyntax is regarded as a core deficit in children with SLI (e.g. Leonard, 1998). As reviewed above, there is no obligatory morphosyntactic element to mark tense, plural, person agreement of verbs and gender of pronouns in Cantonese. Therefore, attention has been devoted to the exploration of other types of morphological markers such as aspect markers and classifiers, in Cantonese-speaking children with SLI (CSLI).

Stokes and Fletcher (2000) compared the use of nouns, verbs and aspect markers in naturalistic speech samples produced by 15 children with CSLI (mean age of 48 months) and 15 language-matched (LM) children. The CSLI group used significantly more noun types than the LM group. However, there was no significant difference between types and tokens of verbs or aspect markers in these two groups. When the findings were examined in more detail, the two groups differed in terms of the degree of collocation diversity of the aspect markers. The use of aspect markers by the CSLI group was restricted to a smaller range of verbs than the LM group. These results were replicated in a subsequent study where the aspect markers used by CSLI children were confined to certain verb types. For example, the perfective markers produced by the CSLI group usually appeared with achievement verbs, while their typically developing (TD) peers showed more diverse and productive use of perfective markers (Stokes & Fletcher, 2003). Using an experimental task, Fletcher et al. (2005) reported a more robust pattern of morphosyntactic deficit in CSLI. In their study, the CSLI group produced significantly fewer aspect markers than their age peers and younger LM peers. In addition, Fletcher et al. also provided evidence that the difficulties in using aspect markers in CSLI are not due to their lack of temporal concepts.

Stokes and So (1997) examined classifiers using an experimental paradigm. The CSLI group performed similarly to their age-matched TD peers in their accuracy on the use of shape classifiers but they differed in their error patterns. The age-matched TD group tended to use the general classifier 個 /kɔ3/ to substitute for a specific classifier while the CSLI group were more likely to completely drop the classifier or to substitute another specific but incorrect classifier. These qualitative differences again suggested that similar to their English-speaking counterparts, CSLI children also showed deficits in the area of morphosyntax.

English-speaking children with SLI are reported to have restricted lexical diversity especially in the word class of verbs. Conti-Ramsden and Jones (1997) reported fewer verb types and tokens in a group of English-speaking children with SLI when compared to their TD peers. Yam (1999) compared the types and tokens of different word classes in the spontaneous speech of children with CSLI and their LM peers. Words were categorized into four types: nouns, verbs, other open-class (e.g. adjectives and adverbs that allow new words to be coined and included in the word class) and closed-class (e.g. pronouns, prepositions, connectives) tokens. The CSLI group used a significantly higher proportion of noun tokens. The more frequent use of noun tokens in the CSLI group was at the expense of other grammatical categories. That means, they showed fewer 'other' open-class tokens and closed-class tokens than the LM group. The nominal preference may reflect that nouns are more easily learned by children with CSLI because they are more concrete. Surprisingly, there was no difference in verb tokens and types between the CSLI and the LM groups. The author suggested that the absence of a significant difference may be due to the relatively simple verbal marking in Chinese. This explanation was used to explain the higher proportion of verbs than nouns in TD Mandarin Chinese-speaking children in spontaneous speech, unlike their English counterparts who used more nouns than verbs (Tardif, 1996). The sparse verb markings may enhance verb production in the Chinese-speaking children and account for the lack of significant differences between the token and types of verbs between the CSLI group and the LM group.

In another study, Klee *et al.* (2004) compared the lexical diversity (including all word classes) in a group of preschool CSLI children and their typical age peers and receptive LM typical peers. Children with CSLI produced significantly less diverse vocabularies than their typical age peers. At an individual level, a combination of measures including vocabulary diversity, mean length of utterances (MLU) and age significantly discriminated children with language impairment from the other two typical groups.

In a recent large-scale study, To *et al.* (2010) established a normative benchmark for assessing the narrative ability of Cantonese-speaking, school-age children aged between 5 and 12. In appraising the validity, a group of 55 children with CSLI was compared against a group of age- and gender-matched children with reference to four narrative measures, namely, (a) semantic score, which is an indicator of vocabulary used to convey the story content; (b) syntactic complexity, which measures the tokens of four advanced syntactic structures in Cantonese; (c) referencing, which evaluates the use of appropriate and clear personal reference; and (d) connectives, which refers to the total number of connectives used. The results showed that although the semantic score was the most developmentally sensitive, it was the measure of syntactic complexity that best discriminated children with and without SLI.

Fletcher *et al.* (2009) concluded that in a language where some syntactic markers are grammatically optional, the manifestations of language impairment may be realized as qualitative differences such as productivity and error patterns rather than merely quantitative differences at the utterance level. In narratives, children's difficulties may be realized as the restricted deployment of more advanced syntactic structures and sophisticated vocabulary. On the whole, morphosyntax and lexical diversity are vulnerable in children with CSLI, similar to their English-speaking counterparts.

Dyslexia

According to the International Dyslexia Association (2002: 1), dyslexia is 'characterized by difficulties with accurate and/or fluent word recognition and by poor spelling and decoding abilities. These difficulties typically result from a deficit in the phonological component of language that is often unexpected in relation to other cognitive abilities and the provision of effective classroom instruction'. Phonological awareness skills in the reading literature refer to one's awareness of the phonological structure of spoken words and the ability to manipulate sound segments. English-speaking children with dyslexia exhibit specific deficits in phonological processing with poor performance in phonological awareness tasks such as rhyme detection and alliteration (Bradley & Byrant, 1983; Rack, 1985).

The orthographic system in Chinese has attracted much research interest in the development of character reading and developmental dyslexia in Chinese-speaking children since the mid-1990s. Broadly speaking, the general developmental trajectory of character reading in Chinese children is parallel to their counterparts learning an alphabetic writing system (Klingebiel & Weekes, 2009). During a very early stage, Chinese children's visual skills are important as they learn a small set of characters by rote memory. In the next stage, the phonological stage, Chinese-children start to form systematic connections between print and pronunciation and meaning as opposed to only rote whole-symbol connections. They become aware that certain components with consistent pronunciations exist across characters. For characters with a phonetic component, children can induce script-sound rules after they have acquired a sufficient number of characters containing the same phonetic component (Ho & Bryant, 1997). The children are able to pronounce new characters with the same pronunciation using these rules. Studies demonstrated that Chinese children in Hong Kong at the early grades performed much better in reading characters with their pronunciations being identical to the phonetic components than reading characters that share partial or no cue from their phonetic components (Ho & Bryant, 1997). Shu *et al.* (2000) reported similar observations in Mandarin Chinese children in Beijing. The final stage is described as the logographic stage when children process the logograms and then the character as a whole automatically.

Phonological awareness skills were assumed to be required in the phonological stage in Chinese character reading by some scholars. Researchers have investigated the relationship between phonological awareness and Chinese character reading, which appears to be parallel to English word reading in normal readers and children with dyslexia. It was found that syllable awareness, onset/rime awareness and tone awareness are associated with learning to read Chinese characters (e.g. Huang & Hanley, 1995; McBride-Chang & Ho, 2000; So & Siegel, 1997). In addition, Chinese children with dyslexia showed significantly weaker phonological awareness skills than the control group (Ho et al., 2002, 2004).

Although these findings may point to the possibility of a phonological basis for dyslexia in Chinese, the link between phonological awareness skills and reading Chinese script is not clear. The phonetic elements in Chinese characters refer to the pronunciation of the whole word, rather than to individual phonemes. Chen et al. (2003) claimed that the role of phonological awareness skills in Chinese character reading might be related to Chinese children's sensitivity to extract and encode the information from the phonetic components when reading phonetic–semantic compounds. In other words, phonological awareness required in Chinese is at the orthographic level for the analysis of phonetic and semantic components in compounds. So the phonological skills that are involved in reading Chinese are not identical to the phonemic awareness knowledge related to decoding and spelling skills in alphabetic writing systems such as English.

Cheung (1999) devised a series of experimental tasks to test the relationship between phonological awareness and Chinese character reading. Three groups of participants were recruited: a group of normal Cantonese-speaking adults literate in Chinese character reading, a group of children with dyslexia and an age-matched control group for the dyslexia group. All the participants were tested on four aspects of ability: phonological awareness, orthographic analysis, orthographic-lexical analysis and character reading skills. There were six phonological awareness tasks targeting syllabic and phonemic levels: (1) syllable number judgment, (2) syllable deletion, (3) phoneme similarity judgment, (4) rime judgment, (5) onset judgment and (6) pitch level judgment. Cheung (1999) replicated the pattern that children with dyslexia showed significantly worse performance in the phonological awareness tasks of syllable deletion, rime judgment, onset judgment and pitch judgment. In addition, the adult groups demonstrated a clear dissociable pattern for phonological awareness and character reading skills. Within the adult group, Cheung found that some adults with weak phonological awareness were not necessarily poor at Chinese character reading. Meanwhile, some adults with good phonological awareness did not outperform those with weak phonological awareness in character reading. The pattern is understandable – even if a person is good at phonological awareness, he or she is unable to use this ability directly to analyze Chinese in the same way that he or she can analyze an alphabetic script. Based on this dissociable pattern, it was concluded that there is an association between phonological awareness and dyslexia in Chinese but the claim for a causal link of Chinese dyslexia or that weak phonological awareness is the crux of children's reading deficit was weak.

Orthographic processing and learning to read Chinese characters involve concepts of the component constituents of the characters, the form of the components and knowledge about the corresponding phonetic and semantic compounds. Other studies on Chinese character reading have focused on various factors that are associated with developmental dyslexia in Chinese. Ho and Bryant (1997) reported that the visual perceptual skills in TD children better predict early reading skills while prereading phonological awareness ability, including rhyme and homophone detection, was a significant predictor of later reading performance after controlling for children's age, IQ and maternal education. In a study of Cantonese children with dyslexia, Ho et al. (2004) comprehensively examined the cognitive profiles of 147 primary school children. Besides phonological awareness and phonological memory, Ho et al. included measures of visual perception, visual memory, orthographic processing and rapid automatic naming (RAN). Using multiple regression analyses, the contributions of RAN and orthographic processing ability together accounted for the largest amount of variance in children's reading ability (21.8%), while phonological memory only explained a small amount (1.2%) and phonological awareness did not show any significant unique contribution. Ho et al. (2000) therefore concluded that RAN and orthographic processing deficits are the two important features of Cantonese-speaking children associated with dyslexia and revised their earlier claim that a phonological deficit is the main contributing factor of Cantonese dyslexia. Related results were reported in a subsequent study on typical children suggesting RAN showed stronger association with children's reading ability than phonological awareness (Chow et al., 2005).

Subsequent studies include new potential variables that may contribute to developmental dyslexia in Chinese. Shu et al. (2006) suggested that morphological awareness, RAN and vocabulary ability but not visual skills and phonological awareness can significantly differentiate Chinese children with and without dyslexia. Chung et al. (2008) examined more potential variables including auditory temporal processing (ATP) and visual temporal processing (VTP) in addition to the previously studied variables, including RAN, visual-orthographic knowledge and morphological and phonological awareness in dyslexia. They tested 78 children aged from 8;4 to 8;11 with 26 children diagnosed with dyslexia, 26 age-matched controls and 26 reading-level-matched controls. Their results showed that phonological awareness, morphological awareness, RAN and VTP significantly predict Cantonese children's character reading skills after controlling for age, grade and IQ. These four target variables explained a total of 22% of the unique variance. Phonological awareness explained the largest amount (10%), followed by morphological awareness (7%). VTP explained a smaller amount (2%) and RAN explained only 3% variance. Visual orthographic knowledge and ATP did not show any significant unique contribution.

It is expected that the profile of Chinese children with dyslexia reported may keep changing as new findings emerge. With future studies examining biological factors such as neurophysiological and genetic factors, the understanding of developmental dyslexia in Chinese can be further improved (Klingebiel & Weekes, 2009).

Autism spectrum disorders

In Hong Kong, public awareness of ASD has improved remarkably over the last decade. Rehabilitation services for individuals with ASD in Hong Kong are expanding rapidly. Treatment approaches and directions are mainly based on programs developed in Western countries; however, studies specifically investigating Chinese children with ASD are emerging.

Some screening tools for the early identification of ASD have been adapted for the local population. Chu (2000) translated the Checklist for Autism in Toddlers (CHAT; Baron-Cohen et al., 1992), a screening tool developed in the UK for the identification of children with autism at 18 months. It consists of nine questions for parents and five direct observation items for practitioners to test the child. The CHAT was administered to three groups of Cantonese-speaking children (1) with the diagnosis of ASD from a clinical psychologist or a pediatrician ($n = 21$), (2) showing typical development ($n = 40$) and (3) showing non-ASD developmental delay ($n = 39$). Chu (2000) reported that the Cantonese-CHAT accurately discriminated the ASD group from the other two groups and demonstrated satisfactory reliability. In a subsequent study, Wong et al. (2004) examined the sensitivity and specificity of CHAT-23, which was based on the original CHAT and a Modified Checklist for Autism in Toddlers (M-CHAT) developed in the United States, which has higher sensitivity and specificity than the original CHAT. M-CHAT has 14 additional parent questions and does not include the direct observation part of the CHAT. CHAT-23 included the M-CHAT as well as the direct observation part of the original CHAT. CHAT-23 yielded high sensitivity and specificity. The good sensitivity and specificity of the adapted tests for ASD in Cantonese may imply that the realization of autistic features in young children may be similar across cultures.

Li *et al.* (2013) studied the advanced pragmatic skills of older Cantonese-speaking children with and without ASD. The study focused on the appreciation of irony conveyed through prosodic cues and SFPs in a group of Cantonese-speaking school children with high functioning ASD and an LM control group aged between 8;3 and 12;9. Four conditions were generated, namely, (1) condition with SFP, (2) condition with prosodic cues, (3) condition with both SFP and prosodic cues and (4) condition without SFP and prosodic cues. Children were asked to judge character speakers' belief and intention in short stories in the four conditions. Results revealed that the ASD group performed as well as the controls in judging characters' belief but significantly poorer in judging intention in the conditions of SFP, prosodic cues or both. The ability to identify speakers' intention of being ironic in the LM control group was better in the SFP condition and the condition with SFP and prosodic cues than the prosodic cue condition, suggesting that SFP may play a more salient role in encoding irony than prosodic cues in Cantonese. There were no significant differences among conditions for the ASD group. The poorer performance of the ASD group compared with controls in identifying intention with SFP, intonation or both types of cues suggests that no matter what linguistic devices a language uses to encode pragmatic functions, the problem of children with ASD lies in identifying the pragmatic information in interaction.

There is another ongoing study examining Cantonese-speaking children's theory of mind (ToM) skills (To *et al.*, in preparation). This study is clinically motivated by the fact that some high-functioning children with ASD can pass various standardized first-order false belief ToM tests but still exhibit traces of autistic behaviors. In particular, some high-functioning children with ASD demonstrated above average structural language skills and may be overestimated as functioning well beyond the norm in other areas (Bolick, 2005). Advanced ToM would be a vulnerable aspect for high-functioning individuals with ASD (Attwood, 2005). This study is expected to inform us whether language and culture affect Cantonese-speaking children's ToM development. Based on previous findings, it is predicted that Cantonese-speaking children would follow the same developmental progression as children speaking other languages and that children with ASD may perform differently from their typical peers.

Assessment and Intervention Considerations

This section discusses cultural and linguistic considerations for assessment and intervention when working with clients from a Chinese background. The focus is on implications for clinicians working with immigrant children whose L1 is Cantonese and who are learning English, which is the majority language of their society upon school entry.

Linguistic diversity

Chinese immigrant children are a heterogeneous group with different language backgrounds. When working with clients and families of Chinese ethnicity, it is important to know the dialect(s) they speak. Although various Chinese dialects share one writing system and similar cultures, the oral forms are mutually unintelligible to each other. For example, monolingual Cantonese speakers are not able to communicate with monolingual Shanghainese speakers using only verbal means, even though both are of Chinese ethnicity. When an interpreter is needed, clinicians should ensure that the clients and the interpreter are speakers of the same dialect. For example, clinicians may ask the parents and the interpreter, 'What dialects do you (or your child) speak, Mandarin, Cantonese, Shanghainese or Hakka?'. Then, the clinicians would know if the two parties' oral languages are intelligible to each other.

Chinese English language learners (ELLs) with speech and language problems may present different challenges to clinicians. In the early stage of acquiring a second language (L2), even typical ELLs undergo a silent period during which they may not initiate talking using their L2 in L2 environments. These children may give an impression of being not responsive. Instead, they are learning the language through listening. Typical ELLs will pass through this stage and after sufficient exposure to the new language, will begin to talk in their L2. Their speech may still be characterized by features of influence from their L1. When assessing bilingual children with suspected language problems, it is essential to evaluate both languages they are learning so that clinicians can differentiate between language differences and language disorders in these children, i.e. whether children's language difficulties are the result of a faulty intrinsic system in learning language or limited proficiency in an L2 (Cheng, 2012).

When compared to standardized assessments, language sample analysis in the two languages is more reliable (e.g. Gutiérrez-Clellen & Simon-Cereijido, 2009). Clinicians can collect a speech sample of the child and the parent interacting in contexts such as looking at picture books. After transcription, clinicians can analyze the non-adult-like patterns noticed from the child's speech. Scholars have documented some common English 'errors' manifested by ELLs with Cantonese L1 backgrounds (e.g. Chan & Li, 2000; Cheng, 2012; Fung & Roseberry-McKibbin, 1999). Tables 6.3 and 6.4 summarize the common phonological patterns and language patterns noted in typical Cantonese speakers who are learning English in Hong Kong (Bunton, 1991). The information is helpful for clinicians to identify language impairment – the realizations of *only* these patterns may not necessarily indicate a language learning problem.

Table 6.3 Some common phonological patterns produced by Cantonese-speaking English learners

English targets	Position	Pattern	Realization	Examples
/b, d, g/	Final	Devoicing	[p̚, t̚, k̚]	robe /ɹəʊb/ → rope [ɹəʊp]
/p, t, k/	Final	Unreleased	[p̚, t̚, k̚]	put /pʊt/ → [pʊt̚]
/v/	Initial	Gliding	[w]	van /væn/ → [wæn]
/v/	Final	Devoicing	[f]	live /laɪv/ → life [laɪf]
/z/	Initial	Devoicing	[s]	zip /zɪp/ → sip [sɪp]
/θ, ð/	Initial/final	Substitution	[f]	thin /θɪn/ → fin [fɪn]
			[s]	three /θriː/ → free [sriː]
			[t]	the /ðœ/ → [tœ]
/ʃ/	Initial/final	Fronting	[s]	ship /ʃɪp/ → sip [sɪp]
/ʒ/	Medial	Fronting and devoicing	[s]	measure /meʒə/ → [mesə]
/tʃ/	Initial	Fronting	[ts]	cheap /tʃiːp/ → [tsiːp]
/dʒ/	Initial	Fronting	[dz]	jump /dʒʌmp/ → [dzʌmp]
/ɹ/	Initial	Gliding	[w]	ride /ɹaɪd/ → [waɪd]
		Lateralization	[l]	ride /ɹaɪd/ → [laɪd]
/n/	Initial	Substitution	[l]	nine /naɪn/ → [laɪn]
/n/	Final	Deletion	Ø	mine /maɪn/ → [maɪ]
/l/	Final	Vocalization	[u]	will /wɪl/ → [wɪu]
/ɪ, iː/	Initial	Addition of a glide	[ji]	easy /iːzɪ/ → [jiːzɪ]
/æ/	Medial	Substitution	[ɛ]	man /mæn/ → [mɛn]
/ɔɪ/	Medial	Reduction	[ɒ]	point /pɔɪnt/ → [pɒnt]
/eə/	Medial	Reduction	[e] or [æ]	pair /peər/ → [pæ] or [pe]
/eɪ/	Medial	Reduction	[e]	fail /feɪl/ → [fel]
/st/	Final	Deletion of [t]	[s]	list /lɪst/ → [lɪs]
/pɹ/	Initial	Deletion of [ɹ]		produce /pɹədjuːs/ → [pədjuːs]

Consonant clusters

Source: Adapted from Bunton (1991).

Table 6.4 Common English errors made by Cantonese-speaking English learners

Language error	Example
(1) Past-tense error	* She _talk_ a lot during class.
(2) Subject/verb disagreement	* The children _is_ happy.
(3) Fragmented sentence	* The performers who visited our school.
(4) Article errors	* Can you give me _pen_?
(5) Semantic mismatch	go to school →* _return_ to school
(6) Collocation	turn on the light →* _open_ the light
(7) Word class	* China is a _communism_ country
(8) Active and passive verbs	* a man _was_ appeared

Source: Adapted from Bunton (1991).

In addition to language sampling, dynamic assessment (DA) can come into play to examine children's ability to learn new language structures, vocabulary and discourse structures (Gutiérrez-Clellen & Peña, 2001; Kapantzoglou et al., 2012). DA has been widely used as an evaluation method for bilingual children with a suspected language problem. It measures children's learning ability instead of their static performance by examining the _change_ in children's performance after a pretest–teaching–posttest process. In DA, SLPs evaluate how 'modifiable' a child is by considering how much the child gains from the intervention, the strategies the child employs and the amount and type of cues the child uses (Lidz, 1991). It is a more reliable and valid way to examine whether a child shows a real language learning problem or he or she is a typical language learner whose delayed performance is due to the lack of adequate exposure to a particular language when compared to standardized language tests (Peña et al., 2001, 2006).

Cultural diversity

In addition to linguistic diversity issues, information on child-rearing practices, education and interpersonal communication presented earlier in this chapter can help clinicians who are not familiar with traditional Chinese families anticipate some adaptations in their assumptions and communication strategies that they might need to make. A number of scholars have provided very practical suggestions when working with Asian clients including those from Chinese backgrounds (Cheng, 2012; Fung & Roseberry-McKibbin, 1999; Lee & Ballard, 2011). Table 6.5 lists some considerations for general interactions, assessment and intervention when working with Chinese clients.

Table 6.5 Suggestions when working with clients from Chinese cultures

Cultural characteristics	Implications
Considerations for general interaction	
• Chinese used to be relatively more formal and contained.	Clinicians can address parents using their surnames and title (e.g. Mrs Wong) while the first name or nickname can be used for the child.
	Parents generally do not hug or kiss when greeting. They prefer shaking hands, waving hands or verbal greetings.
	Parents may not be comfortable sitting on the floor during assessment or therapy, either at home or in the clinic. Parents may prefer having clinicians play with their child on a mattress on the floor while they are sitting on a chair. Sometimes, they may prefer the child sitting on their lap near a table.
	Parents may not maintain the expected degree of eye contact with clinicians. This is not a sign of impoliteness but only unfamiliarity.
• Chinese children are expected to be obedient, well disciplined and listen attentively.	Children may be unwilling to respond when they are not confident about their answers. Clinicians can provide more time to establish rapport and more encouragement for their effort.
	Children may not be comfortable in talking to unfamiliar adults. Clinicians may consider starting with some comprehension tasks in a session followed by tasks requiring more talking.
	Clinicians can observe children's interaction with other familiar communication partners such as siblings or peers (lower authority) and in different contexts. Children may behave very differently in these contexts.
Assessment considerations	
• Examinations and testing are important.	Parents are concerned about the outcomes of testing and assessment. They may unintentionally provide the answers and hints to children during assessment. Clinicians can explain to parents what they would like the parents to do or not do at the beginning of the session.

• Play is not highly valued.	Clinicians can interview parents about children's play by asking, 'What does your child usually play with?' and then followed by 'Does s/he play on his own, or with your or other children?'. If the parents reply that the child plays on his or her own, then the parents may find it difficult to show their interaction skills in a free play session. Clinicians may consider other contexts for collecting speech samples such as having another child as the playmate, or clinicians may request parents to record speech samples in some daily life context such as mealtime.

Intervention considerations

• Teachers are authorities and should be highly regarded.	Parents usually regard clinicians as teachers and show high respect to them. Parents may think that they should not disturb the treatment process and try to sit back. Clinicians can invite siblings or other children to engage in the therapy session as they can also facilitate the child's language learning. Clinicians can also ease the parents into the intervention process by providing more encouragement to the parents. Clinicians may anticipate that this will take time and may not be effective early on in the therapeutic processes.
• Chinese adults often learn through observations.	Parents may appear to be passive in therapy sessions. Clinicians can couple verbal instructions with demonstrations to match parents' observational approach to learning.
• Living arrangements are multigenerational.	Grandparents are sometimes the primary caregivers of young children. Language programs emphasizing parents' interaction skills may need adaption.
• Adults are relatively directive and authoritative to their children.	Parents do not regard their role to be equal conversational partners or playmates with their children. Using reciprocal interaction as a strategy to facilitate children's language is a new interaction style to them and recommended interaction strategies may require adapting to be appropriate for the family.
• Children are taught to follow rules and listen.	Chinese children, particularly in the school years, appear to be passive and seldom initiate a conversation. Clinicians can be explicit in inviting children to participate and can involve peers as models in the intervention process.

Conclusions

Clients with different cultural and linguistic backgrounds vary in their values, beliefs, family structure and style of living. This chapter highlights the linguistic characteristics of Cantonese when compared to English, as well as the manifestations of developmental language disorders in the language. Moreover, it also brings insights regarding the Confucian influence on Chinese children's learning style, parent–child relationships and interpersonal interactions. The information can assist SLPs' decision-making during assessment and intervention planning for Chinese children with language disorders.

References

Attwood, T. (2005) Theory of mind and Asperger's syndrome. In L.J. Baker and L.A. Welkowitz (eds) *Asperger's Syndrome: Intervening in Schools, Clinics, and Communities* (pp. 11–41). Mahwah, NJ: Lawrence Erlbaum Associates.

Baron-Cohen, S., Allen, J. and Gillberg, C. (1992) Can autism be detected at 18 months? The needle, the haystack, and the CHAT. *British Journal of Psychiatry* 161, 839–843.

Bolick, T. (2005) Cognitive assessment of preschool and elementary school students. In L.J. Baker and L.A. Welkowitz (eds) *Asperger's Syndrome: Intervening in Schools, Clinics, and Communities* (pp. 85–113). Mahwah, NJ: Lawrence Erlbaum Associates.

Bradley, L.L. and Bryant, P.E. (1983) Categorizing sounds and learning to read: A causal connection. *Nature* 301, 419–421.

Bunton, D. (1991) A comparison of English errors made by Hong Kong students and those made by non-native English learners internationally. *Institute of Language in Education Journal* 2, 9–23.

Census and Statistics Department (2012) 2011 Population census – summary results. Hong Kong. See http://www.census2011.gov.hk/pdf/summary-results.pdf (accessed 15 July 2012).

Chan, A.Y.W. and Li, D.C.S. (2000) English and Cantonese phonology in contrast: Explaining Cantonese ESL learners' English pronunciation problems. *Language, Culture and Curriculum* 13 (1), 67–85.

Chan, M.K.M. (1996) Gender-marked speech in Cantonese: The case of sentence-final particles *je* and *jek*. *Studies in the Linguistic Sciences* 26, 1–38.

Chan, M.K.M. (2001) Gender-related use of sentence-final particles in Cantonese. In M. Hellinger and H. Bussmann (eds) *Gender Across Languages: The Linguistic Representation of Women and Men* (pp. 57–72). Amsterdam: John Benjamins.

Chao, Y.R. (1968) *A Grammar of Spoken Chinese*. Berkeley, CA: University of California Press.

Chen, X., Shu, H., Wu, N. and Anderson, R.C. (2003) Stages in learning to pronounce Chinese characters. *Psychology in the Schools* 40 (1), 115–124.

Cheng, L.L. (1989) Service delivery to Asian/Pacific LEP children: A cross-cultural framework. *Topics in Language Disorders* 9, 1–14.

Cheng, L.L. (2012) Asian and Pacific American languages and cultures. In D.E. Battle (ed.) *Communication Disorders in Multicultural and International Populations* (4th edn, pp. 37–60). St. Louis, MO: Elsevier.

Cheng, T.K. (1987) *Zhong Hua Min Zu Wen Hua Shi Lun* (*This History of Chinese Culture*). Hong Kong: Joint Publishing Co. Ltd.

Cheung, P.S.P. (1999) The characteristics of dyslexia in Cantonese-speaking children in Hong Kong. Unpublished master thesis, City University of Hong Kong.

Chow, B.W.Y., McBride-Chang, C. and Burgess, S. (2005) Phonological processing skills and early reading abilities in Hong Kong Chinese kindergarteners learning to read English as a second language. *Journal of Education Psychology* 97, 81–87.

Chu, K.L.J. (2000) Validity and reliability of the Cantonese version of the checklist for autism in toddlers (CHAT): A preliminary study. Unpublished master thesis, The University of Hong Kong.

Chung, K., McBride-Chang, C., Wong, S.W.L., Cheung, H., Penney, T.B. and Ho, C.S.H. (2008) The role of visual and auditory temporal processing for Chinese children with developmental dyslexia. *Annuals of Dyslexia* 58, 15–35.

Conti-Ramsden, G. and Jones, M. (1997) Verb use in specific language impairment. *Journal of Speech, Language and Hearing Research* 40, 1298–1313.

Fletcher, P., Leonard, L., Stokes, S. and Wong, A.M.-Y. (2005) The expression of aspect in Cantonese-speaking children with specific language impairment. *Journal of Speech and Hearing Research* 48, 621–634.

Fletcher, P., Leonard, L.B., Stokes, S.F. and Wong, A.M-Y. (2009) Morphosyntactic deficits in Cantonese-speaking children with specific language impairment. In S-P. Law, B.S. Weekes and A.M-Y. Wong (eds) *Language Disorders in Speakers of Chinese* (pp. 75–88). Bristol: Multilingual Matters.

Fung, F. and Roseberry-McKibbin, C. (1999) Service delivery considerations in working with clients from Cantonese-speaking backgrounds. *American Journal of Speech-Language Pathology* 8, 309–318.

Gutiérrez-Clellen, V.F. and Peña, E.D. (2001) Dynamic assessment of diverse children: A tutorial. *Language, Speech, and Hearing Services in Schools* 32, 212–224.

Gutiérrez-Clellen, V.F. and Simon-Cereijido, G. (2009) Bilingual children: Challenges and future directions. *Seminars in Speech and Language* 30 (4), 234–245.

Harris, M. and Coltheart, M. (1986) *Language Processing in Children and Adults: An Introduction.* London: Routledge & Kegan Paul.

Ho, D.Y.F. (1986) Chinese patterns of socialization: A critical review. In M.H. Bond (ed.) *The Psychological Character of the Chinese People* (pp. 1–37). Hong Kong: Oxford University Press.

Ho, C.S.H. and Bryant, P. (1997) Phonological skills are important in learning to read Chinese. *Developmental Psychology* 33, 946–951.

Ho, C.S.-H., Law, T.P.S. and Ng, P.M. (2000) The phonological deficit hypothesis in Chinese developmental dyslexia. *Reading and Writing: An Interdisciplinary Journal* 13, 57–79.

Ho, C.S.H., Chan, D.W.O., Tsang, S.M. and Lee, S.H. (2002) The cognitive profile and multiple-deficit hypothesis in Chinese developmental dyslexia. *Developmental Psychology* 38, 543–553.

Ho, C.S.H., Chan, D.W.O., Lee, S.H., Tsang, S.M. and Luan, V.H. (2004) Cognitive profiling and preliminary subtyping in Chinese developmental dyslexia. *Cognition* 91, 43–75.

Hoosain, R. (1991) *Psycholinguistic Implications for Linguistic Relativity: A Case Study of Chinese.* Hillsdale, NJ: Lawrence Erlbaum Associates.

Huang, G.H.-C. and Gove, M. (2012) Confucianism and Chinese families: Values and practices in education. *International Journal of Humanities and Social Science* 2 (3), 10–14.

Huang, H.S. and Hanley, J.R. (1995) Phonological awareness and visual skills in learning to read Chinese and English. *Cognition* 54, 73–98.

International Dyslexia Association (2002) What is dyslexia? See http://www.interdys.org/FAQWhatIs.htm (accessed 30 December 2014).

Johnston, J.R. and Wong, M.Y.A. (2002) Cultural differences in beliefs and practices concerning talk to children. *Journal of Speech, Language and Hearing Research* 45, 916–926.

Kapantzoglou, M., Restrepo, M.A. and Thompson, M. (2012) Dynamic assessment of word learning skills: Identifying language impairment in bilingual children. *Language, Speech, and Hearing Services in Schools* 43, 81–96.

Klee, T., Stokes, S., Wong, A., Fletcher, P. and Gavin, W. (2004) Utterance length and lexical diversity in Cantonese-speaking children with and without language impairment. *Journal of Speech, Language and Hearing Research* 47, 1396–1410.

Klingebiel, K. and Weekes, B.S. (2009) Developmental dyslexia in Chinese: Behavioral, genetic and neuropsychological issues. In S.P. Law, B.S. Weekes and A.M-Y. Wong (eds) *Language Disorders in Speakers of Chinese* (pp. 138–168). Bristol: Multilingual Matters.

Kwok, H. (1984) *Sentence Particles in Cantonese*. Hong Kong: Centre of Asian Studies, The University of Hong Kong.

LaPolla, R.J. (1990) Grammatical relations in Chinese: Synchronic and diachronic considerations. Unpublished doctoral thesis, University of California.

Lee, T.H.T. and Law, A. (2001) Epistemic modality and the acquisition of Cantonese final particles. In M. Nakayama (ed.) *Issues in East Asian Language Acquisition* (pp. 67–128). Tokyo: Kurosio Publishers.

Lee, T.Y. and Ballard, E. (2011) Working with Mandarin-speaking clients: Linguistic and cultural considerations. *Acquiring Knowledge in Speech, Language and Hearing* 13 (3), 132–140.

Leonard, L.B. (1998) *Children with Specific Language Impairment*. Cambridge, MA: The MIT Press.

Leong, C.K. (1986) What does accessing a morphemic script tell us about reading and reading disorders in an alphabetic script? *Annals of Dyslexia* 36, 82–102.

Leung, C-S. (1992) A study of the utterance particles in Cantonese as spoken in Hong Kong. Unpublished master's thesis, Hong Kong Polytechnic.

Leung, F.K.S. (2002) Behind the high achievement of East Asian students. *Educational Research and Evaluation* 8 (1), 87–108.

Lewis, M.P. (2009) *Ethnologue: Languages of the World* (16th edn). Dallas, TX: SIL International. See http://www.ethnologue.com/ for online version.

Li, J.P.W., Law, T., Lam, G.Y.H. and To, C.K.S. (2013) Role of sentence final particles and prosodic cues in irony comprehension in Cantonese-speaking children with and without ASD. *Clinical Linguistics & Phonetics* 27 (1), 18–32.

Li, X.-K., Huang, J.-J. Shi, Q.-S., Mai, Y. and Chen, D.-F. (1995) *The Study of the Guangzhou Dialect*. Shaoguan: Guangdong Renmin Chubanshe.

Lidz, C.S. (1991) *Practitioner's Guide to Dynamic Assessment*. New York: Guilford Press.

Luke, K.K. (1990) *Utterance Particles in Cantonese Conversation*. Amsterdam/Philadelphia, PA: John Benjamins Publishing Company.

Lynch, E. and Hanson, M. (1998) *Developing Cross-Cultural Competence: A Guide for Working with Young Children and Their Families* (2nd edn). Baltimore, MD: Paul H. Brookes.

Lyons, J. (1977) *Semantics*. Cambridge: Cambridge University Press.

Matthews, S. and Yip, V. (1994) *Cantonese: A Comprehensive Grammar.* London: Routledge.

McBride-Chang, C. and Ho, C.S.-H. (2000) Developmental issues in Chinese children's character acquisition. *Journal of Educational Psychology* 92, 50–55.

Moneta, G.B. (2004) The flow model of intrinsic motivation in Chinese cultural and personal moderators. *Journal of Happiness Studies* 5, 181–217.

Ng, R.S.Y. and Ingram, S.C. (1989) *Chinese Culture in Hong Kong*. Hong Kong: Asia 2000 Ltd.

Peña, E., Iglesias, A. and Lidz, C. (2001) Reducing test bias through dynamic assessment of children's word learning ability. *American Journal of Speech-Language Pathology* 10, 138–154.

Peña, E., Gillam, R., Malek, M., Ruiz-Felter, R., Resendiz, M., Fiestas, C. and Sabel, T. (2006) Dynamic assessment of school-age children's narrative ability: An experimental investigation of classification accuracy. *Journal of Speech, Language, and Hearing Research* 49, 1037–1057.

Rack, J. (1985) Orthographic and phonetic coding in normal and dyslexic readers. *British Journal of Psychology* 76, 325–340.

Shu, H., Anderson, R.C. and Wu, N. (2000) Phonetic awareness: Knowledge of orthography–phonology relationships in the character acquisition of Chinese children. *Journal of Educational Psychology* 92, 56–62.

Shu, H., McBride-Chang, C., Wu, S. and Liu, H. (2006) Understanding Chinese developmental dyslexia: Morphological awareness as a core cognitive construct. *Journal of Educational Psychology* 98, 122–133.

So, D. and Siegel, L.S. (1997) Learning to read Chinese: Semantic, syntactic, phonological and working memory skills in normally achieving and poor Chinese readers. *Reading and Writing: An Interdisciplinary Journal* 9, 1–21.

Stokes, S.F. and So, L.K. (1997) Classifier use by language-disordered and age matched Cantonese-speaking children. *Asia Pacific Journal of Speech, Language and Hearing* 2 (1), 83–101.

Stokes, S.F. and Fletcher, P. (2000) Lexical diversity and productivity in Cantonese-speaking children with specific language impairment. *International Journal of Language and Communication Disorders* 35, 527–541.

Stokes, S.F. and Fletcher, P. (2003) Aspectual forms in Cantonese-speaking children with specific language impairment. *Linguistics* 41, 381–406.

Tai, J. (1994) Chinese classifier systems and human categorization. In M. Chen and O. Tseng (eds) *In Honor of Professor William S-Y. Wang: Interdisciplinary Studies on Language and Language Change* (pp. 479–494). Taiwan: Pyramid Publishing Company.

Tardif, T. (1996) Nouns are not always learned before verbs: Evidence from Mandarin speakers' early vocabularies. *Developmental Psychology* 32, 492–504.

Tardif, T., Shatz, M. and Naigles, L. (1997) Caregiver speech and children's use of nouns versus verbs: A comparison of English, Italian, and Mandarin. *Journal of Child Language* 24 (3), 535–565.

To, C.K.S., Stokes, S., Cheung, H-T. and T'sou, B. (2010) Narrative assessment for Cantonese-speaking children. *Journal of Speech, Language & Hearing Research* 53, 648–669.

To, C.K.S., Woo, E., Cheung, P.S.P., Lam, L.L., Sheh, A. and Wong, A. (in preparation) *Assessing Theory of Mind Skills in Chinese Children.*

van Kleeck, A. (1994) Potential cultural bias in training parents as conversational partners with their children who have delays in language development. *American Journal of Speech-Language Pathology* 3, 67–77.

Wong, V., Hui, L.H.S., Lee, W.C., Leung, L.S.J., Ho, P.K.P., Lau, W.L.C., Fung, C.W. and Chung, B. (2004) A modified screening tool for autism (Checklist for Autism in Toddlers [CHAT-23]) for children. *Pediatrics* 114 (2), 166–175.

Yam, C.K.W. (1999) *Lexical Diversity in Cantonese Speaking Children with Specific Language Impairment.* Hong Kong: The University of Hong Kong.

7 Perspectives on Working with Preschool Children from Panjabi-, Gujarati- and Bengali-Speaking Families

Jane Stokes and Nita Madhani

This chapter presents a framework for speech-language pathology practice with multilingual populations, giving specific information about the linguistic communities in East London with which the authors are familiar: Panjabi, Gujarati and Bengali. Cultural and linguistic considerations are introduced and an approach to assessment that entails the building of a child's profile is described and exemplified by a case study. Intervention options are also considered.

The focus of this chapter is the preschool population, which, in the UK, tends to mean 0–5 years of age where the statutory school age is 5 years old. Many children in London now attend preschool education programs where they are introduced to English as the main, and mostly only language used. More than 40% of schoolchildren in London speak English as a second language (L2). In Tower Hamlets, one of the boroughs in East London, almost 75% of schoolchildren speak English as an L2. In London's schools, 233 languages are spoken, with Bengali, Urdu and Somali currently the most widely spoken after English. Panjabi, Gujarati, Arabic, Turkish, Tamil, Yoruba and French are also in the top 10, and European languages are also common, with Polish and Russian being increasingly widely spoken (Eversley *et al.*, 2010).

A Broad Framework for Practice

The chapter includes observations and recommendations for practice that draw on a more sociocultural than purely linguistic foundation (Martin & Stokes, 2009). The authors have been influenced by approaches to the provision of speech and language therapy which

- focus less on the expert model and more on partnership, working with families in supporting the child's development and learning (Pappas & McLeod, 2008); and
- involve less emphasis on the diagnosis of a medical or quasi-medical condition and more on shared coproduction, with the family, of meanings and practices related to living with communication difficulties in the context of a culturally and linguistically diverse environment (Cruz-Ferreira, 2012; Martin, 2009).

Specific Focus on Three Languages

This section describes the three languages most commonly used in East London, namely Panjabi, Gujarati and Bengali (Sylheti variety). Key features of these languages are provided in order to support the practicing speech and language therapist when finding out about the home language of the family. In this way, we hope to make the therapist aware of aspects of syntax and vocabulary that may be relevant in the early stages of the intervention process. The information presented will allow the therapist to make some initial analysis based on his or her observations and will allow for some comparison of the language observed with what is known about the structure and features of the language. We also present some basic information about the early language development of Panjabi, Gujarati and Bengali (Sylheti) based on the work we have done with communities in East London. For speech and language therapists working with these language communities, information such as this will be useful in analyzing language samples, interpreting the stages of development observed and planning activities appropriate to the different language features.

We recognize that many speech and language therapists may read chapters such as this, as a source of factual information, facts about particular cultures which may be applied to all families from that culture. We would caution against this approach, which has inherent dangers of the speech and language therapist adopting a 'cookbook' attitude to the area of cultural and linguistic diversity. The information provided here should be seen as a starting point for talking with families about their unique circumstances. Hand (2011) as cited in Fourie (2011) says that

> Speech-language therapists are experts in communication. However, this does not mean they are necessarily any better than other groups in cross-cultural communication. When professionals get serious about working with diversity, it is easier to deal with facts than it is to deal with discourses, or interactions. However, there may be great value for us in looking at discourse, and the analysis of our professional

discourses, for the insights and the recommendations they may provide. (Hand, 2011; as cited in Fourie, 2011: 82)

Cruz-Ferreira (2012: 19) discusses the 'fundamental inadequacy of descriptive accounts of single languages to approach multilingualism...the issue concerns the uses that children make (or not) of their overall linguistic resources'. She calls on 'adults working with multilingual children...to raise awareness of sociolinguistic and cultural variability and to exercise analytical flexibility' (Cruz-Ferreira, 2012: 20). We would echo this call, and ask the reader to do so too, when reviewing what are described below as features of the different languages. We introduce practicing speech and language therapists to some key features to be aware of and offer guiding principles in approaching linguistic assessment. If one wants to really understand the nature of a language, there is no substitute for learning that language, and native speakers of a language are the best guides. We strongly encourage speech and language therapists working in linguistically diverse communities to explore and understand the origins, structure and use of the languages encountered. This will stimulate reflective practice and deepen understanding of the linguistic structures of different languages as well as support the assessment and information-gathering process.

While there are considerable similarities across Panjabi, Gujarati and Bengali, there are some differences. We concentrate less on the detailed syntactic distinctions between them and more on the features that the languages share. Within each of these language communities, there will be language variations, dialects and regional varieties. As with all languages, colloquialisms prevail in different generations. The linguistic influences engendered by migration patterns and living among other language speakers must be considered in any description of the language. Each of these language communities has a rich and diverse culture in the UK while maintaining strong links with India, Pakistan and Bangladesh, and East Africa.

General information about the communities

Speakers of Panjabi, Gujarati and Bengali are of North Indian heritage. Significant numbers in the Gujarati and smaller numbers in the Panjabi communities are from families who emigrated from northern India to East Africa in the 20th century, and from there to the UK beginning in the 1950s and onward.

Many Panjabi speakers have family origins in northwest Pakistan – Mirpur and Azad Kashmir. Pakistani men came to the UK in the 1950s to work in the cotton industry and settled in the UK with wives and families. There are two distinct groups of Panjabi speakers. When working with a family, it is important to ascertain which group they belong to and the beliefs they may hold. Those from Mirpur and Azad Kashmir generally follow Islam and speak Mirpuri and Urdu. Their written language is Urdu (Arabic script). There are also Panjabi speakers from Punjab in India and these families speak, read and write Panjabi and mostly follow Sikhism. Panjabi is written in Gurmukhi script, an alphabetic script which originates from Devanagari script, with a characteristic horizontal bar from which letters are suspended. It is used primarily in the northern Indian state of Punjab where it is also the official script.

Bengali is the national language of Bangladesh and of West Bengal, the part of India that borders Bangladesh. Sylheti is the regional variety spoken by people from the Sylhet region of Bangladesh. People from the Sylhet region comprise the majority of Bangladeshi emigrants, and large numbers settled in East London from the 1950s onward (Kershen, 2005). Sylheti shares many of the words of standard Bengali, but there are considerable differences in morphosyntax (e.g. in word endings), lexicon and phonology. Whether standard Bengali and Sylheti are mutually intelligible is a question that provokes a variable response. Sylheti speakers can generally understand standard Bengali, but Bengali speakers unfamiliar with Sylheti may find difficulty in understanding it. The alphabetic script used for Bengali is characterized by a horizontal line from which the letters hang and vowels are indicated by the use of diacritics attached to the consonants.

Gujarati is the main language spoken in the state of Gujarat in Western India. Over the last 150 years, significant numbers of Gujarati people left India for East Africa and other countries around the world. The largest expatriate Gujarati populations are in the United States, Canada and the UK. The majority of Gujarati speakers are Hindus or Jains, with smaller numbers practicing different faiths like Islam and Zoroastrianism. Gujarati script is also a version of Devanagari script, an alphabetic script, written like other North Indian languages from left to right but without the horizontal line.

Characteristics of the Panjabi, Gujarati and Bengali languages

These languages are classified as Indo-Aryan, from the Indo-European group of languages, and originate from Sanskrit. They differ from the Dravidian group of languages spoken in southern India.

Features of the three languages are presented in Table 7.1 and are contrasted with English to help the therapist develop a framework for language analysis and to structure the questions that can be asked of the family in gathering further information about the range of syntactic structures used by the child. More detailed texts and websites can be referred to, but we provide some of the salient information relating to basic grammatical features and the early stages of language development.

Table 7.1 Grammatical features of Panjabi, Gujarati and Bengali

Grammatical aspects	Panjabi	Gujarati	Bengali	Contrast with English
Word order	SOV	SOV	SOV	SVO
Gender	M/F	M/F/N	Not a feature	Only marked in pronouns
Case markers	On noun endings	On noun endings	Not a feature	Not a feature
Plurals	Marked and requires gender agreement	Marked and requires gender agreement	Marked but no gender agreement required	Plurals marked but not gender
Questions	Question signaled by particle or intonation	Question signaled by particle or intonation	Question signaled by particle or intonation	Question often requires change in word order and insertion of auxiliary 'do'/'does'
Negatives	Negative signaled by particle before verb	Negative signaled by particle before verb	Negative signaled by particle after verb	Negative often requires change in word order and insertion of auxiliary 'does'
Adjectives	Requires agreement for gender and number	Requires agreement for gender and number	Requires agreement for number	No agreement required
Pronouns	Third-person pronoun has no gender distinction	Third-person pronoun has no gender distinction	Third-person pronoun has no gender distinction	For third-person distinction made between male, female neutral gender
Time, manner, place	Expressed by suffix or postposition	Expressed by suffix or postposition	Expressed by suffix or postposition	Expressed by prepositions

Grammatical features

The word order is subject-object-verb (SOV; in contrast to the English word order subject-verb-object [SVO]). If adjectives are present, they precede the noun. The subject of a sentence can often be inferred from the word ending on the verb and is often omitted.

Verbs are expressed by a verb root and word endings to mark aspect and agreement. Postpositions, similar in meaning to prepositions in English, follow the noun rather than precede it. In English, we say 'the ball in the box', whereas in North Indian languages the order of constituents literally translated is 'the ball the box in'. Location also may be expressed by a suffix rather than by a postposition. When saying 'to the hotel' in Bengali (Sylheti) the 'to' can be expressed as an '-o' ending on the word 'hotel' to make 'hotelo'. Gender is expressed in Gujarati (male, female and neuter) and Panjabi (male and female), but gender is not expressed in Bengali. Plural markers are not mandatory in all contexts. In most cases, definite or indefinite articles are not used, and determiners are not obligatory, although words to indicate number are included. Questions do not require altered word order, but are indicated either by intonation alone, or by the insertion of a question particle or question word.

Language development

There is very limited research on the stages of language development in these languages. Based on the work that was done in East London in the 1980s by the authors on Panjabi (Madhani as cited in Duncan, 1989) and Bengali (Sylheti) (Stokes as cited in Duncan, 1989; Stokes as cited in Ball *et al.* 2012), we can say that:

- One-word utterances are followed by two-word utterances, and so on, but in view of the differences in morphology, it is possible for a seven-word utterance in English to be translated by a two-word utterance in a North Indian language. For example, 'I don't want to eat any rice' can be translated into Bengali (Sylheti) by just two words *'baat khaina'*. This translates literally as 'rice (*baat*) I will not eat (*khaina*)' where the negative is expressed by the ending *'na'* and 'I will' is expressed by the form of the verb *'khai'*.
- Negatives appear earlier than in English, as the structure is simpler with a negative particle being added to the statement.
- Questions can be formed earlier, again as the structure is simpler, with the insertion of a question particle.
- Kinship terms are more developed than in English with specific words for, for example, maternal uncle and paternal grandfather, and these vocabulary items are learned early.

- Many English nouns appear in the vocabulary of children brought up in London which may be pronounced differently or given inflections corresponding to the speaker's first language (L1).

Although there is a need for further research, knowledge of these features of language development will influence the practice of speech and language therapists in various ways. For example, the question 'How many words does the child put together?' will not be useful when, as in the example above, a seven-word sentence in English can be translated by two words in Bengali (Sylheti). Similarly, children may have more adult-like negative and question forms in North Indian languages earlier than in English. In addition, assessment of the vocabulary used by a child who speaks more than one language should consider the child's total lexicon.

Bilingualism

In working in contexts where a child is being brought up bilingually, it is essential for the speech and language therapist to explore the nature of that bilingualism. Some children may be exposed to two or more languages from birth, whereas others' first encounter with English occurs when they start preschool or school. The pattern of language use must be taken into consideration along with the attitudes toward bilingualism within the family.

Bilingualism must be seen as one of the variables alongside other variables such as gender, social class, learning ability and medical and family history. The language environment of the child and the relative exposure of the different languages involved will all be relevant in building a picture of the child. These all contribute to the uniqueness of the child involved.

A number of misconceptions are prevalent about the possible deleterious effect of bilingualism and these need to be countered with reference to the abundance of literature that confirms the potentially positive influence of bilingualism on cognitive development (e.g. Baker, 1995; Engel de Abreu et al., 2012). Speech and language therapists should be aware of their role in potentially discussing issues of language choice with respect to maintaining the L1 and considering parental expectations. It is essential for the therapist to be aware of family language choices and to be prepared to discuss these openly and with consideration for each family's unique set of circumstances. Language choices may change through the life of the child, and be affected by the child's different environments. The therapist must be prepared to provide parents with information based on sound research and may well encounter anxieties about whether a child with communication difficulties may be disadvantaged by being exposed to two languages. Baker (1995), De Houwer (2009) and Genesee et al. (2004) are useful sources for more detailed discussion of these arguments. See also Chapters 2 and 3, this book.

The therapist may need to consider the role played by code-switching. Miccio *et al.* (2009) define code-switching as alternations between languages that conform to the grammatical principles of the languages in question. Code-switching may be inter-sentential, occurring between sentences, or intra-sentential, occurring within a single sentence.

An example of inter-sentential code-switching in Panjabi would be if the child changed languages from one sentence to the next:

'*Usi roti khai* (we ate dinner). Then we played football'.

An example of intra-sentential code-switching would be if the child, when asked in Panjabi 'what did the boy do?', replies:

'*Mundene pen bag wich pai*' (literally translates as 'boy pen bag in' = the boy put the pen in the bag).

Here we see the child using English vocabulary within the sentence and Panjabi word order and a postposition marker to express 'in'.

Pert and Letts (2006) found that code-switching was established in the community of Mirpuri English speakers in Rochdale, UK, by the age of three and a half. Code-switching should not be seen as a deficit form of language or a sign of language disorder (Martin, 2009). It should not be seen as indicating linguistic confusion. Code-switching does not occur at random but rather requires the speaker to have an ability to apply grammatical and pragmatic rules to his or her use of language. Indeed, it is evident that in order to code-switch the child needs to have an understanding of pragmatics and syntax. As in the above example, the bilingual Panjabi–English child may use the word order of Panjabi and one or more vocabulary items from another language. Miccio *et al.* (2009: 252) state that code-switching is a sign of 'proficiency in two languages and should not be considered deviant or be discouraged as a form of self-expression'.

An important point to note here is that spoken English is constantly undergoing changes and adaptations in response to the influence of its minority languages. The language of multiracial adolescents in a British working-class community is described vividly in Rampton (1995), where he describes the mix of Creole, Panjabi and Asian English. The exposure that any child has to the mix of different languages in his or her community will be unique to that child's experience. The development of the language of children growing up in a majority English-speaking society changes all the time in response to the influence of English from the environment and popular television, and the influence of older siblings coming home from school speaking English. In the absence of extensive research on the development of the languages being discussed, it can be challenging for the speech and language therapist to make reference to what can be termed typical behavior. The need for analytical flexibility is key.

Clinical Contexts and Terminology

As diagnostic categories differ across languages and cultures, we provide a brief overview of the terms currently used with preschool clinical populations referred to speech and language therapy services in the UK. Terminology is shaped by research and clinical experience and terms used by speech and language therapists shift over time and in different contexts (Speech Pathology Association of Australia, 2008). Speech and language therapists have frequent cause to question their own and others' diagnostic criteria, resulting in a complex process of diagnosis and classification with children from families where more than one language is spoken.

In spite of these challenges, diagnostic classification categories may be necessary for some aspects of clinical practices. A diagnosis may provide access to resources in some situations or the therapist may be seeking a diagnosis in order to decide on the appropriate *care pathway*. In the UK, this term is commonly used as part of a methodology for the mutual decision-making and organization of care for a well-defined group of people during a well-defined period (definition adapted from the European Pathway Association; www.e-p-a.org). Many speech and language therapy services have developed care pathways, taking into account the evidence base and best practice guidelines. The allocation of a child to a care pathway leads to decisions about how often the child is to be seen, by whom, where and for what length of time. There has been limited application of care pathway methodology to children who speak languages additional to English, and the monolingual is often seen as the typical client.

A brief overview of the definitions as used currently by the authors is presented below, with discussion of considerations that should be taken into account when applying the terms to multilingual populations.

Developmental language delay: the term is used to describe a child who is developing language along typical lines, but more slowly than other children of the same age. These children are also referred to as 'late talkers' and constitute a significant number of children referred to speech and language therapy.

Developmental language disorder: this describes a child whose language is not developing typically. Key features of this language profile are weaknesses in grammar and range of vocabulary. Many clinicians use developmental language disorder interchangeably with the term *specific language impairment* (SLI). The definition excludes children with language delays due to intellectual impairment, physical disability, hearing loss, emotional problems or environmental deprivation. It is used for children whose difficulties are with language only or with speech and language only (Tomblin, 2011).

Autism spectrum disorders: this is the term commonly used to cover the whole range of conditions that have in common the triad of impairment of social interaction, social communication and social imagination (http://www.autism.org.uk).

Speech sound disorders, encompassing phonological delay and disorder: again, the terminology is used inconsistently by those in practice, and researchers continue to debate the different classification systems. According to Bowen (http://speech-language-therapy.com), 'Speech sound disorder (SSD) involves difficulty with and/or slowness in the development of a child's speech. The term "speech sound disorder(s)" is an umbrella heading under which there are several sub-categories that include articulation disorder, phonological disorder and childhood apraxia of speech. Speech sound disorder is sometimes called "speech impairment" or "speech difficulties"'.

When applying these terms to children from families where more than one language is used, there are significant challenges. The absence of a clear and shared understanding of what these terms mean when describing a bilingual/multilingual individual results in the situation where clinicians make assumptions and come to clinical decisions which should be, but are often not, critically analyzed. For example, as we have seen earlier, North Indian languages do not mark the third-person pronoun for gender, so no distinction is made between 'he' and 'she'. A child in a preschool setting may present at an early stage of learning English, and may only use the pronoun 'he' for all third-person references. This might be seen as an indication of disordered language development. Similarly, the inconsistent use or omission of the definite article 'the' is a feature of many L2 English speakers. Remediating these kinds of features would not be of therapeutic value. They would more properly be viewed as an English teaching target than a speech and language therapy target.

Service Delivery Issues

In a large majority of cases, both in the UK and in the United States, a challenge that speech and language therapists report is that of being a monolingual dealing with a child from a different language background to their own (Stokes, 2000). There is extensive research on English language acquisition, and there are countless standardized and non-standardized assessments for monolingual English-speaking children. By contrast, there is a paucity of information available to English-speaking speech and language therapists when faced with understanding and interpreting data gathered from children speaking languages other than English. Monolingual speech and language therapists in the UK, working with bilingual or multilingual communities, report feelings of fear, inadequacy, anxiety, loss of control, lack of knowledge and confusion (Stokes, 2000). Many report that they have not been prepared for this kind of work by their pre-registration education. Monolingual English-speaking speech and language therapists will be required to take an eclectic and pragmatic approach to assessing a child from a different language background to their own. When assessing children from different linguistic and cultural backgrounds, the speech and language therapist needs to take a holistic view, and should consider not only developmental features but also sociocultural and linguistic factors.

Team working

Faced with unfamiliar languages, speech and language therapists can support each other in teams by collaborating, mentoring, using video and observing experienced therapists. Teams working regularly in bilingual communities should ensure that there is appropriate supervision, training and study time to give staff the confidence and skills to engage with families with whom they do not share the language. As specialists in communication, speech and language therapists are well positioned to make close and accurate observations, even when they do not understand the language, of a child's non-verbal behavior and understanding. A child's communication is by no means solely dependent on knowledge of the syntax and vocabulary of a language.

In some services, the responsibility for working with bilingual or potentially bilingual clients has been allocated to a specialist. While there is benefit in this approach, there is a danger that knowledge of cultural and linguistic diversity is viewed as a specialist subsection of service delivery. Knowledge of cultural and linguistic diversity should be integral to professional practice for all practitioners. Working as a team, staff should engage in jointly writing policies to support the provision of equitable services. On a profession-wide level, the regulatory and professional bodies provide direction in the form of guidelines and best practice information (see RCSLT, 2007).

Resources

Team leaders can encourage the collection of relevant information on languages and on cultural practices. If the team has a commitment to an equitable approach, it would be appropriate for them to develop a bank of resources that could support the therapists, about the different community languages spoken in the area in which the service is based. The London Special Interest Group on Bilingualism, a group of speech and language therapists with particular experience of working with bilingual families, has created a series of language guides, available online at www. londonsigbilingualism.co.uk. In addition, there needs to be a recognition that working with languages and cultures that are not familiar to the therapist requires more time and additional resources.

Access to local bilingual personnel

There are different models of accessing bilingual support, ranging from the creation of posts of bilingual coworkers – trained by the speech and language therapy team – bilingual interpreters employed across a local geographical area and bilingual assistants available in different childcare and educational settings. It is important to note that working with interpreters is a skill to be developed. Barnett as cited in Duncan (1989) discusses the value and efficiencies of working with bilingual personnel. The skills involved in interpreting specialist areas such as communication disorders are considerable, and it is our view that establishing good relationships with the available interpreting services is crucial in communities where there are large numbers of families speaking languages other than, or additional to, English.

The importance of making such connections with the language communities where one works is illustrated by the following example. In one of the author's experience, a close working relationship was set up between the speech and language therapy clinic and a local Vietnamese mother and toddler group. This facilitated work with Vietnamese-speaking children referred to speech and language therapy and resulted in the development of a locally produced language support resource co-created by the community organization and the speech and language therapy team. It is in the interest of the team to seek out key contacts in order to ensure that the service provided is fair and accessible. This may require developing relationships over a number of years.

Cultural and Social Factors

A sociocultural perspective broadens our understanding of disabilities. For example, Ochs et al. (2004) have looked at autism from an anthropological perspective, articulating a sociocultural approach to autism. They underline the importance of viewing people with autism not only as individuals in relation to other individuals but also as members of social communities. They advocate that understanding autism can be enhanced through adopting anthropological concepts. Considering the broader social community also will aid the therapist in understanding how best to support the family and the wider community in addressing the needs of the child.

The values and beliefs held by the family will be important influences in the way that disability is construed. Jegatheesan *et al.* (2010) found that parents with religious beliefs drew on their faith to help them make sense of and construct meanings around disability. Families may have different values and religious beliefs to that of the therapist, and this may require varied approaches in order to develop shared respect and understanding. People will not tend to act on advice and suggestions given without respect to the belief systems they hold. Other family beliefs also may affect intervention. For example, Stow *et al.* (2012: 27) state that 'parents may fail to engage in therapy activities, as they perceive the child's difficulties to have a medical basis and would prefer an overtly medical solution'.

Cultural differences in interaction patterns must also be considered. Stow *et al.* (2012: 26) make the point that 'assessment and therapy is a formal form of adult-child interaction developed within a western context'. For example, within different cultural groups, it may not be expected that children initiate communication with adults and non-verbal responses may have different cultural connotations. An understanding of interaction patterns from a sociocultural perspective will inform clinical activities and facilitate the engagement of the family in the process of assessment and the provision of therapy.

Assessment

We have now set the context for the North Indian languages most commonly found in inner cities in the UK and discussed the challenges facing teams working with diverse populations. With this context, we will now take the reader through our recommendations for approaching assessment, followed by a discussion of intervention considerations. We present an example of using this framework with a two-year-old child from a bilingual background whose parents/caregivers are concerned about his language ability.

Assessment may serve multiple purposes. For example, discussion with the family and others in the team may indicate that a diagnosis is needed to unlock resources, or the therapist may be seeking a diagnosis in order to decide on the appropriate care pathway. It may be important for the family to find explanations or answers in order to help them support the child. In this chapter, our focus is on assessment for the purpose of identifying the child's current skills.

In our approach, the speech and language therapist constructs a profile of the child's skills, without requiring detailed knowledge of the syntax, semantics and pragmatics of the family's L1. The procedure draws on the skills of the therapist who obtains information about the child's communication in partnership with people who know the child, rather than relying on standardized assessments or developmental checklists of typical communication behaviors. The therapist builds a profile of the child's communication abilities, using a detailed case history and observations, including information about the child's use and understanding of L1 and, where appropriate, the child's L2. Information about the L1 may require the assistance of a trained coworker or interpreter. Colleagues from other disciplines – health, education and social care professionals – may be involved in the development of the profile of the child's communication.

The therapist can use a simple framework, regardless of the language used, for collecting information, drawing on the areas of

- patterns of language use in the family;
- attention and general listening skills;
- play;
- non-verbal communication;
- understanding of language; and
- expressive language.

Parent interview

We turn now to a discussion of parent interviews, a critical foundation for accurate assessment and appropriate intervention decisions in bilingual children. In conducting the parent interview, the speech and language therapist needs to give careful thought to questions relating to the child's language development. Therapists will need to draw on available resources about different languages, such as that provided in Table 7.1, which will help guide the monolingual therapist in devising relevant questions about the child's language development.

As with asking questions about language development, when asking questions about the child's developmental milestones, the therapist needs to proceed cautiously. Experiences of gross and fine motor skill development may vary across cultures and families. Some families may be happy continuing to carry children close to the parent, there may be differing attitudes to the use of baby walkers and differing expectations of toilet training may affect the timeline of diaper use. Different attitudes to weaning or to the introduction of solid food may affect the development of eating and swallowing. Religious customs and personal belief systems may affect the use of hot and cold food, and eating patterns vary across families and cultures.

In all these areas, it is our experience that instead of the therapist feeling that she or he needs to have an encyclopedic knowledge of every culturally influenced behavior, the key to success will be an open mind and a willingness to learn. In getting to know any family, regardless of whether the therapist shares the language or the culture, the therapist is required continually to work on and maintain a non-judgmental, anti-discriminatory approach. While it may be unconventional to be guided by the lyrics of a song, it is the authors' view that the words of the Australian songwriter Shane Howard, made famous by the Irish singer, Mary Black, are relevant, when she sings:

Oh come on walk with me, talk with me
Tell me your stories
I'll do my very best to understand you...

And later

There's a thousand things to do
So let's start here with me and you
Gonna take a little time
Let's see what we can find... ©Shane Howard

For us, this seems to reflect the essential aspects of the taking of a case history; the acknowledgment that it will take time, and that it will entail the telling of stories, and that it is the therapist who will do his or her best to understand. There is also here an explicit statement that the case history starts with 'me' and 'you'; i.e. that in taking the case history the therapist necessarily brings his or her own understandings of children and of this child into the 'space' which is created in the interaction between the parent(s) and the child. The cultural dimension of case history taking is not a one-way street. Unless the therapist is able to recognize that he or she is bringing his or her own culturally informed ideas and opinions to the interaction, the nature of what is discussed will not be honest and open. For example, when asking the routine questions about behavior, the therapist needs to have an awareness of his or her own personal view of, for example, discipline and chastisement in the home.

Building a profile

In the creation of the profile, the speech and language therapist will draw on a range of different methods and tools for collecting information. The parent interview is the primary source of information, but assessments will include observation and recording of non-verbal and verbal communication, possibly in collaboration with an interpreter. Parent interviews will include questions that may not be featured in interviews with monolingual families such as attitudes to bilingualism and other cultural and linguistic considerations.

In building a profile, the therapist invites the parents to describe patterns and behaviors in context, and verifies each point, checking with the parent that he or she has understood what the parent is conveying. This process is facilitated by the therapist but led by the parent's observations and concerns. Information about the child is gathered as part of a shared understanding between the therapist and the parent. In contrast to a more traditional approach of using a standard case history format, the therapist continually monitors his or her impressions, shares his or her questions with the family and others and is ready to revise and review initial hypotheses. This collaborative approach will foster positive rapport and build trust.

During this process, the therapist will need to gather information about the child's patterns of language use, listening and attention, non-verbal communication, play, understanding of language and expressive language. When there is not a shared cultural and linguistic background, it becomes more important for the therapist to contextualize the information gathered. It is essential to relate every aspect of the child's behavior to the family's linguistic and cultural context, including relationships with extended family and participation in cultural activities and festivals. More detailed information on building a profile is presented below with examples relating to a young child from a Gujarati-speaking family, described in Box 7.1.

Box 7.1

Kirit, a boy from a Gujarati-speaking background, was referred to speech and language therapy and seen for initial assessment by an English-speaking speech and language therapist, when he was 2 years and 2 months old. His parents were concerned that he was not 'talking more'. It was reported that he did not respond to his name. The speech and language therapist gathered information through taking a case history during a drop-in session in a children's center environment. The father acted as interpreter, with the mother providing much of the information. The case history revealed that Kirit has no delay in his physical development. The parents report that Kirit does not like to chew any solid food and his mother feeds him when he is distracted, while watching television.

Both parents speak Gujarati to Kirit and to their older daughter who is nearly 4 years old. They say that they use some basic phrases in English like 'come on Kirit' and 'good boy Kirit', but generally they address him in Gujarati. His sister uses mainly Gujarati with him. Kirit's mother reports that he uses some single words – some were in English such as 'daddy' and 'juice', words commonly used in Gujarati families in England, plus words like 'up' and 'down'. Kirit's mother reports that Kirit does not respond verbally or non-verbally to Gujarati instructions like 'get your shoes' or 'show me your hands'. She reports that he uses some Gujarati phrases like 'hurry up'.

Kirit's mother reports that the child can understand some routines. When somebody picks up the remote control for the television, he will climb on the settee and get ready to watch. He is reported to laugh when watching TV.

Kirit's mother reports that he takes no notice of his older sister when she reaches to give him a cuddle. His mother feels Kirit does not notice other children in other settings. She takes Kirit to a mother and toddler drop-in group at the children's center. There are a couple of other children there who speak Gujarati, and Kirit's mother has noticed that they are saying more than Kirit.

Kirit does not look for things or fetch things when requested. When his mother hides his ball and a musical toy in an obvious place in a box under the table, Kirit does not look for them. Kirit does not show frustration or anger and will only cry occasionally. Kirit's mother feels that when he cries there is something wrong, but she can't tell what is wrong and she cannot comfort him.

In the assessment session, Kirit did not respond to his name or look at his mother. He did not look up when the phone rang during the session. He did not identify everyday common objects in response to either his mother's Gujarati requests, or the speech and language therapist's English requests. Kirit's mother and father spoke to him in Gujarati but Kirit did not respond.

During the session, Kirit repeated some words like 'up' when the bilingual speech and language therapy assistant played with a toy model of Superman and made it jump. He appeared to like being chased by Superman (the assistant was holding the toy), which made him smile and laugh. When the assistant put the doll down, Kirit picked it up and gave it to her without looking at her.

At the end of the session, Kirit's parents were given activities to develop his social interaction and to get him to seek things including food rewards and favorite things. The family was encouraged to use their home language, Gujarati, as this is the language his mother is most comfortable with. She reports she sings nursery rhymes and other popular Indian songs and she says that Kirit likes to listen to these.

Three months after the initial assessment and advice session, when he was 2 years and 5 months old, Kirit's parents took him to India. While there, they took him to spiritual healers and medical doctors. Kirit was in the country for 2 months, and exposed solely to Gujarati, which was used by family members exclusively. There were opportunities for him to interact with children and adults across a wide range of ages.

(Continued)

> Kirit was seen in the clinic again when he was 2 years and 9 months old. By this time, he had had a full developmental check, including vision and hearing, which were found to be normal. On this occasion, Kirit was tolerant of parallel play but did not respond to his name. Kirit did not follow instructions from his mother in Gujarati, or from the speech and language therapist in English. At this second appointment, Kirit's mother reported other areas of concern including irregular sleep patterns.
>
> He explored objects and showed some interest in cause-and-effect toys, and in bubbles and tactile play (sand and water). He showed a preference for smooth metal things like a spoon and a key but did not use them functionally. He was seen to mouth these objects and explored objects by touching them with his lips. There was no evidence of him using symbolic or representational play in relation to himself or others using familiar, culturally appropriate objects like a comb, a spoon, a key or a car.

Pattern of language use

The therapist will need to ask questions and make observations about the pattern of language use in the home and outside the home. Here, the therapist can ask the broad question 'who speaks what language to whom', which can then be followed up with more detailed questions and observations about the relative amounts of exposure to the different languages. It is important to describe the child as potentially bilingual although at any particular time, it is not necessarily accurate to describe a child as bilingual.

In Kirit's case, exposure to English at the time of initial assessment was very limited; however, as he lived in England and was due to attend school in London, the child has the potential to be bilingual. For Kirit, his L1 is Gujarati and his L2 is English. At home, the mother speaks Gujarati to Kirit, and the parents speak Gujarati to each other. Kirit's father generally speaks Gujarati to the children at home, as the parents are keen for their children to learn their home language. Some English words are used at home, and the older daughter is now being formally exposed to English through attendance at preschool. Kirit's sister usually speaks in Gujarati at home; however, with increasing exposure to English, she is likely to bring more English back into the home. It is a commonly observed pattern that once children have started at school, they may understand the home language but respond in English when addressed in their L1. When Kirit is at the mother–toddler group, Kirit's mother uses English with other parents and with the group leader, and Kirit hears English in the formal parts of the morning where drinks are given out, and when instructions are given.

The family used Gujarati exclusively during their trip to India, where the children heard a wide range of different relatives and friends using their home language in all contexts.

Attention and general listening skills

Assessment of the child's attention and listening skills includes looking at the ability to listen and respond to familiar everyday sounds, associating, for example, the noise of a tap running with bath time or the call of the muezzin on the radio to prayer time. The child's ability to engage with an adult, switching attention from his or her choice of activity to the adult's choice of activity will be relevant in any assessment of communication. The child may have greater difficulties in listening to an unfamiliar language. There may be other cultural variations related to child-rearing and family routines that may impact on the child's attention and listening abilities. The therapist will need to take into consideration, for example, whether shared reading and joint play with adults or older siblings form part of a family's regular activity. When assessing attention and listening, it is important to ask about family expectations. In some families, a nickname may be more commonly used than the official name used in the referral, and the therapist must be aware of this to avoid making premature judgments about the ability of the child to respond. If the child is known by a different name at home, his or her lack of response in the clinic may not indicate a difficulty in listening or understanding, just an inappropriate use of the name less familiar to the child.

According to Kirit's mother, he engages for extended periods of time with an activity of his choice such as water play or bubbles. When a new activity is introduced, Kirit needs visual cueing and reduced stimulation if he is to attend. His mother reported that Kirit does not respond to his name and, unlike his sister, Kirit does not look up or run to the front door when the doorbell rings. Kirit has shown interest in rhythm and does like simple jingles and rhymes. His mother reported that he listens when the prayer tape cassette is playing, as it is repetitive chant.

Non-verbal communication skills

Therapists are advised to be cautious in the process of untangling clinical observation and cultural stereotype. This can be illustrated by the example of eye contact, which is variable across different cultures and situations. Reduced eye contact, as evidence of a social communication difficulty, needs to be distinguished from the deferential uses of eye contact typical in some cultures when children are talking to adults. This will require experience, and discussion with the families involved. The input of trained bilingual staff from the same linguistic and cultural community as the family can help develop the therapist's understanding of the cultural context of these complex non-verbal behaviors. Therapists should guard against attributing limited eye contact either to cultural variation or to social communication difficulties without exploring this in more depth with the family and with colleagues within and outside their profession.

In spite of cultural differences in specific behaviors such as eye contact, children from all cultures present broadly similar behaviors in relation to seeking comfort, signaling distress, signaling hunger – initially through crying, vocalizing and gesturing, and then verbalizing. In Kirit's case, this developmental progression is missing. His mother cannot identify the reason for him crying and cannot comfort him. Kirit indicates some needs non-verbally by pulling his mother's clothing, and he has been observed to take an adult's hand to help him access activities that motivate him. For example, he takes an adult's hand to a water tap as he enjoys playing with water. Kirit does not use eye contact as expected by his family and he does not vocalize consistently to communicate his need or intention. In his case, lack of eye contact should be seen as part of his overall delays in communication behaviors.

Language understanding

In the UK, speech and language therapists have been using terms influenced by the Derbyshire Language Scheme (Knowles & Masidlover, 1982), which describes a child's level of understanding of language in terms of the number of information-carrying words level. There are benefits to this approach, but the therapist needs to be aware that it can be difficult to translate this way of describing comprehension from English into other languages. As discussed earlier, North Indian languages may express meanings through word endings rather than through separate words, so the assumption that an instruction such as 'put the shoes under the chair' will be translated into Gujarati using the same number of words is misguided.

Together with parent interviews and through observation, the therapist can explore the child's ability to understand by asking questions about the child's responses to simple instructions in everyday routines. The therapist can ask about the child's understanding of the functions of objects, everyday verbs and who, what, why questions.

More in-depth assessment of the child's understanding of language will require collaboration with a trained interpreter experienced in working with speech and language therapists. Working with an L1 speaker to assess a child's language will help the therapist understand more about the structure of that language. Literal translations of instructions or assessment questions may be inappropriate particularly in longer, more complex instructions. For example, the passive sentence in English 'the boy was chased by the dog' cannot be literally translated in Panjabi. The interpreter would need to convert it to an active sentence. He or she can point out to the therapist that it is not possible to make a passive sentence and this is not an appropriate focus for investigation.

With regard to vocabulary or language use, a skilled interpreter will be able to adapt the translations required by the therapist, bearing in mind what is typically used in the local community. There may be vocabulary items that are never used in the child's home language but only in English. For example, although the word 'kitchen' can be translated into Gujarati, many families in the UK would use the English form. The influence of Kirit's sister, coming back from an English-speaking school environment, may affect the vocabulary used, as for example a word such as 'rucksack' may only be used in English to describe the bag which she takes to school.

The assessment of understanding of a bilingual child's L1 will be similar to the assessment of a monolingual English-speaking child with the therapist asking the same kinds of questions about his or her ability to follow simple instructions or to point to objects on request. In Kirit's case, the therapist has obtained useful information about his ability to understand some familiar routines in context, and his difficulty in following instructions in Gujarati. Kirit does not follow instructions or single-word commands in Gujarati consistently. When asked to point to objects within close reach, he is sometimes able to point to them, but at other times he does not show any interest. He can pick up an item when he has a visual cue such as pointing, or when he is shown a matching item.

Expressive language

The speech and language therapist makes a record, in collaboration with the parents, of the actual words, phrases and sentences used by the child. In responding to questions or requests for vocabulary items, the child's correct response should be accepted in either language as it demonstrates understanding of the concept. The assistance of a bilingual colleague will be invaluable in recording either orthographically or phonetically what the child is saying and in what situations. The therapist can refer to Table 7.1 to structure the analysis of what the child says. The therapist should take into account the fact that just counting the number of words used by a child in a sentence may not give an accurate picture of the stage of language development. As we have seen earlier, a seven-word utterance in English can be expressed as a two-word utterance in Bengali, so the therapist should be cautious of using number of words as a measure. Discussion should then ensue with the parents about whether the language demonstrated by the child is commensurate with their expectations, and how it compares with the language of other children in the family or in their social circle. The accurate recording of language is something that the therapist can work on together with the family and bilingual colleagues, where available. For example, the family can use a mobile phone to record a clip of the child communicating at home. The clip can then be analyzed together with the parents and a bilingual colleague to examine the range of words used, the vocabulary items and the meanings attached to these. It can form a useful joint project that will both develop the family's awareness of their child's communication strengths and weaknesses and contribute to useful data for the child.

Kirit's mother reported that he uses a few meaningful single words related to activities which he finds motivating. He will say 'bubbles' in English as he enjoys this activity and will use the word as a request at home. He also says *'pani'* in Gujarati, meaning 'water', which he uses when he is playing with water, but not as a request for water. He uses jargon words which are not understandable to Gujarati or English speakers. Kirit repeats words that he has heard previously but uses these without attaching meaning and out of context. The speech and language therapist has heard some vocalizations directed toward an adult but these are not consistent in form or use.

Play

Similar detailed observation and recording of play preferences should be made. With an awareness of the culturally specific nature of play, the therapist should explore the different play experiences encountered in the family and the different attitudes to supporting play. The therapist is advised to explore together with the parents their feelings about the nature of their child's play experiences. It has proved useful to ask the family a broad question such as 'In what way is your child's experience of play different from your own when you were growing up?'. This has led to opportunities for the therapist to understand more fully the expectations of the parents, and a context to discuss play and its importance for language development. With this shared information, the therapist can be guided by the parents on the choice of play activities which will resonate best with the family's customs and culture.

In Kirit's case, it has been observed that he likes exploring toys by touching and mouthing them. He will engage with simple cause-and-effect toys that offer immediate gratification. He has shown some functional use of everyday objects – he placed a toy mobile phone next to his ear momentarily.

During the assessment process, a picture of the child's profile of communication strengths and needs emerges based on information from interviews and observations designed to address the six areas of assessment: pattern of language use, attention and listening, non-verbal communication skills, understanding, expressive language and play. By listening carefully to the information provided by the family, much useful information is available in the absence of more formal standardized testing procedures.

This information will guide the therapist in making intervention decisions, in collaboration with the family and with the support of bilingual personnel if available.

Intervention Considerations

In line with our commitment to collaboration with the family, a family-centered approach is advocated in this case. There will be better engagement with families when their views about the important aspects of their child's development are integrated into the intervention plan. It is also important to explain the different possible interventions available and develop a relationship of trust and mutual support in the decision-making surrounding the child. In order to discuss intervention options with the family, the therapist may need to consider the use of an interpreter, a bilingual coworker or an advocate. For example, Kirit's father speaks English but his mother, having come to the UK as an adult, may find it helpful to have access to an independent person who shares her language. This will aid her ability to express herself to the therapist.

The ways in which information is imparted to the family need serious consideration. It may not be appropriate to simply translate existing leaflets or reports into the family's home language, without finding out if this is a helpful method of providing information on, for example, communication disorders, or advice on playing with their child. If service providers ask families how they would like to be given information and kept up to date with current therapy approaches, the answers will inform the style of information exchange. Translation of documents may seem to be an effective way of sharing information but should be approached with caution, taking into account the literacy levels of the communities involved, the competence of the translators and the effectiveness of this method of communication. For example, the demonstration of therapy techniques is likely to be more effective than the distribution of translated written activity sheets.

In Kirit's case, the family was happy to be given advice leaflets written in English on supporting their child's language, as long as their content was fully discussed and examples modeled in Gujarati. The leaflet referred to the importance of supporting children through simple use of language, and identifying and using visual cues and key motivators to form part of their daily routine. The family then made notes as to how they would be implementing the advice with key words in the English leaflet being written in Gujarati by the interpreter, in discussion with the speech and language therapist.

In discussing intervention strategies, the speech and language therapist will play a key role in:

- providing evidence-based information on the phenomenon of bilingualism and how this will impact on the child's language development; and
- supporting the family in making informed decisions about language choices.

The speech and language therapist needs to be aware and informed about the overall benefits and importance of promoting bilingualism to all parents, especially when parents are doubting themselves. This can be done by supporting the parents and acknowledging the importance of their culture and language, as well as sharing with the family the results of research which shows that bilingualism confers cognitive and social advantages. There is no evidence to support the widely held belief that if families use more than one language this will cause confusion for the child with communication difficulties (Guiberson, 2013). Well-meaning advice from health and education professionals is sometimes given to parents that they should concentrate just on one language, and it is important for the speech and language therapist to be able to counter this.

In designing intervention for bilingual children, one of the key considerations is the language(s) of intervention. There is limited research on the efficacy of interventions with bilingual children, but there is some evidence for the view that interventions that focus on both languages are superior to those that focus on one (Elin Thordardottir, 2010). Recommendations about language use must be informed by the individual situation of different families. For children from bilingual homes, both languages will need supporting. For children who encounter English as an L2 at school, it will be important to also support their L1 through therapy activities. Where the family is committed to bringing up their child bilingually and continuing to expose the child to the culture of their L1, then it is the role of the speech and language therapist to support this. In the case of Kirit, the speech and language therapist supported both Gujarati and English in intervention. The therapist had access to a Gujarati-speaking assistant, but if she had not been available the therapist might have been able to find useful colleagues among the local Gujarati community organizations, schools and social networks.

The therapist needs to discuss with the parents what their preferences are for the languages used at home, in the clinical situation and in the preschool settings. The role of siblings in supporting the child's language development should also be taken into account in discussions and decisions about the language(s) of intervention. There is clinical evidence that older children spend more time interacting with their siblings than parents do (Stow et al., 2012). This is the pattern of language use particular to Kirit where his sister uses English when interacting with him.

The therapist needs to help the parents make informed choices not only about verbal language and about bilingualism, but also, as in Kirit's case, about using alternative communication systems across two languages and cultures. Sensitive and well-managed dialogue with parents will maintain ongoing commitment from the parents and establish their trust in the speech and language therapist to maximize the communication and language potential of their child. The reader is advised to consult the information provided by the London SIG in bilingualism on their website www.londonsigbilingualism.co.uk for further advice for parents.

In addition to providing information on bilingualism and supporting the parents' language choices, intervention strategies should also be consistent with the family's cultural beliefs, values and practices. In the case of Kirit, the behaviors of the child in relation to faith-based activities, such as prayer, and the influence of belief systems on the family's approach to having a child with a disability can be usefully examined from a sociocultural perspective. This will aid the therapist in understanding how best to support the family and the wider community in addressing the needs of the child. It will be important to respect the family's preferences for intervention which may include the involvement of religious practices and the inclusion of religious belief systems about disability.

Intervention and assessment are continuous and evolving processes and the therapist will need to respond to the situations that develop during the course of getting to know the family. When one of the authors was working with a Bengali family who had just returned from Bangladesh after a six-month stay, the father described a sorting game that the children had enjoyed, using pebbles and feathers. This then led to the therapist using pebbles and feathers brought by the family in developing the child's pattern recognition, as well as vocabulary relating to size, color and texture. The father related better to this activity than to the use of plastic figures in the clinic setting and the nature of the interaction between parent and child was therefore richer.

So, in considering how to design intervention, the speech and language therapist should situate decisions within a collaborative family-centered framework. Where applicable, both languages should be supported and intervention should incorporate culturally relevant activities and be aligned to the family's cultural values and beliefs.

Conclusions

We hope that the discussions in this chapter may help therapists who do not share the language of the child, to overcome their apprehensions about the challenge of this area of work. We are convinced that adopting a family-centered model of working and building a profile of children's abilities is a sound way to proceed in assessment and intervention with bilingual or potentially bilingual children.

The intention has been to share our experience with an emphasis on the richness of working with culturally and linguistically diverse groups. We speak from a UK perspective, however, through attendance at international conferences and contacts with colleagues, we know that these issues are common to many settings parallel to our own, where speech and language therapists work, yet do not share the language of their client. With the paucity of research in this area, much of what we have covered is drawn from the development of models of service delivery, based on good practice. We believe that working in the environments we describe in London has benefited us hugely and has affected the way that we work as speech and language therapists with all families, including those where we do share the language of the child. It has been a rewarding and stimulating area of work and there is certainly more to be learned and shared.

References

Baker, C. (1995) *A Parents' and Teachers' Guide to Bilingualism* (1st edn). Clevedon: Multilingual Matters.

Ball, M., Crystal, D. and Fletcher, P. (2012) *Assessing Grammar: The Languages of LARSP*. Bristol: Multilingual Matters.

Cruz-Ferreira, M. (2012) Sociolinguistic and cultural considerations when working with multilingual children. In S. McLeod and B. Goldstein (eds) *Multilingual Aspects of Speech Sound Disorders in Children* (pp. 13–23). Bristol: Multilingual Matters.

De Houwer, A. (2009) *Bilingual First Language Acquisition*. Bristol: Multilingual Matters.

Duncan, D.M. (ed.) (1989) *Working with Bilingual Language Disability*. London: Chapman and Hall.

Elin Thordardottir (2010) Towards evidence-based practice in language intervention for bilingual children. *Journal of Communication Disorders* 43, 523–537.

Engel de Abreu, P.M.J., Cruz-Santos, A., Tourinho, C.J., Martin, R. and Bialystok, E. (2012) Bilingualism enriches the poor: Enhanced cognitive control in low-income minority children. *Psychological Science* 23, 1364–1371.

Eversley, J., Mehmedbogovic, D., Sanderson, A., Tinsley, T., von Ahn, M. and Wiggins, R.D. (2010) *Language Capital, Mapping the Languages of London's Schoolchildren*. London: CILT National Centre for Languages.

Fourie, R.J. (2011) *Therapeutic Processes for Communication Disorders: A Guide for Clinicians and Students*. Hove: Psychology Press.

Genesee, F., Paradis, J. and Crago, M. (2004) *Dual Language Development and Disorders: A Handbook on Bilingualism and Second Language Learning*. Baltimore, MD: Paul H Brookes.

Guiberson, M. (2013) Bilingual myth-busters series: Language confusion in bilingual children. *Perspectives on Communication Disorders and Sciences in Culturally and Linguistically Diverse Populations* 20, 5–14.

Howard, S. (1993) Flesh and Blood [recorded by Mary Black]. On The Holy Ground [CD]. London: Grapevine.

Jegatheesan, B., Miller, P.J. and Fowler, S. (2010) Autism from a religious perspective: A study of parental beliefs in South Asian Muslim immigrant families. *Focus on Autism and other Developmental Disabilities* 25, 98–109.

Kershen, A.J. (2005) *Strangers, Aliens and Asians: Huguenots, Jews and Bangladeshis in Spitalfields 1660–2000.* London: Routledge.

Knowles, W. and Masidlover, M. (1982) *The Derbyshire Language Scheme.* Nottingham: Derbyshire County Council.

Madhani, N. (1989) First language Panjabi development. In D.M. Duncan (ed.) *Working With Bilingual Language Disability* (pp. 50–59). London: Chapman and Hall.

Martin, D. (2009) *Language Disabilities in Cultural and Linguistic Diversity.* Bristol: Multilingual Matters.

Martin, D. and Stokes, J. (2009) Researching language socialization of multilingual language disability. Proceedings of International Association of Logopedics and Phoniatrics 3rd Symposium on Communication Disorders in Multilingual Populations. Agros, Cyprus.

Miccio, A.W., Hammer, C.S. and Rodriguez, B. (2009) Code-switching and language disorders in bilingual children. In B.E. Bullock and A.J. Toribio (eds) *The Cambridge Handbook of Linguistic Code-Switching* (pp. 241–252). Cambridge: Cambridge University Press.

Ochs, E., Kremer-Sadlik, T., Gainer Sirota, K. and Solomon, O. (2004) Autism and the social world: An anthropological perspective. *Discourse Studies* 6, 147–183.

Pappas, N.W. and McLeod, S. (2008) *Working with Families in Speech-Language Pathology.* San Diego, CA: Plural Publishers.

Pert, S. and Letts, C. (2006) Codeswitching in Mirpuri speaking Pakistani heritage preschool children. Bilingual language acquisition. *International Journal of Bilingualism* 10, 349–374.

Rampton, B. (1995) *Crossing: Language and Ethnicity Among Adolescents.* Manchester: St Jerome.

Royal College of Speech and Language Therapists (2007) Good practice for speech and language therapists working with clients from linguistic minority communities. See www.rcslt.org (accessed 8 August 2015).

Speech Pathology Association of Australia Ltd. (2008) Criteria for the analysis of speech pathology terms: Challenges and a methodology. Final publication of the Terminology Frameworks Project. Melbourne, Victoria, Australia.

Stokes, J. (1989) First language Bengali development. In D.M. Duncan (ed.) *Working With Bilingual Language Disability* (pp. 60–74). London: Chapman and Hall.

Stokes, J. (2000) Strategies for working with clients from monolingual backgrounds. Proceedings of International Association of Logopedics and Phoniatrics 2nd International Symposium on Communication Disorders in bilingual populations, Johannesburg, South Africa.

Stokes, J. (2012) An investigation of syntax in children of Bengali (Sylheti)-speaking families. In M.J. Ball, D. Crystal and P. Fletcher (eds) *Assessing Grammar: The Languages of LARSP* (pp. 139–148). Bristol: Multilingual Matters.

Stow, C., Pert, S. and Khattab, G. (2012) Translation to practice: Sociolinguistic and cultural considerations when working with the Pakistani heritage community in England, UK. In S. McLeod and. B. Goldstein (eds) *Multilingual Aspects of Speech Sound Disorders in Children* (pp. 24–27). Bristol: Multilingual Matters.

Tomblin, B. (2011) Co-morbidity of autism and SLI: Kinds, kin and complexity. *International Journal of Language & Communication Disorders* 46, 127–137.

8 Typical Language Development and Primary Language Impairment in Monolingual French-Speaking Children

Elin Thordardottir

This chapter surveys aspects of the typical development of spoken French in native speakers of preschool and early school age, the manifestation of primary language impairment (PLI)[1] in French-speaking children and assessment methods for the evaluation of language level and the identification of language impairment. We begin with highlights of some of the characteristics of the French language, focusing on aspects that impact on cross-linguistic comparisons that have been prominent in the discussion of the manifestation and underlying nature of PLI. We then present normative data on the development of French and continue with a discussion of the manifestation of PLI in French-speaking children, and the assessment tools and methods available for its identification. The studies surveyed in this chapter focus both on Quebec French and on European French.

Highlights of the Characteristics of French in Acquisition

Grammatical morphology is among the aspects of language frequently targeted in language assessment and intervention and has played a prominent role in research on the underlying nature of PLI, both in English and in French (e.g. Jakubowicz, 2003; Rice & Wexler, 1996). French is considered to be a moderately inflected language. It is substantially more inflected than English, but less inflected than a number of other languages

Table 8.1 Summary of French grammatical morphology

	Tense	Person	Mood	Number	Gender
Verbs	Various simple and composite tenses	Three persons of singular Three persons of plural	Indicative Imperative Conditional Subjunctive Participles	Past participle[a]	Past participle[a]
Nouns				Singular Plural	Masculine Feminine
Adjectives				Singular Plural	Masculine Feminine
Pronouns		Personal pronouns		Singular Plural	Masculine Feminine

[a] The past participle of composite tense verbs must agree in number and gender with the subject or complement under certain circumstances.

such as Russian or Icelandic, which also feature case marking. Table 8.1 provides an overview of French grammatical inflectional morphology.

Noun phrase morphology

French noun gender (masculine or feminine) is marked primarily by the determiner (such as the indefinite or definite article *un/une, le/la*). To some extent, the form of a noun gives an indication as to its gender, as in *chanteur/chanteuse* – male singer/female singer. However, the majority of words do not provide such cues by their form, and gender therefore needs to be memorized for each word. For example, these rhyming words have different genders: *la table* (the table), *le sable* (the sand). Young children are reported to have some sensitivity to forms that are strongly associated with either gender, for example, judging non-words such as *forsienne* to be feminine and *bicron* to be masculine (review in Hickmann, 1997). For most nouns, the only audible plural marker in spoken language is the determiner. The singular determiners *le* and *la* become plural *les*, and the singular determiners *un* and *une* become plural *des*. In the written form, an *–s* is added at the end of the word, which is silent except in some contexts discussed below. A small subclass of irregular nouns undergo a change in the word ending in the plural (e.g. *cheval, chevaux* – horse, horses). For these words, the plural is marked in two ways, by the determiner and the change in ending.

Pronouns and adjectives must agree in gender and number with the noun to which they refer. Although many common adjectives assume irregular forms with distinct gender forms (*beau, belle* – beautiful; *vieux, vieille* – old), the feminine gender is generally formed by affixing an *–e* to the masculine form of the adjective. Similarly, many pronouns form the feminine by the addition of an *–e* to the masculine form (*quel, quelle* – who, what, which; *certain, certaine* – certain), whereas other pronouns assume more distinct forms (*ce, cette* – this). The plural of adjectives is generally formed by the addition of an *–s*. As is the case of noun plurals, the gender and plural marking of adjectives may be audible or inaudible depending on the form of the word and the context in which it is produced. If the masculine form ends in a silent consonant, that consonant becomes audible in the feminine form, resulting in distinct masculine and feminine forms in spoken language (e.g. the masculine and feminine forms of 'green' are *vert* /vɛʁ/ and *verte* /vɛʁt/). In contrast, the pronunciation of the feminine and masculine form does not differ for adjectives in which the final consonant is pronounced in the masculine form (e.g. 'red' is *rouge* /ʁuʒ/ for both genders). There is some dialectal variation as well in whether slight vowel changes occur between forms such as *vert* and *verte* and the extent to which the final *–e* may be pronounced. A further complication is that silent markers become audible depending on the context of the word. When a word ending in a silent consonant is followed by a word with an initial vowel, the two words may be linked such that the silent consonant becomes audible. For example, the word-final /s/ of *gros* is silent in *l'ours est gros* (the bear is fat), but is audible in *le gro**s** ours* (the fat bear). This linking phenomenon, referred to as *'liaison'*, in some cases obligatory and in other cases optional, is receiving increased research interest by acquisition researchers (Chevrot *et al.*, 2009). Analysis systems of French vary in how they deal with these silent gender and plural markings (Rondal, 2003; Elin Thordardottir, 2005).

Verb morphology

French lexical verbs fall into three inflectional groups. The first group includes all verbs whose infinitive form ends in *–er* except the verb *aller* (to go). Examples are *aimer* (to love) and *dessiner* (to draw). This is by far the largest group of lexical verbs. The second group comprises verbs whose infinitive ends in *–ir* and whose gerund form ends in *–issant* (e.g. *finir, finissant* – to end). The third group is by far the smallest, but includes a variety of verbs with infinitives ending in *–re* (*vendre, conduire* – to buy, to drive), *–oir* (*recevoir*, to receive), *–ir* with the gerund form *–ant* (*partir-partant*, to leave) and the verb *aller* (to go). In spite of the variability, the conjugation is fairly predictable with the third group of verbs falling into five families based on phonological similarity (Nicoladis & Paradis, 2012).

French verbs are inflected for person, tense and mood. There are three persons of the singular (first, second and third) and three persons of the plural. French has a number of simple and compound verb tenses marking present, past and future. At later stages of development when sentences express more complex thoughts, verbs also assume different moods, including the conditional and subjunctive in addition to the indicative. The number of different verb forms is tempered by the fact that a large number of verb forms are homophonous in their spoken form (though differences exist in the spelled forms). For example, all three persons of the singular and the third-person plural of the present of the most common verb group (–er verbs) are homophonous: *j'aime, tu aimes, il aime, ils/ells aiment*, and the same is true of the imperfect past (imparfait): *j'aimais, tu aimais, il aimait, ils aimaient*. In addition, the past participle and infinitive of this verb group are also homophonous although they have distinct written forms (*aimer, aimé* – to love, loved). The remaining three verb groups have less, but still important homophony between inflectional forms but they have distinct infinitive and past participle forms (e.g. *prendre, pris* – to take, taken; *finir, fini* – to finish, finished).

Overregularization errors

Overregularization errors have played an important role in accounts of grammatical acquisition. In English as well as other Germanic languages, the incorrect application of the regular past tense to irregular verbs has been used to test theoretical accounts such as how the regular past tense rule comes to be. According to a dual mechanism account (Marcus, 1996), the regular past tense is applied to verbs once the regular past tense rule stemming from a dedicated rule mechanism becomes active. A second mechanism is required to memorize those verbs to which the rule does not apply and to block the application of the rule for those verbs. In contrast, a single mechanism view holds that the ability to apply the regular past tense to new verbs does not derive from a rule mechanism separate from the lexicon. Instead, the regularity is extracted from the resemblance among a critical mass of stored verb items (Marchman & Bates, 1994; Elin Thordardottir *et al.*, 2002). These types of accounts have been tested by linking the emergence of overregularization errors to chronological age (maturation of a grammatical mechanism) versus verb vocabulary size (critical mass), taking advantage of the very clear distinction in Germanic languages between verbs that form the past tense with the regular affix versus a stem change without affixation. Such a clear distinction between regular and clearly irregular verb patterns does not exist in French, as the three different verb groups each use verb consistent endings and some use stem changes as well to mark tense and person. The verb groups do, however, differ in how many other verbs have the same pattern and therefore, how strongly predictable the pattern is. Nevertheless, various examples of overregularization errors have been reported in French (review in Hickmann, 1997). For verbs, such errors frequently involve overapplication of the common –er verb group form of the infinitive or past participle (*rier* for *rire* – to laugh; *prendé* for *pris* – taken; *metté* for *mis* – put).

However, errors can also involve the overuse of other, less common verb groups (*prendu* for *pris* – taken; *tiendre* for *tenir* – to hold; *viendre* for *venir* – to come; *éteindu* for *éteint* – extinguished).

In spite of not being as clear-cut as in English, overregularization errors have been used to test theoretical accounts in French. Nicoladis and Paradis (2012) tested the single mechanism and dual route accounts in bilingual French–English-speaking children. They defined overregularization in French as the overapplication of the most common verb form, *er* verbs. In contrast, overapplication of the less common verb forms was considered in this study to be irregularization. The study found more accurate production of regular than irregular verbs across both languages and that the percentage correct use was correlated with vocabulary size in that language – both findings are more consistent with a single mechanism view. Royle and Elin Thordardottir (2008) observed that typically developing (TD) monolingual French-speaking children age 3–5 years produced many –*er* group overgeneralizations when attempting the passé composé (perfect past) of verbs from other groups, whereas their counterparts with PLI did not, suggesting that the children with PLI might not yet have formed as strong a preference for this most common verb group as their unimpaired peers.

Variable word orders

Another notable characteristic of French is the variety of word orders that are permitted and frequently used. French speakers frequently employ left and right dislocations, whereby subjects and verb object complements are dislocated to the right or to the left and sometimes repeated in the form of a pronoun. For example, all of the following sentences with subject dislocations have the same meaning: *la fille dort* (the girl sleeps), *elle dort la fille* (she sleeps the girl) or *la fille elle dort* (the girl she sleeps). Maillart and Parisse (2008) have proposed that there are developmental stages in children's tendency to produce subject dislocations. This word order variation introduces a level of optionality which may complicate or prolong the time it takes children to learn certain structures. One of these may be the object clitic – a structure that has been implicated in PLI in French as particularly problematic (Grüter, 2005; Jakubowicz et al., 1998). The object clitic is the pronominal form of the direct object of a verb. The direct object can be expressed by a lexical item or by a pronoun. The following examples illustrate the variety of places in the sentences the lexical and clitic object may appear, including sentences that use both: *j'ai vu la baleine* (I saw the whale), *je l'ai vue* (I saw it), *je l'ai vue, la baleine* (I saw it, the whale), *la baleine, je l'ai vue* (the whale, I saw it). Matthews et al. (1997) showed that French-speaking children were less likely to express both lexical and pronominal objects than their English-speaking counterparts were, and their findings suggested that word order variations influenced the likelihood that French-speaking children expressed either form of the object of transitive verbs.

Normative Reference Bases for French Language Development

The typical sequence of acquisition of many early-acquired French grammatical structures has been inferred from longitudinal case studies of a small number of children (see overview in Hickmann, 1997). Large-scale normative studies of French development have been scarce, but have increased in number in recent years and have started to document the typical ages at which mastery is reached. Recent studies have extended the investigation to the early school years. Detailed longitudinal studies are able to document low-frequency behaviors, and will thus often document sporadic use of grammatical structures at young ages, before these structures can be expected to be encountered in fairly short clinical samples and across children. Therefore, although there is overall good agreement between longitudinal and cross-sectional studies as to the sequence of acquisition, cross-sectional studies give a better estimate of the typical ages at which milestones are reached. Both types of studies show French-speaking children to use grammatical morphology quite correctly from an early age. However, the observation of early correct use does not necessarily indicate full mastery. Many forms used correctly early on in simple structures undergo more diverse and complex use later in development with associated error patterns. For example, even though the definite article is used correctly by young children in simple contexts, problems can arise later, with the use of the partitive article: *de l'eau* (water, definite article required), *un peu d'eau* (a little water, no definite article with *un peu*).

Longitudinal as well as cross-sectional studies have shown that gender and plural markings are used correctly in spontaneous language early on (Elin Thordardottir, 2005; Zesiger *et al.*, 2010). Using longitudinal data, Bassano (2000) showed that the use of determiners develops in a gradual process. The stages of acquisition involve the use of 'fillers', or pseudodeterminers with an ambiguous form preceding the use of true determiners and a long period during which such fillers and true determiners coexist. Further, a developmental sequence was identified involving the correct use of determinerless nouns (proper nouns), incorrect determinerless nouns (obligatory determiner omitted), nouns preceded by a filler and correct adult use of determiners. Bassano *et al.* (2008) showed that monosyllabic words were more likely than multisyllabic words to be preceded by a filler, creating an iambic pattern (two-syllable pattern with greater stress on the second syllable), indicating that the development of determiner use is influenced by a number of factors, including prosodic ones. As for verbs, longitudinal corpus studies and cross-sectional studies agree that the earliest tenses to appear beyond the present of the indicative are compound tenses *passé composé* (perfect past) and *futur proche* (periphrastic future). Other studies have noted that the full acquisition of grammatical morphology extends well into the school years, with the appearance of late-developing structures such as the subjunctive mood (Elin Thordardottir *et al.*, 2005).

Large-sample studies of lexical development

Lexical development in young children has been studied with French versions of the MacArthur–Bates Communicative Development Inventory (CDI) both in France (Kern, 2007) and in Quebec (Trudeau *et al.*, 1999), resulting in descriptions of the lexicon in terms of size, lexical and grammatical composition and phonological characteristics. In the version developed in France (Gayraud & Kern, 2007), large variability was noted, but scores increased systematically with age. Nouns were found to predominate in both comprehension and production throughout this early period. This is in line with Bassano (2000), who documented an early noun bias in French acquisition in language sample data, although she also reported that verbs were more frequent in French compared to same-age English-speaking children. In the French CDI, the most advanced children used predicates and function words as well. Gesture use was found to be highly correlated with comprehension skills. In the Quebec version of the MacArthur–Bates CDI (Boudreault *et al.*, 2007; Trudeau & Sutton, 2011), scores increased systematically with age, however without a noticeable vocabulary spurt. In terms of lexical composition, nouns predominated throughout the age range of the study; however, their frequency relative to other word classes initially increased and then decreased somewhat. In contrast, the relative frequency of verbs increased steadily throughout the period, as did the use of grammatical words. At age 17 months, half of the children were reported to produce word combinations, and at age 21 months, 90% of the children did.

Versions of the MacArthur–Bates CDI are available in a number of languages, and are often viewed as providing a means of making cross-linguistic comparisons. However, normative data have revealed significant differences that show that versions of the CDI are not identical across languages. Obvious changes occur in the grammatical sections, reflecting structural differences between languages. Trudeau and Sutton (2011) reported that even their most advanced children did not approach ceiling scores on the section on grammatical morphology, which is quite detailed in the Quebec French version and produces different scores than the English version. Cross-linguistic differences are found in vocabulary as well. Elin Thordardottir (2005) found that French-speaking children had significantly smaller vocabularies than their English-speaking age matches both on the CDI parent report and in language samples – a finding confirmed by Trudeau and Sutton for the CDI. Small but significant gender differences up to age 30 months, favoring girls, have been reported for both forms of the French CDI (Bouchard *et al.*, 2009; Kern, 2007) and for language sample data (Le Normand *et al.*, 2008).

Large-sample studies of morphosyntactic development

Normative data on syntactic and morphosyntactic production in spontaneous language have been reported by Rondal (2003), Elin Thordardottir (2005), Elin Thordardottir *et al.* (2005) and Le Normand *et al.* (2008). Rondal reported data on mean length of utterance in words (MLUw) and in morphemes (MLUm) for a single child (Grégoire) from age 2 to 3 years. Le Normand *et al.* collected language samples on 316 French Parisian children in nine age groups ranging from 24 to 48 months using a standard set of toys in a 20-minute interaction with the parent or familiar adult. Measures reported include MLUw, total number of words, number of different words and type-token ratio (TTR). In addition, the corpus was coded for certain word classes and grammatical words by an automatic part-of-speech tagger. Detailed descriptive measures by age group are reported for each of the measures, which are shown to increase systematically with age. The study also reported a strong effect of socioeconomic status on language development.

Elin Thordardottir (2005) developed a systematic analysis method for French based on Systematic Analysis of Language Transcripts (SALT) conventions (Miller & Chapman, 1984–2002). The French conventions are available in the online version of SALT analysis software and in the 2005 article. This analysis can be computerized or done by hand. The French SALT coding conventions are not directly based on the English ones in the sense of coding the same forms. Rather, it follows a parallel procedure, respecting the characteristics of the French language, in particular, its greater inflectional complexity. Grammatical morphemes are coded for verb person, verb tense, verb mood, noun, adjective and pronoun plural marking, and gender marking on adjectives and pronouns. Unlike the English SALT coding system, the French system targets production regardless of presumed productivity. For example, English SALT does not code irregular past tenses because it is presumed that young children do not associate forms such as *bring* and *brought* to the same lexical item. Given the considerably larger number of grammatical morphemes in French than in English, decisions on when to assume productivity for each morpheme are complicated and bound to be subject to a high degree of error. For that reason, target forms that are produced correctly are coded, even if they are homophonous with other inflectional forms. This system, allowing for the coding of any verb tense and mood, has the advantage that it can be applied to varied language levels. This coding system has been used in several studies targeting children of different ages.

Normative data using this analysis approach involving language samples of 100 utterances collected in a conversational context with an examiner have been published for MLUw and MLUm, morphological diversity and lexical development in children age 24–43 months (Elin Thordardottir, 2005), and for MLUw and MLUm in children age 4;6–5:6 years (Elin Thordardottir *et al.*, 2010). MLU data on groups of children with TD and PLI are available from two additional studies (Elin Thordardottir & Namazi, 2007; Elin Thordardottir *et al.*, 2011). The MLU data from these various studies are reported in Table 8.2, together covering groups of children ranging in age from 24 to 66 months, and including a total of 127 children. The table shows a systematic increase in both MLU measures with age. All these studies were conducted in the same lab using the same data collection and transcription method (described in Elin Thordardottir, 2005) as well as rigorous reliability checks which were reported in each of the published studies.

The systematic coding of grammatical morphemes in the samples provides cross-sectional data on the typical development of French inflectional morphology, including the sequence of acquisition of grammatical morphemes and the age at which they are typically acquired. Elin Thordardottir (2005) reported, for each morpheme coded, the age group and MLU level at which emergence and mastery are reached, from sporadic use (use by at least one child in the group), to more consistent use (by at

Table 8.2 Group means and (standard deviations) for mean length of utterance in words (MLUw) and morphemes (MLUm) in conversational samples of 100 utterances in monolingual French-speaking children with and without PLI from age 24 to 66 months (using the coding procedure developed by Elin Thordardottir [2005])

	TD		PLI	
	MLUw	MLUm	MLUw	MLUm
24 months[a]	1.9 (0.3)	2.2 (0.5)		
32 months[a]	2.8 (0.9)	3.6 (1.0)		
43 months[a]	3.3 (1.0)	4.3 (1.2)		
45 months[b]	3.5 (0.6)	4.5 (0.8)	2.0 (0.4)	2.4 (0.5)
52 months[c]	4.0 (1.1)	5.2 (1.3)		
60 months[c]		4.7 (1.1)	5.9 (1.4)	
61 months[d]			3.5 (0.9)	4.3 (1.1)
66 months[c]		5.9 (1.7)	7.6 (2.3)	

[a] Elin Thordardottir (2005, *n* = 19).
[b] Elin Thordardottir and Namazi (1997, *n* = 12 per TD and PLI groups).
[c] Elin Thordardottir *et al.* (2010, *n* = 78).
[d] Elin Thordardottir *et al.* (2011, *n* = 14 in PLI group).

least half of the children in the group) and productive use (use with two different words by half or more of the children in the group). The resulting graphs revealed a more systematic progression toward mastery when morphemes were plotted against MLU than against age. Figure 8.1 provides data of the same kind for a sample of children age 4;6–5;6 ($n = 57$), plotted as a function of MLUm groups ranging from 4.0 to 8+. All the children were monolingual speakers of French with typical development, and all scored within normal limits on non-verbal cognition (Elin Thordardottir et al., 2005). This analysis confirms the order of acquisition of early morphemes

MOOD	Past participle					
	Present participle					
	Conditional mood					
	Subjunctive mood					
	Imperative mood					
TENSE	Passé simple					
	Futur simple					
	Plus-que-parfait					
	Imparfait					
	Futur périphrastique					
	Passé composé					
PERSON	2nd person plural					
	1st person plural					
	3rd person plural					
	3rd person "on"					
	3rd person sing					
	2nd person sing					
	1st person sing					
NOUNS	Pronoun plural					
	Adjective plural					
	Adjective gender					
	Pronoun gender					
	Noun plural					
	MLU LEVEL	4.0-4.99	5.0-5.99	6.0-6.99	7.0-7.99	8.0+

	Morpheme did not appear in any sample
	Morpheme was used by fewer than half of the children in the group
	Morpheme was used at least once in samples of half or more of the group
	Morpheme was used with at least two different words by half or more of the group

Figure 8.1 Use of grammatical morphology by monolingual French-speaking children at MLUm levels of 4 to 8+ (Elin Thordardottir et al., 2005)

previously described by longitudinal case studies, such as an early preference for composite tenses (Bassano, 2000) with the passé composé (perfect) and imparfait (imperfect) past tenses and the futur proche (periphrastic future) well mastered at an MLU of 4.0. The analysis adds information on later acquired morphemes, showing that the futur simple (simple future) and plus-que-parfait (pluperfect), appear only sporadically up to an MLU of 7.0, and do not reach productive use by half of the children in any MLU group. Similarly, the conditional and subjunctive moods appear, but are not yet mastered by any group. Overall, these cross-sectional data are in good agreement with longitudinal case studies covering the first years of life. They also extend the study of morphological development into the early school years, revealing that while morphological acquisition starts early, with many morphemes produced correctly early on, this development also follows a protracted course, with many morphemes not appearing until the late preschool or early school years, and with morphological acquisition not being complete at that point.

It is evident that the morphological development of French not only starts early but also extends longer than it does in English. Very young French-speaking children demonstrate correct use of many morphemes, including person marking, and gender marking of adjectives. At age 5;6, when English morphology is largely considered to be acquired by most children, French-speaking children are still adding verb tenses and moods to their repertoire. MLUm in French is significantly higher than that of English-speaking counterparts, whereas MLUw is comparable between languages, at least at early stages (Elin Thordardottir, 2005). At the same time, vocabulary diversity is smaller in French whether measured in spontaneous language or by parent report (Elin Thordardottir, 2005). These differences reflect not only the nature of the morphosyntactic coding conventions, but also a difference in the structures used by each of the languages to convey meaning. These differences have important implications for the interpretation of cross-linguistic comparisons for the purpose of matching participants in research and in the assessment of bilingual children (Elin Thordardottir *et al.*, 2006).

Primary Language Impairment in French

A developmental language impairment that manifests primarily in the area of language with normal findings on clinical tests of non-verbal cognition and sensory function is termed *dysphasie* in French (Le Normand, 2003). The conceptual definition of this diagnostic category is similar to that of specific language impairment (SLI) or PLI (Leonard, 1998) and is similarly formulated in terms of inclusionary and exclusionary criteria. However, the clinical identification of *dysphasie* requires a more severe language deficit than does PLI, affecting both language comprehension and production. Some authors are explicit in stating that PLI does not fall within the same category as *dysphasie*, but rather falls in the category of what is termed *retard* (delay) in French (Le Normand, 2003). Therefore, in spite of the resemblance in the conceptual definition, children identified clinically as having *dysphasie* in French-speaking areas and *SLI/PLI* in English-speaking areas result in groups with only partial overlap (see discussion in Elin Thordardottir *et al.*, 2011). In studies on French that are published in English, the term *PLI* is frequently used to refer to children who were recruited clinically as having *dysphasie*. Other studies deliberately use criteria in line with PLI to increase cross-linguistic comparability, but in so doing, these studies do not directly represent the clinical population identified according to local criteria. This must be kept in mind when the results of studies are compared cross-linguistically between French and English as well as by clinicians who wish to apply research findings to children on their caseloads. In Quebec, a new definition of *Trouble Primaire du Langage* (primary language impairment) has been proposed which is more in line with the more mainstream international definition of PLI (OOAQ, 2004). However, the more traditional definition of *dysphasie* is still in effect for official purposes.

A fair number of studies have examined the manifestation of *dysphasie* or PLI in French-speaking children. Early studies focused nearly exclusively on aspects of grammatical morphology, verbs in particular, under the widely held assumption at the time that this is an area of particular vulnerability across languages. Many studies were conducted from the perspective of a linguistic deficit as the underlying cause of PLI; some starting with a pattern observed in English and seeking to verify their applicability to French, other studies testing predictions based on the structural complexity of French. These studies documented lower performance by children with *dysphasie* as compared to unimpaired control children in various aspects of morphology, including certain verb tenses (Jakubowicz, 2003), grammatical function categories (Jakubowicz *et al.*, 1998) and the use of finite verb morphology (Hamann *et al.*, 2003; Paradis & Crago, 2001).

The practical implications of these studies for clinical diagnosis or intervention are generally unclear. First, although many of the studies comment on clinical implications related to the potential utility of a particular grammatical morphology as clinical markers of language impairment, most of the studies were not undertaken with a clinical purpose in mind, but rather to test theoretical issues. The utility of the purported clinical markers must be viewed as tentative at best in studies that did not go beyond documenting a group difference between impaired and unimpaired groups and that had a narrow focus on selected language structures. Concluding that a particular area of language is one of disproportionate difficulty requires comparison with other areas of language. Similarly, careful documentation of the overall language level is required to ascertain whether failure to produce a particular structure results from specific difficulty with that structure or rather from a more general language delay. Furthermore, diagnostic accuracy can be low even when group differences are significant; therefore, further verification of the sensitivity and specificity of potential clinical markers is needed (Bortolini *et al.*, 2006; Elin Thordardottir *et al.*, 2011). Yet another factor to consider is that studies differ in recruitment methods, diagnostic criteria, the extent to which participant characteristics are documented and how control groups are selected. In some cases, TD controls involve single children for whom longitudinal data are available, but who are not directly matched to the SLI group on any particular variable.

The extended optional infinitive (EOI) account (Rice & Wexler, 1996) was among the most prominent accounts in PLI research for many years. In this account, the optional infinitive (OI) period seen in typical development in English and some other languages is extended compared to TD peers. During the OI period, children tend to use non-finite verbs in finite contexts as if they regard finiteness as optional rather than obligatory. Paradis and Crago (2001) examined whether the EOI account could be applied to PLI (*dysphasie*) in French. In spontaneous language samples in an interview context in which questions were used to elicit sentences with present, past and future tenses, 7-year-old children with PLI made significantly more errors than 3-year-old TD controls, with the majority of errors involving tense. However, finiteness errors were different from those observed in English in that they tended to involve bare stem forms rather than the infinitive. In English, the infinitive has the same form as the bare stem of a verb. In French, this is not the case. Instead, for the most frequent verbs (*–er* verbs), the bare stem is homophonous with the correctly inflected forms of the singular persons of the indicative present. Paradis and Crago proposed that children with PLI used such bare stems as default forms. Therefore, while the EOI stage in English is characterized by the use of bare stems that are incorrect in a finite context, the French equivalent of this stage would, according to these authors, involve bare stem forms which also happen to be the correct conjugated form in finite contexts for a large number of French verbs. These results illustrate the implications of the homophony of French verb forms for the interpretation of French error patterns in relation to prominent accounts of PLI.

Other studies examining early patterns of verb use in French have reported early primitive sentences involving 'root infinitives', which are bare past participles or infinitives generally produced without a subject. As infinitives and past participles are homophonous for many French verbs, context is used to decide which one is more likely, examples: *tombé* (fallen), *aller là* (go there) (Bassano, 2000; Hamann *et al.*, 2003; Elin Thordardottir & Namazi, 2007). Subject omissions are reported to occur also in sentences with finite verbs (*est par terre* – is on the floor; *a tout mangé* – ate everything)

(Hamann *et al.*, 2003). Bassano reported from a longitudinal case study from age 1 to 2;6 years that 62% of infinitives occurred alone and 38% in compound tenses, with corresponding numbers for the past participle at 71% and 29%. All of these could occur with or without a subject. Utterances with a subject and a non-finite verb, which would be more directly analogous to English EOI errors, have been reported by Paradis and Crago (2001), whereas other studies on verb inflection in French generally do not report on non-finite forms in clauses that have an overt subject (Hamann *et al.*, 1996, 2003; Jakubowicz , 2003). Hamann *et al.* (1996) reported that of 278 instances of the subject clitic pronoun in a longitudinal corpus, all but five occurred in tensed clauses. This suggests that once children move from subjectless root infinitives to sentences involving a subject, they also move to using a finite form of the verb. Hamann *et al.* (2003) examined aspects of morphology in spontaneous language samples of children with PLI younger and older than 5 years. Strong subject pronoun (*moi, toi*) were rarely seen without the subject clitic (*moi, je vais jouer* – me, I'm going to play, where *moi* is the strong subject pronoun, and *je* the clitic pronoun) and overall, subject omissions diminished with age, such that the root infinitive stage was reported to finish for children with PLI by age 6 years. Overall, the authors concluded that an OI stage directly analogous to the OI stage in English does not occur in the acquisition of French.

Some accounts focusing on linguistic deficits in PLI have focused separately on tense and agreement (Clahsen, 1989; Rice & Wexler, 1996). In French, tense and agreement can be disentangled to a greater extent than is possible in English – however, not entirely because of homophony of certain forms. For example, the first-, second- and third-person singular and third-person plural forms are homophonous for many verbs within a given tense. To illustrate, for the verb *aimer*, these persons are *aime, aimes, aime, aiment* in the present (all pronounced the same), but *aimais, aimais, aimait, aimaient* in the imperfect (pronounced the same, but differently from the present). Greater differentiation of these persons occurs in the future tense: *aimerai, aimeras, aimera, aimeront*, of which only the second- and third-persons singular are homophonous. In each of these cases, the tense distinction is clear. A further difference in French and English tense marking is that tense in French is used to denote both temporal relations and aspect, but only in the past. Thus, the passé composé (perfect past) is used to refer to resultative events whereas the imparfait denotes progressive or habitual events. French-speaking children's first use of these tenses denotes aspect rather than tense (review in Hickman, 1997).

As another example of prominent research on PLI in French from a linguistic deficit approach, Jakubowicz (2003) proposed the Computational Complexity Hypothesis (CCH). The CCH posits that functional categories that involve more operations are more complex, are acquired later and are more vulnerable in PLI than categories that involve fewer operations.

The particular categories that are most complex vary across languages. For French, the hypothesis was tested by comparing the production of two compound past tenses, the passé composé (perfect past, *j'ai mangé*, I have eaten) and the plus-que-parfait (pluperfect, *j'avais mangé*, I had eaten) using an elicitation task. According to this account, the pluperfect would be more difficult grammatically than the perfect because it involves more operations: for the pluperfect, the auxiliary must be in the past tense, whereas in the passé composé, the auxiliary is present tense. However, from a conceptual point of view, the pluperfect is seen as more transparent precisely because the auxiliary is in the past tense whereas for the passé composé, the present tense auxiliary might be misleading. Results confirmed the CCH in that children with PLI ages 5–9 years produced very few pluperfect responses and tended to produce the perfect in its place. However, because the study participants covered a fairly large age range, an alternative explanation might be that the less linguistically advanced children had not yet mastered the pluperfect due to a generally low language level, and thus that the pluperfect might not have been a specific area of deficit. As noted in another section, the perfect is the first tense to appear after the present tense, significantly earlier than the pluperfect.

In addition to verb inflections, a grammatical form that has received research attention in French PLI as well as in other Romance languages (Bortolini *et al.*, 2006) is the object clitic, discussed in a previous section of this chapter in relation to variations in word order. It will be recalled that the object clitic is the pronominal form of the direct object. Whereas the lexical direct object normally appears after the verb, the object clitic moves before the verb (*je mange la pomme, je la mange* – I eat the apple, I eat it). In an early study, Jakubowicz *et al.* (1998) compared the use of determiners and object clitics (which are homophonous) in an elicitation task in children with PLI age 5–13 years and TD children age 5 years. Children with PLI had significantly more difficulty with the object clitic than the determiner, suggesting that the problem was not related to the low surface substance of these elements (Leonard, 1989) but rather their grammatical function. Good performance on the determiner has also been reported by Le Normand *et al.* (1993). Paradis *et al.* (2009) found significantly low use of the object clitic by 7-year-olds with PLI. Grüter (2005) extended the study of object clitics to comprehension as well as production, documenting low use by children with PLI, but adequate comprehension. The typical development of the object clitic can help make sense of these various results. Studies on the object clitic in spontaneous language show that it emerges late in children with TD. Several studies have reported low use of the clitic by both children with PLI and TD children (Hamann, 2003; Hamann *et al.*, 2003; Elin Thordardottir & Namazi, 2007), suggesting that its non-use may not be indicative of a problem except in older children whose language level supports more frequent use. Children's use of the object clitic in French has also been shown to be influenced by task, such as spontaneous versus elicited contexts, and modality (comprehension and production). The likelihood that object clitics are used has also been shown to be influenced by whether the verb in the sentence is in the first, second or third person (Pirvulescu & Hill, 2012), and clitic omissions have been related to particular sentence types involving dislocations (Pérez-Leroux *et al.*, 2011). One of the difficulties in establishing a percentage correct rate of use of object clitics in spontaneous language is that it is often difficult to decide with certainty whether use of the clitic is truly obligatory in a given context. To date, research on the French object clitic has not provided solid evidence that it possesses high precision as a clinical marker of PLI.

Beyond grammatical morphology in PLI research

In stark contrast to these studies documenting morphological deficits in French-speaking children with PLI, Elin Thordardottir and Namazi (2007) detected very few morphological errors in the spontaneous speech of French-speaking preschool children with PLI. In this study, participants were clinically referred but inclusionary criteria were based on the mainstream diagnostic criteria for PLI (rather than *dysphasie*) to ensure comparability with previous studies on English. Verb and noun inflection accuracy rates ranged from 94% to 100%. Error types observed included bare infinitives, past participles, auxiliary omissions, incorrect verb tense and incorrect verb person. However, each of these occurred very infrequently. In that sense, the language pattern of the children with PLI mirrored that of younger French-speaking children with typical development (Elin Thordardottir, 2005), consistent with the cross-linguistic observation that error patterns in PLI generally involve the same types of errors as those seen in typical development, but may occur at increased rates. The use of the object clitic in this study was not problematic for children with PLI – in fact, they resembled the age-matched group rather than the MLU-matched group in this respect – but overall use of the object clitic was low in all groups of participants. This study also examined lexical composition. Children with PLI had a smaller vocabulary than unimpaired controls. In terms of composition, they differed from younger MLU-matched controls in that they had a lower proportion of function words and a greater proportion of social words, which may point to a syntactic weakness, but one which did not manifest in morphological errors.

In recent years, studies on PLI in French-speaking children have examined a much wider range of linguistic behaviors and have investigated PLI from more varied theoretical perspectives, notably from the standpoint of processing limitations as a contributing underlying factor. In that vein, Pizzioli and Schelstraete (2008) examined the effect of argument structure complexity on the accuracy of grammatical morphology in 9-year-old children with PLI. In an elicitation task, children with PLI were more likely to omit auxiliaries and the article of the direct object of the verb than non-impaired control children were, and they were more likely to do so with transitive than intransitive verbs. In contrast, sentence length as such had no effect on accuracy rates. It was concluded that cognitive resources play a role in accuracy rates in PLI. Elin Thordardottir *et al.* (2011) investigated the performance of children with PLI on tasks that target linguistic processing, namely non-word repetition and sentence imitation, finding these areas to be of significant difficulty for these children, as they have been found to be for English-speaking children and children speaking a variety of other languages (e.g. Ellis Weismer *et al.*, 2000; Elin Thordardottir, 2008). The study also documented a significant general delay across lexical and grammatical domains of language. The study went on to document the diagnostic accuracy of various measures for the identification of PLI in 5-year-old French-speaking children – those results are presented in more detail in a later section on assessment. Recent studies on French-speaking children have also looked at the influence of more global skills such as serial procedural learning of non-linguistic materials, which was found to be unimpaired (Gabriel *et al.*, 2011) and non-linguistic analogic reasoning skills, on which children with PLI were found to be deficient (Leroy *et al.*, 2012). In the area of phonology, Maillart and Parisse (2006) documented a developmental effect in the phonological abilities of French-speaking children with PLI in two age groups, 4 and 8 years, such that a significant group difference in phonological ability between children with and without PLI was found only for the older age group. The older children with PLI demonstrated phonological difficulties at the phoneme and syllable level, which exceeded their general language difficulty. Zourou *et al.* (2010) investigated phonological awareness (PA) skills in children with PLI in a longitudinal intervention study, and found that reading instruction resulted in increased PA skills in the children with PLI. However, the better PA skills did not transfer to more complex tasks such as reading and spelling ability. It was concluded that PA skills are fragile in children with PLI but that further research is needed to examine the contribution of other related skills such as vocabulary development and the acquisition of grammatical rules.

Summary of studies on the manifestation of PLI in French

It is evident from this review that the research base on PLI in French-speaking children is considerable and growing, and that it has evolved and diversified greatly over the years, similar to the research on PLI in other languages. Early studies focused heavily on grammatical morphology, frequently starting with an a priori assumption that this was the most likely locus of difficulty, consistent with prominent views at the time. Many of these studies concluded that particular deficits existed in that area, however, typically without measurement of or direct comparison to other areas of language. In addition, in early studies, participants frequently spanned large age ranges and comparison groups were not necessarily matched with the PLI group on precise criteria such as age or language level. Increasingly in more recent studies, these methodological variables are more tightly controlled, background variables are documented in more detail and diagnostic criteria are carefully specified. Further, recent studies increasingly adopt diagnostic criteria in line with mainstream definitions of PLI rather than *dysphasie*, which helps make meaningful cross-linguistic comparisons, but decreases the studies' applicability to clinical populations identified according to the traditional criteria.

Due to these methodological considerations and to structural differences between French and English, it is difficult to form a conclusive picture of PLI in French or to compare its manifestation directly with that seen in English. One aspect that is clearly similar in both languages is that deficits are evident across many domains of language, including vocabulary, length of utterance, morphology, phonology and language processing tasks. Whether one or more of these areas present particular difficulty beyond other areas is hard to determine. Those studies that have directly compared various areas within the same children do not single out a particular area (Elin Thordardottir & Namazi, 2007; Elin Thordardottir *et al.*, 2011).

Morphological error patterns appear to differ between French and English both in the particular error types, the error rates and the timing of vulnerability of particular linguistic structures. Morphological deficits in English PLI manifest most strongly around ages 4–6 years and are largely mastered around 10 years of age (Rice *et al.*, 2004; Rice & Wexler, 1996). In contrast, the studies on French that have proposed morphological difficulties have primarily focused on school-age children (Grüter, 2005; Jakubowicz, 2003; Jakubowicz *et al.*, 1998; Maillart & Parisse, 2006; Paradis & Crago, 2001) with few grammatical errors observed for preschool children (Elin Thordardottir & Namazi, 2007). Whether these age differences reflect a real difference in the manifestation of PLI in the two languages or are the result of methodological differences, including diagnostic criteria, the matching of control groups and the scope of the studies can only be determined by further research. The manifestation of PLI in the two languages is similar in that it involves a general language delay across domains of language, with performance significantly below that of unimpaired children of the same age.

Assessment of Language Abilities in French-speaking Children

The clinical evaluation of the language skills of French-speaking children has employed various methods, including qualitative observations, formal tests, informal measures and spontaneous language sampling. Far fewer standardized tests are available for French than for English, and as a result, the use of such tests has not played as prominent a role in the clinical assessment of French and diagnostic criteria have generally not been defined in terms of cutoff scores in relation to normative data. A greater number of standardized tests have been developed for French in Europe than in Canada. An overview of assessment measures currently available for use with French-speaking children is presented in Table 8.3. This overview is not meant to provide an exhaustive list of available tests for the assessment of French, nor to recommend particular tests beyond others that may have been omitted in this review, but rather to illustrate that such tests are increasingly being developed and their use is becoming more commonplace. Examples of tests assessing oral language skills include the ELO (Étude des stratégies de compréhension orale; Khomsi, 1987), the N-EEL (Nouvelles épreuves pour l'examen du langage; Chevrie-Muller & Plaza, 2001) and the L2MA-2 (La batterie langage oral, langage écrit, mémoire, attention; Chevrie-Muller et al., 2010). These widely used tests, which were developed and normed expressly for French, survey various aspects of language by means of subtests. Tests have also been developed for French to assess aspects of literacy skills, including spelling: Chronodictées (Baneath et al., 2006), oral and written language skills: BALE (Batterie Analytique du Langage Écrit; Jacquier-Roux et al., 2010) and reading: Alouette (Lefavrais, 1965–2005) and La forme noire (Maeder, 2011).

Table 8.3 Frequently used assessment tests in French

Test, Authors	Area of language	Age range	Origin	Adapted from English?
MacArthur–Bates CDI Kern (2007)	Gestures, vocabulary, grammar	8–30 months	France	Yes
MacArthur–Bates CDI Trudeau et al. (1999)	Gestures, vocabulary, grammar	8–30 months	Quebec	Yes
Test de concepts de base Boehm Boehm (1990)	Comprehension of basic concepts	3–5 years	France	Yes
N-EEL Chevrie-Muller and Plaza (2001)	Vocabulary, grammar, morphology, phonology	3–8 years	France	No
Carrow (TACL) Groupe coopératif (1999) and Elin Thordardottir et al. (2010)	Receptive language	K children 4;6–5;6	Quebec	Yes

(Continued)

Test, Authors	Area of language	Age range	Origin	Adapted from English?
ENNI Elin Thordardottir et al. (2010)	Narrative story grammar, cohesive ties	4;6–5;6	Quebec	Yes (but uses wordless picture stimuli)
Non-word repetition Elin Thordardottir et al. (2010, 2011)	Phonological short-term memory	4;6–5;6	Quebec	No
Systematic language sample analysis Elin Thordardottir (2005) and Table 8.1 and Figure 8.1 this chapter	Mean length of utterance in words and morphemes, morphological diversity	24–66 months	Quebec	Yes (analysis prin-ciples based on English tradition)
ELO Khomsi (1987)	Vocabulary, grammar	4–11 years	France	No
L2MA2 Chevrie-Muller et al. (2010)	Vocabulary, morphology, pro-cessing, reading, spelling	7–11 years	France	No
ECOSSE Lecocq (1996)	Semantic and syntactic comprehension	4–13 years	France	Yes
EVIP Dunn et al. (1997)	Receptive vocabulary	2;6–18 years	Canada	Yes
CELF-CDN-F Semel et al. (2009)	Vocabulary, gram-mar, language processing	4–16 years, depending on subtest	Quebec	Yes
Alouette Lefavrais (1965–2005)	Reading	6–6 years	France	No
Chronodictées Baneath et al. (2006)	Spelling	7–15 years	France	No
BALE Jacquier-Leroux et al. (2010)	Oral and written language	7– years	France	No
La forme noire Maeder (2010)	Reading comprehension	9–12 years	France and Quebec	No

Other published tests are available that have been adapted from tests originally constructed in English. These tests generally involve substantial modifications to account for linguistic differences as well as renorming in French. Examples of such tests are the France and the Quebec versions of the MacArthur–Bates CDI (Kern, 2007; Trudeau et al., 1999), the French version of the Boehm Test of Basic Concepts (Boehm, 1990), the Canadian EVIP (Échelle de vocabulaire en images; Peabody et al., 1993) – counterpart of the English PPVT (Dunn & Dunn, 1997), the Canadian French version of the CELF-4 (Évaluation Clinique des notions langagières fondamentales; Semel et al., 2009) and the ECOSSE (Épreuve de compréhension syntaxico-sémantique; Lecocq, 1996) – a French adaptation of the TROG (Test for Reception of Grammar; Bishop, 1982). In addition to the MacArthur CDI, another French parent report form, the DLPF (Développement du langage de production en français), which addresses lexical, grammatical and pragmatic development and covers a more extended age range, has been developed by Bassano et al. (2005). Norms on age of acquisition (AoA) have been reported for a set of 230 French words, obtained by objective testing on 280 French schoolchildren age 2;6–7 years and by a rating procedure (Chalard et al., 2003).

In addition to these commercially available tests, other test materials have been developed for French in research settings, which are available in published articles or from the research labs where they were developed, such as a French non-word repetition test with preliminary norms which appears in an appendix in Elin Thordardottir et al. (2011), and a test of phonological awareness for preschoolers (Lefebvre et al., 2008). Systematic analysis methods for spontaneous language samples with corresponding norms have been developed for French as well, including SALT analysis guidelines developed by Elin Thordardottir (2005) and a French version of the LARSP procedure (Maillart et al., 2012).

Normative data on French-speaking Quebec children ($n = 78$) in three age groups around 5 years of age (4;6, 5;0 and 5;6) targeting various aspects of language development were reported by Elin Thordardottir et al. (2010) in an effort to facilitate the clinical evaluation of five-year-old children. The selection of measures for this study was inspired by previous studies on areas to include in a complete clinical assessment conducted in English (Conti-Ramsden, 2003; Conti-Ramsden et al., 1997, 2001; Dollaghan & Campbell, 1998; Ellis Weismer et al., 2000; Tomblin et al., 1996). The areas included receptive vocabulary, receptive language, conversational MLU and narratives as well as measures targeting aspects of language processing: non-word repetition, sentence imitation, following directions, forward and backward digit span and rapid automatized naming. The specific measures included existing formal tests and measures adapted or developed expressly for this study. Receptive language was measured by the EVIP vocabulary test and the 'Carrow' (a Quebec French adaptation of the Test of Auditory

Comprehension of Language; Carrow-Woolfolk, 1985; Groupe coopératif, 1999). Measures developed for this study included a sentence imitation test adapted from the Clinical Evaluation of Language Fundamentals-Preschool (Wiig *et al.*, 1992, adapted by Royle & Elin Thordardottir, 2003) and a test of non-word repetition, adapted from a larger non-word list developed by Courcy (2000). In addition, a Canadian test of narrative ability, the Edmonton Narrative Norms Instrument (ENNI), originally developed for English by Schneider *et al.* (2002–2006) at the University of Alberta, was first adapted to French within this study. This test employs a series of wordless picture storybooks with stories of increasing length and complexity of story grammar. The stories told by the children as they view the books are transcribed and scored for Story Grammar, or the extent to which the children include the main elements of the story, for First Mentions, a measure of the children's ability to provide sufficient information as characters are first introduced, and for syntactic and morphological use.

The results of this study were provided in terms of descriptive data, including means and standard deviations for each of the measures for each of the age groups. Scores on each of the measures increased with age. Correlational analysis revealed associations of varying strengths between the measures. Only MLU had no significant association with any of the other measures, suggesting that it taps into a different linguistic skill than the other measures, which in turn overlapped somewhat in the skills they assess. In another study, MacLeod *et al.* (2010) reported normative data on the acquisition of consonants by Quebec French children age 20–53 months ($n = 156$). The measures were collected using a picture naming task and include consonant inventory, consonant accuracy, consonant acquisition and a comparison to English. The diagnostic accuracy of each of these measures for 5-year-old children was examined (see section on diagnostic criteria).

The adaptation of standardized English tests to French is surrounded by controversy. Table 8.3 specifies whether the tests were developed for French or involve a translation and/or adaptation of a test originally constructed in English. Some of the adapted tests have undergone validation studies that support their applicability to francophone children. For example, for the French CDI, Kern (2007) reported on the comprehension and production of vocabulary as well as gesture use of French-speaking children ages 8–16 months ($n = 548$). Boudreault *et al.* (2007) presented a validation and norming study of the Quebec version of the MacArthur–Bates, including 777 children between 8 and 30 months of age. Trudeau and Sutton (2011) provided further developmental milestones for lexical production in the 16–30 month range ($n = 826$). Other tests are modified to various extents based on theoretical criteria which may contribute to their construct validity. However, most of them are not subjected to further validation studies such as concurrent or predictive validity, nor is information on their diagnostic accuracy available in their manuals. The practice of adapting tests to French without proper revalidation has been criticized by Bouchard *et al.* (2009), who note that many tests are adapted which do not have good validity or psychometric properties even in their original version. An issue of equal concern is that even for a test of high quality in English, the properties of the translated version cannot be assumed without verification. In fact, any modified test is likely to be of lower quality than a test developed expressly for the language in which it is to be used.

The tests also vary in the geographical area and dialectal group for which they were developed, such that within a given region, tests may not be available that cover all areas of language in need of assessment. To some degree, tests developed in one geographical area are used in other areas. However, many problems are noted with such transfer reflecting linguistic and cultural differences. As an example, vocabulary items on the N-EEL, developed in France, include the colors brown and purple, which children in France and Quebec label, respectively, as *marron* or *brun* and *violet* or *mauve*. Another picture item on this test depicts an accordion, which Quebec children generally do not recognize and label as *piano*. Issues of this kind are generally relatively easy to deal with by small changes in the scoring criteria. However, other differences that involve more subtle grammatical, pragmatic or cultural differences may be harder to predict or to account for, with the result that their effect on the test score is unknown. Interestingly, Quebec speech-language pathologists vary in whether they prefer to use tests developed originally for another dialect of French or a test translated from English into Quebec French. Some state that they prefer the latter because they see North American tests as more fitting for cultural reasons. No systematic studies are available examining the extent to which the use of tests from Europe can provide an accurate assessment of Quebec children or vice versa. Given the current lack of a full set of ideal assessment procedures in either location, such an examination could help guide the choice of the most adequate test materials from those available.

The suitability of test items and norms also has to be carefully considered even when tests are used within the same country in which they were developed. An example of this is the EVIP test of receptive vocabulary and standardized on a pan-Canadian sample of French-speaking children, many of whom are bilingual to varying degrees, speaking French as their first or as their second language. Subsequent research involving large samples of monolingual French speakers from Quebec have revealed that these children perform substantially better than the published norms, by as much as a standard deviation (Godard & Labelle, 1995; Elin Thordardottir *et al.*, 2010). As a result, the French-Canadian norms of the EVIP are inappropriate for use with monolingual French speakers in Quebec and due to the large variation in language status in the norming sample, it is not clear which linguistic groups within Canada are adequately represented by the norms. The finding on the EVIP underscores the need for careful consideration of norming issues. French-speaking children in Canada range from monolingual native speakers to children having received significant exposure to French, often within French immersion educational settings, but for whom French is a second language. On the EVIP, the differences between these groups are clearly sufficiently large to call for separate norms. With the present norms, there is a substantial risk of underidentifying PLI in monolingual French speakers from Quebec and overidentifying PLI in bilingual children. Indeed, in a study on the diagnostic accuracy of the EVIP among other measures for the identification of PLI in monolingual French speakers in Quebec, a standard score of 100 (the mean score of the norms) was considered a failure on screening, calling for the need for further assessment. Similar to the EVIP, the norming sample of the CELF-CDN-F, although conducted entirely in Quebec, included both native monolingual speakers and children speaking French as their second language, having resided in Quebec as little as two years and being exposed to French as little as 50% of the time. For a more in-depth discussion of the effect of the amount of bilingual exposure on performance on language measures in French, the reader is referred to Elin Thordardottir (2011) and Elin Thordardottir and Brandeker (2013).

The translated versions of English tests may be more widespread in Canadian than European contexts given the lack of tests developed expressly for Canadian French and the proximity of an English-speaking community. In some cases, such versions of tests involve some modification and adaptation and some local norms have been developed (Groupe coopératif, 1999; Elin Thordardottir et al., 2010). Other tests used in clinical settings are simple 'in-house' translations, which are often used as descriptive measures only. However, the practice of applying the English norms is also fairly common, often with the caveat that this is done for information purposes only. Such a practice must be strongly discouraged given that providing this comparison in a clinical report increases the likelihood that it will be interpreted in some way regardless of the expressed caveat. Structural differences between French and English affect both lexical and grammatical measures (see e.g. Bassano, 2000; Elin Thordardottir, 2005; Trudeau & Sutton, 2011) and result in marked differences in the sequence of acquisition of particular structures as well as their vulnerability in children with language impairment. Therefore, a comparison with norms in a different language can be highly misrepresentative and should not be done. It should be noted also that the use of translated tests even if limited to a descriptive interpretation is problematic as well, for the same reasons. A test that is not developed for the language to be assessed produces a skewed picture of the child's development, which increases the risk of misdiagnosis. In addition, it draws the examiner's attention to aspects of language that are of relevance in the language of the test but may not be of equal relevance in the language being tested, which can misdirect intervention efforts.

Diagnostic accuracy and criteria for French PLI

Language assessment is conducted clinically for various purposes – one being the identification of language impairment. The identification involves a yes/no decision – the ruling in or ruling out of the disorder. However, the definition of *dysphasie* in French has not been associated with a clear set of criteria for clinical identification in terms of the areas of language that should be assessed, the specific tests, the cutoff criteria or other clinical markers (Le Normand, 2003). The traditional definition of *dysphasie* (Le Normand, 2003) is definitely different from that of SLI/ PLI. It is broader in that it includes children with dyspraxia and children with semantic–pragmatic disorder, who are not included in the definition of PLI. At the same time, it is narrower in that it includes only children with severe deficits that affect both comprehension and production. It is hard, however, to find specific guidelines on identification criteria. Clinical criteria may involve the observation of severe communicative difficulty, along with qualitative markers, many of which have emerged from clinical experience rather than systematic research. A systematic overview of such observations and criteria was developed by the Quebec Association of Speech-Language Pathologists and Audiologists (Ordre des orthophonistes et audiologistes du Québec; OOAQ, 2004) in an attempt to promote consistency across clinics, but these methods await systematic validation by research.

Elin Thordardottir *et al.* (2011) undertook an examination of the diagnostic accuracy of a number of clinical markers for the identification of PLI in Quebec French-speaking five-year-olds. This study used measures for which normative data were collected previously (Elin Thordardottir *et al.*, 2010): receptive vocabulary, receptive grammar, grammatical production in spontaneous language, narrative story grammar, rapid automatized naming, non-word repetition, sentence imitation and following directions (see previous section on assessment). In order to test for the diagnostic accuracy of each of these measures, a group of children with PLI were recruited to serve as the gold standard against which the accuracy of the language measures would be compared. For this purpose, given the differences between *dysphasie* and PLI and recent efforts in Quebec to move toward a revised definition, the study adopted a definition in line with that of PLI. Accordingly, clinical referral included children identified as having *dysphasie* except the subtypes manifesting primarily as dyspraxia or semantic pragmatic disorder. In addition, children manifesting strong signs of a persistent language impairment but not quite meeting the strict Quebec government criteria for *dysphasie* were included. Fourteen children with PLI thus identified were tested on each of the clinical measures. The 78 children in the normative study conducted previously served as children identified as having typical language development. They had been recruited based on no previous diagnosis of development impairment of any kind and no serious concerns about development.

Three diagnostic criteria frequently used in clinical identification were used: –1 SD, –1.3 SD (corresponding to the tenth percentile) and –2 SD (the criterion generally applied in Quebec when standardized tests are employed). Results revealed that the –2 SD criterion yielded perfect or near-perfect specificity for almost all of the measures, but very low levels of sensitivity, most in the range of 0–0.44. The measure with the highest sensitivity at this cutoff point was non-word repetition, at 0.77, which is considered unacceptably low (Plante & Vance, 1994). In other words, overdiagnosis had almost no likelihood of occurring at –2 SD, but the cost was that the majority (almost all) of children with PLI were missed. Moving the cutoff score closer to the mean increases sensitivity. However, clinically, the fear is typically that this results in unacceptable levels of false positives, meaning low levels of specificity. In this study, it was found that, of the three cutoff scores tested, the best combination of sensitivity and specificity was obtained at –1 SD, with several measures yielding sensitivity levels above 0.85 (EVIP, sentence imitation, non-word repetition), and one as high as 0.93 (following directions). Specificity for each of these measures remained as high as their sensitivity. Therefore, sensitivity was gained without significant loss of specificity. Logistic regression was used to examine whether any combination of two measures yielded higher accuracy levels than the best of the measures used singly. The only combination that achieved this was that of non-word repetition and the EVIP (receptive vocabulary).

It is important to note that the measures varied greatly in their diagnostic accuracy. Measures focusing on language processing (non-word repetition, sentence imitation, following directions) were generally more accurate in identifying PLI in the French-speaking children than measures of accumulated knowledge such as receptive vocabulary, grammar or spontaneous language, although the EVIP did well on its own. Some of the measures yielded asymmetric results. MLU proved to have fairly good specificity but unacceptably low sensitivity. The clinical implication is that a low MLU suggests a high likelihood of PLI, whereas an MLU within the normal range is uninformative and does not help much in ruling out PLI. This underscores the need for the careful examination of diagnostic accuracy across different measures and across different age groups. The validation of a measure as being developmentally sensitive and having appropriate norms for the population to be tested does not guarantee diagnostic accuracy. The goal of assessment should also be kept in mind. Some measures are better suited for the identification of impairment, whereas other measures may be more informative for in-depth assessment and intervention planning.

The results of this study have important implications for the clinical identification of PLI in French-speaking children as well as theoretical implications concerning its underlying nature. Clinically, it is important to note that the different measures of language varied considerably in their diagnostic accuracy, as documented previously for English measures (Plante & Vance, 1994). A common complaint among clinicians assessing French-speaking children is the lack of appropriate norms. The findings of this study are a useful reminder of the fact that collecting norms is necessary but not sufficient. The interpretation of the norm-referenced data needs to be guided by systematic study of the distribution of scores in groups of children with TD and PLI, which establishes the discriminant validity of the measure. On that note, it should be specified clearly that the present results on French refer to children age 5 years, and that it may be that different measures or areas of languages are most sensitive to PLI in other age groups. Information of this kind is still unavailable for a large number of English measures that are in wide clinical use. However, several studies on English have compared the diagnostic accuracy of a series of language measures (Conti-Ramsden et al., 1997, 2001; Tomblin et al., 1996). The French results are generally in good agreement with the English findings in that they show that various standardized tests can provide an accurate means of identification of PLI and that measures that target language processing are overall the most accurate. This in turn suggests that in spite of differences in the type and severity of morphosyntactic error patterns documented in the literature, PLI in both languages presents as a generalized delay in language development touching many areas of language and that language processing skills are involved as well.

Other potential assessment measures include linguistic markers that have been proposed in the research literature as potential clinical markers of PLI in French, including aspects of verb inflection and omission of the object clitic (Grüter, 2005; Hamann, 2003; Jakubowicz, 2003; Jakubowicz et al., 1998; Paradis & Crago, 2001). These were reviewed in a previous section. As mentioned there, the diagnostic accuracy of these potential markers has been suggested by the finding of group differences between children with PLI and children with TD, but it has not been adequately verified by testing the extent to which these markers correctly identify individual children as having or not having PLI. Before these markers can be applied clinically, further research is needed into the clinical utility of these clinical markers and the age ranges in which they are most accurate. Similarly, systematic research has not been carried out to establish the most appropriate cutoff levels for particular standardized tests in French in relation to *dysphasie* or PLI.

Concluding Remarks

A comparison of language development and manifestation of PLI across languages is a good exercise in reflecting on which aspects of what we consider general truths about language development are universal and which ones must be rediscovered for each language. This is particularly relevant for clinicians who were trained in one language but work in another, and for clinicians who wonder to what extent research findings obtained in one language can be applied to another language. The great majority of the research literature on language development and developmental language disorders has focused on English, in spite of increasing cross-linguistic research. Therefore, many clinicians find themselves faced with these very questions.

The research reviewed in this chapter has revealed that the structure and acquisition of French differs in many important ways from English as does the manifestation of PLI in terms of which language structures are vulnerable at different ages and in terms of error rates and patterns. Grammatical morphology is more complex in French – its acquisition starts earlier than in English and also takes longer; however, it is not as severely affected by PLI as it is in English. The review also indicates many general similarities between the languages. For example, in English and French, language development follows a typical sequence across children, although the sequence is not the same in the two languages. Measures such as vocabulary size, MLU, morphological diversity and other norm-referenced measures can be used to document individual children's language level and compare it to that of other children of the same age or same language level, and to compare the child's performance across domains of language to identify strengths and weaknesses. Further, normative measures of accumulated language knowledge and in particular measures of language processing such as non-word repetition lead to the accurate identification of PLI in both languages. Both languages are similar, therefore, in that children with PLI evidence deficits in language processing and manifest a linguistic profile similar to that of younger children with TD speaking that same language; however, this profile differs in important ways between the languages.

Note

(1)   The term *primary language impairment* (PLI) is used in this chapter synonymously with specific language impairment (SLI). PLI is preferred here as it more clearly denotes an impairment manifesting *primarily* rather than *exclusively* in the area of language. These terms, however, refer to the same group of children and imply no differences in diagnostic criteria.

References

Baneath, B., Alberti, C. and Boutard, C. (2006) *Chronodictées: outils d'évaluation des performances orthographiques avec et sans contrainte temporelle.* Isbergues: Ortho Édition.

Bassano, D. (2000) Early development of nouns and verbs and verbs in French: Exploring the interface between lexicon and grammar. *Journal of Child Language* 27, 521–559.

Bassano, D., Labrell, F., Champaud, C., Lemetayer, F. and Bonnet, P. (2005) Le DLPF: un nouvel outil pour l'évaluation du développement du langage de production en français. *Enfance* 57, 171–208.

Bassano, D., Maillochon, I. and Mottet, S. (2008) Noun grammaticalization and determiner use in French children's speech: A gradual development with prosodic and lexical influences. *Journal of Child Language* 35, 403–438.

Bishop, D.M.V. (1982) *Test of Reception of Grammar (TROG).* Oxford: Pearson.

Boehm, A.E. (1990) *Test des concepts de base de Boehm, version pré-scolaire* Éditions du Centre de Psychologie Appliquée. Paris, France.

Bortolini, U. Arfé, B., Caselli, C., Degasperi, L., Deevy, P. and Leonard, L. (2006) Clinical markers for specific language impairment in Italian: The contribution of clitics and nonword repetition. *International Journal of Language and Communication Disorders* 41, 695–712.

Bouchard, M.-E., Fitzpatrick, E. and Olds, J. (2009) Psychometric analysis of assessment tools using with francophone children. *Canadian Journal of Speech-Language Pathology and Audiology* 33, 129–138.

Bouchard, C., Trudeau, N., Sutton, A., Boudreault, M.-C. and Deneault, J. (2009) Gender differences in language development in French Canadian children between 8 and 30 months of age. *Applied Psycholinguistics* 30, 685–707.

Boudreault, M.-C., Cabirol, É.-A., Trudeau, N., Poulin-Dubois, D. and Sutton, A. (2007) Les inventaires MacArthur du développement de la communication: validité et données normatives préliminaires. *Canadian Journal of Speech-Language Pathology and Audiology* 31, 27–37.

Carrow-Woolfolk, E. (1985) *Test for the Auditory Comprehension of Language – Revised.* Allen, TX: DLM Teaching Resources.

Chalard, M., Bonin, P., Méot, A., Boyer, B. and Fayol, M. (2003) Objective age-of-acquisition (AoA) norms for a set of 230 object names in French: Relationships with psycho-linguistic variables, the English data from Morrison et al. (1997) and naming latencies. *European Journal of Cognitive Psychology* 15, 209–245.

Chevrie-Muller, C. and Plaza, M. (2001) *Nouvelles Epreuves Pour L'Examen du Langage* Editions du Centre de Psychologie Appliquée. Paris, France.

Chevrie-Muller, C., Maillart, C., Simon, A.-M. and Fournier, S. (2010) *La batterie language oral, langage écrit, mémoire, attention, L2MA2* (2nd edn). Toronto: Pearson.

Chevrot. J.-P., Dugua, C. and Fayol, M. (2009) Liaison acquisition, word segmentation and construction in French: A usage based account. *Journal of Child Language* 36, 557–596.

Clahsen, H. (1989) The grammatical characterization of developmental dysphasia. *Linguistics* 27, 897–920.

Conti-Ramsden, G. (2003) Processing and linguistic markers in young children with specific language impairment. *Journal of Speech, Language and Hearing Research* 46, 1029–1037.

Conti-Ramsden, G., Crutchley, A. and Botting, N. (1997) The extent to which psychometric tests differentiate subgroups of children with SLI. *Journal of Speech, Language and Hearing Research* 40, 765–777.

Conti-Ramsden, G., Botting, N. and Faragher, B. (2001) Psycholinguistic markers for specific language impairment (SLI). *Journal of Speech, Language, and Hearing Research* 46, 1029–1037.

Courcy, A. (2000) Conscience Phonologique et apprentissage de la lecture. Unpublished doctoral dissertation, Université de Montréal.

Dollaghan, C. and Campbell, T. (1998) Nonword repetition and children language impairment. *Journal of Speech, Language and Hearing Research* 41, 1136–1146.

Dunn, L. and Dunn, L. (1997) *Peabody Picture Vocabulary Test – III.* Circle Pines, MN: AGS.

Dunn, L., Thériault-Whalen, C. and Dunn, L. (1993) *Echelle de vocabulaire en images Peabody: Adaptation francaise du Peabody Picture Vocabulary Test.* Toronto, Ontario: PsyCan.

Elin Thordardottir (2005) Early lexical and syntactic development in Quebec French and English: Implications for cross-linguistic and bilingual assessment. *International Journal of Language and Communication Disorders* 40, 243–278.

Elin Thordardottir (2008) Language specific effects of task demands on the manifestation of specific language impairment: A comparison of English and Icelandic. *Journal of Speech, Language, and Hearing Research* 51, 922–937.

Elin Thordardottir (2011) The relationship between bilingual exposure and vocabulary development. *International Journal of Bilingualism* 14 (5), 426–445. DOI: 10.1177/1367006911403202

Elin Thordardottir and Namazi, M. (2007) Specific language impairment in French-speaking children: Beyond grammatical morphology. *Journal of Speech, Language, and Hearing Research* 50, 698–715.

Elin Thordardottir and Brandeker, M. (2013) The effect of bilingual exposure versus language impairment on nonword repetition and sentence imitation scores. *Journal of Communication Disorders* 46, 1–16.

Elin Thordardottir, Ellis Weismer, S. and Evans, J.L. (2002) Continuity in lexical and morphological development in Icelandic and English-speaking 2-year-olds. *First Language* 22, 3–28.

Elin Thordardottir, Rothenberg, A., Rivard, M.-E. and Naves, R. (2006) Bilingual assessment: Can overall proficiency be estimated from separate measurement of two languages? *Journal of Multilingual Communication Disorders* 4 (1), 1–21.

Elin Thordardottir, Kehayia, E., Lessard, N., Sutton, A. and Trudeau, N. (2010) Typical performance on tests of language knowledge and language processing of French-speaking 5-year-olds. *Canadian Journal of Speech Language Pathology and Audiology* 34, 5–16.

Elin Thordardottir, Gagne, A., Levy, J., Kehayia, E., Lessaud, N., Sutton, A. and Trudeau, N. (2005) Spontaneous language sample measures for French-speaking 5-year-olds. Poster presented at the annual ASHA Convention, San Diego, CA, November.

Elin Thordardottir, Kehayia, E., Mazer, B., Lessard, N., Majnemer, A., Sutton, A., Trudeau, N. and Chilingaryan, G. (2011) Sensitivity and specificity of French language and processing measures for the identification of primary language impairment at age 5. *Journal of Speech, Language, and Hearing Research* 54, 580–597.

Ellis Weismer, S., Tomblin, B., Zhang, X., Buckwalter, P., Chynoweth, J. and Jones, M. (2000) Nonword repetition performance in school-age children with and without language impairment. *Journal of Speech, Language, and Hearing Research* 48, 865–878.

Gabriel, A., Maillart, C., Guillaume, M., Stefaniak, N. and Meulemans, T. (2011) Exploration of serial structure procedural learning in children with language impairment. *Journal of International Neuropsychological Society* 17, 336–343.

Gayraud, F. and Kern, S. (2007) Caractéristiques phonologiques des noms en fonction de l'âge d'acquisition. *Enfance* 59, 324–338.

Godard, L. and Labelle, M. (1995) Utilisation de l'EVIP avec une population québecoise. *Fréquences* 7, 18–21.

Groupe coopératif en orthophonie – Région Laval, Laurentides, Lanaudière (1999) Épreuve de compréhension de Carrow-Woolfolk, adaptation du TACL-R (Comprehension measure of Carrow-Woolfolk, adaptation of the TACL-R). Montreal, Quebec: Ordre des orthophonistes et audiologistes du Québec.

Grüter, T. (2005) Comprehension and production of French object clitics by child second language learners and children with specific language impairment. *Applied Psycholinguistics* 26 (3), 363–391.

Hamann, C. (2003) Phenomena in French normal and impaired language acquisition and their implications for hypotheses on language development. *Probus* 15, 91–122.

Hamann, C., Rizzi, L. and Frauenfelder, U. (1996) On the acquisition of subject and object clitics in French. In H. Clahsen (ed.) *Generative Perspectives on Language Acquisition* (pp. 309–334). Amsterdam: John Benjamins.

Hamann, C., Ohayon, S., Dubé, S., Frauenfelder, U., Rizzi, L., Starke, M. and Zesiger, P. (2003) Aspects of grammatical development in young French children with SLI. *Developmental Science* 6, 151–158.

Hickmann, M. (1997) The acquisition of French as a native language: Structural and functional determinants in a crosslinguistic perspective. *Journal of Speech-Language Pathology and Audiology* 21, 236–257.

Jacquier-Roux, M., Lequette, C., Pouget, G., Valdois, S. and Zorman, M. (2010) *BALE: Batterie Analytique du Langage*. Grenoble: Laboratoire des sciences de l'éducatio, UPMF-Grenoble.

Jakubowicz, C. (2003) Computational complexity and the acquisition of functional categories by French-speaking children with SLI. *Linguistics* 41, 175–211.

Jakubowicz, C., Nash, L., Rigaut, C. and Gérard, C.-L. (1998) Determiners and clitic pronouns in French-speaking children with SLI. *Language Acquisition* 7, 113–160.

Kern, S. (2007) Lexicon development in French-speaking infants. *First Language* 27, 227–250.

Khomsi, A. (1987) Épreuve d'evaluation des strategies de comprehension en situation orale, 0-52. *Editions du Centre de Psychologie Appliquée*. Paris, France.

Lecocq, P. (1996) *Epreuve de comprehension syntaxico semantique (ECOSSE)*. Paris: Editions du Septention.

Lefavrais, P. (1965–2005) *Alouette-R*. Paris: ECPA (Les Editions du Centre de Psychologie Appliquée).

Lefebvre, P., Girard, C., Desrosiers, K., Trudeau, N. and Sutton, A. (2008) Phonological awareness tests for French-speaking preschoolers. *Canadian Journal of Speech Language Pathology and Audiology* 32, 158–167.

Le Normand, M.-T. (2003) Retards de langage et dysphasies. In J.A. Rondal and X. Seron (eds) *Trouble du langage: bases théoriques, diagnostic et re-education* (pp. 727–747). Sprimont: Mardaga.

Le Normand, M., Leonard, L.B. and McGregor, K.K. (1993) A cross-linguistic study of article use by children with specific language impairment. *European Journal of Disorders in Communication* 28 (2), 153–163.

Le Normand, M.-T., Parisse, C. and Cohen, H. (2008) Lexical diversity and productivity in French preschoolers: Developmental gender and sociocultural factors. *Clinical Linguistics and Phonetics* 22, 47–58.

Leonard, L. (1989) Language learnability and specific language impairment in children. *Applied Psycholinguistics* 10, 179–202.

Leonard, L. (1998) *Children with Specific Language Impairment*. Cambridge, MA: The MIT Press.

Leroy, S., Parisse, C. and Maillart, C. (2012) Analogical reasoning in children with specific language impairment. *Clinical Linguistics and Phonetics* 26, 380–395.

MacLeod, A., Sutton, A., Trudeau, N. and Elin Thordardottir (2010) Phonological development in quebecois French: A cross-sectional study of preschool age children. *International Journal of Speech-Language Pathology*, Early Online 1–17.

Maeder, C. (2010) *La forme noire: Test de compréhension écrite de récits*. Isbergues: Ortho Édition.

Maillart, C. and Parisse, C. (2006) Phonological deficits in French-speaking children with SLI. *International Journal of Language and Communication Disorders* 41 (3), 253–274.

Maillart, C. and Parisse, C. (2008) Dislocations as a developmental marker in French language: A preliminary study. *Clinical Linguistics and Phonetics* 22, 255–258.

Maillart, C., Parisse, C. and Tommerdahl, J. (2012) F-LARSP 1.0: An adaptation of the LARSP language profile for French. *Clinical Linguistics and Phonetics* 26, 188–198.

Marchman, V. and Bates, E. (1994) Continuity in lexical and morphological development: A test of the critical mass hypothesis. *Journal of Child Language* 21, 339–366.

Marcus, G. (1996) Why do children say 'breaked'? *Current Directions in Psychological Science* 5, 81–85.

Matthews, D., Lieven, E., Theakston, A. and Tomasello, M. (1997) French children's use and correction of weird word orders: A constructivist account. *Journal of Child Language* 34, 381–409.

Miller, J. and Chapman, R. (1984–2002) *Systematic Analysis of Language Transcripts: Software for Analyzing English and Spanish Language Transcripts*. University of Wisconsin, MA: Language Analysis Laboratory.

Nicoladis, E. and Paradis, J. (2012) Acquiring regular and irregular past tense morphemes in English and French: Evidence from bilingual children. *Language Learning* 62, 170–197.

Ordre des orthophonistes et audiologistes du Québec (2004) *Guide et outils cliniques: Trouble primaire du langage, dysphasie (Clinical Guidelines and Tools: Primary Language Impairment, Dysphasia)*. Montreal, Quebec: Author.

Paradis, J. and Crago, M. (2001) The morphosyntax of specific language impairment in French: An extended optional default account. *Language Acquisition* 9, 269–300.

Paradis, J., Crago, M. and Genesee, F. (2009) Domain-general versus domain-specific accounts of specific language impairment: Evidence from bilingual children's acquisition of object pronouns. *Language Acquisition* 13, 33–62.

Pérez-Leroux, A., Pirvulescu, M. and Roberge, Y. (2011) Topicalization and object omission in child language. *First Language* 31, 280–299.

Pirvulescu, M. and Hill, M. (2012) Object clitic omission in French-speaking children: Effects of the elicitation task. *Language Acquisition* 19, 73–81.

Pizzioli, F. and Schelstraete, M.-A. (2008) Argument-structure complexity in children with specific language impairment: Evidence from the use of grammatical morphemes in French. *Journal of Speech, Language, and Hearing Research* 51, 1–16.

Plante, E. and Vance, R. (1994) Diagnostic accuracy of two tests of preschool language. *American Journal of Speech-Language Pathology* 4, 70–76.

Rice, M. and Wexler, K. (1996) Toward tense as a clinical marker for specific language impairment in English-speaking children. *Journal of Speech and Hearing Research* 39, 1239–1257.

Rice, M., Tomblin, B., Hoffman, L., Richman, W. A. and Marquis, J. (2004) Grammatical tense deficits in children with SLI and non-specific language impairment: Longitudinal considerations. *Journal of Speech, Language, and Hearing Research* 47, 816–834.

Rondal, J.-A. (2003) Langage oral. In J.A. Rondal and X. Seron (eds) *Trouble du langage: bases théoriques, diagnostic et re-education* (pp. 375–411). Sprimont: Mardaga.

Royle, P. and Elin Thordardottir (2003) Le grand déménagement. French adaptation of the Recalling Sentences in Context subtest of the CELF-P. Unpublished research tool, McGill University.

Royle, P. and Elin Thordardottir (2008) Elicitation of the passé compose in French preschoolers with and without specific language impairment. *Applied Psycholinguistics* 29, 341–365.

Schneider, P., Dubé, R. and Hayward, D. (2002–2006) The Edmonton Narrative Norms Instrument. University of Alberta Faculty of Rehabilitative Medicine website. http://www.rehabmed.ualberta.ca/spa/enni (accessed 25 May 2015).

Semel, E., Wiig, E., Secord, W., Boulianne, L. and Labelle, M. (2009) *Évaluation clinique des notions langagières fondamentales: Version pour francophones au Canada.* Toronto: Pearson Canada Assessment.

Tomblin, J.B., Records, N. and Zhang, X. (1996) A system for the diagnosis of specific language impairment in kindergarten children. *Journal of Speech and Hearing Research* 39, 1284–1294.

Trudeau, N. and Sutton, A. (2011) Expressive vocabulary and early grammar of 16- to 30-month-old children acquiring Quebec French. *First Language* 31, 480–507.

Trudeau, N., Frank, I. and Poulin-Dubois, D. (1999) Une adaptation en francais québecois du MacArthur Communicative Development Inventory. *Journal of Speech-Language Pathology and Audiology* 23, 31–73.

Wiig, E., Secord, W. and Semel, E. (1992) *Clinical Evaluation of Language Fundamentals, Preschool.* San Antonio, TX: The Psychological Corporation.

Zesiger, P., Zesiger, L., Arabatzi, M., Baranzini, L., Cronel-Ohayon, S., Franck, J. and Frauenfelder, U. (2010) The acquisition of pronouns by French-speaking children: A parallel study of production and comprehension. *Applied Psycholinguistics* 31, 571–603.

Zourou, F., Ecalle, J., Magnan, A. and Sanchez, M. (2010) The fragile nature of phonological awareness in children with specific language impairment: Evidence from literacy development. *Child Language Teaching and Therapy* 26, 347–358.

9 Comparing Measures of Spontaneous Speech of Turkish-Speaking Children With and Without Language Impairment

Seyhun Topbaş and İlknur Maviş

Children with language impairments (LIs) have deficits in one or more of the language areas, including phonology, syntax, morphology, semantics and pragmatics. In Turkey, identification of children with LI has recently been raised as an important issue. Speech-language therapy (SLT) is a young profession in Turkey, although it is growing rapidly (Topbaş, 2006). As part of the new professional law establishing SLT, regulations set forth by the Ministry of Health (2011) in cooperation with the Ministry of National Education (MoNE, 2014) included obligations to offer SLT services to individuals with speech-language impairments. Until a decade ago, the identification of children with LIs (including those who would now be diagnosed with specific language impairment [SLI]) was left to the intuition of doctors or other professionals' opinions. Language disorders were (a) included along with developmental disabilities occurring secondary to hearing impairment, mental retardation, learning disabilities, autism and other organic, neurological or psychiatric disorders; or (b) denied altogether, often by taking a wait-and-see approach for many years. No doubt, many children were inappropriately underdiagnosed or unattended.

According to the results of the first and only countrywide disability survey in Turkey by the State Institute of Statistics & State Planning Organization in 2006, speech impairment occurred in only 0.38% of the Turkish population. This rate did not include language disorders considered to be either primary LI or LI secondary to developmental disabilities, autism, hearing impairment, mental retardation or visual, physical or emotional disabilities. On the other hand, there has been an increase in the caseloads of SLTs, which consist mostly of preschool and school-age children who exhibit delayed language and/or LI with unknown etiologies, i.e. SLI (Topbaş, 2006, 2010b). Families who are now more aware of the SLT profession are seeking help for their children. In light of this situation, the focus of this chapter will be on developing language measures that will identify children with LIs including delayed language development and children with SLIs. In this chapter, a very brief summary of the Turkish language and of typical development will be given, followed by a review of research on atypical language development (ALD). Efforts to develop standardized Turkish language tests are summarized and recent findings comparing the performance of children with and without LI on a variety of measures from language samples are presented.

Major Relevant Characteristics of the Turkish Language and Language Development

Turkish is a highly inflected, agglutinative language, belonging to the Turkic family of the Ural-Altaic group. Inflection appears as suffixation where the derived and inflected suffixes are added to the root of nouns and verbs with rich combinations to create new meanings. Rarely, some prefixes and infixes are also used in foreign adapted words. The order of morphemes is fixed in that derivational morphemes precede the inflectional ones. A word can be a nominal (noun, pronoun, adjective), adverb, verb, postposition, conjunction, interjection or a discourse connective (Göksel & Kerslake, 2005).

The neutral word order is subject-object-verb (SOV), but word order is flexible for the pragmatic purposes of signaling topic-focus (Erguvanlı, 1984). In general, sentence-initial position is the topic position. According to Kornfilt (1997), topicalized constituents move to the sentence-initial position, backgrounded constituents move to the post-verbal position and new information or focused constituents occur immediately before the verb.

Basic grammatical relations depend on the use of inflectional marking on verbs and nouns. Noun phrases (NPs) are made transparent via case marking, permitting word-order variation. Object NPs are often overtly case marked but subject NPs are not. The subject pronouns *ben* (I) and *siz* (you) are typically omitted since inflectional morphemes on verbs (-*ım*, -*sunuz*) indicate the person and number of the subject being marked as predicates. Object nouns may also be omitted depending on the context of utterance. Gender is not expressed in nouns or pronouns and it does not affect agreement; thus, gender is not expressed grammatically in Turkish (for a brief review, see Yavaş, 2010).

The course of language development is summarized based on the comprehensive review of Aksu-Koç (2010). With respect to *timing and order of acquisition in Turkish*, the rich and regular morphology is acquired from 1;6 onward. By age 2;6, children command verb and noun inflections in simple sentences. There is a simultaneous emergence of verb and noun inflections, but nominal inflections are more subject to errors than verb inflections. Case marking follows a pattern of dative < accusative < locative < genitive < ablative < instrumental (Topbaş *et al.*, 2007). Among those, the dative and accusative markers appear much earlier and are more frequent than the other cases, but they are produced with more errors in some contexts. Because they are core cases in syntactic relations, they might be subject to more constraints that arise from the particular properties of the verbs with which they are used as arguments. Other factors that may cause difficulty are the complex interaction of the syntactic function of the accusative as a direct object marker with the pragmatic functions of word order, and the semantic features of objects such as specificity and referentiality. To sum up, in general, grammatical morphology in simple sentences is acquired at an early stage, although mastery necessarily waits upon further developments in complex syntax and semantics in the following years (Aksu-Koç, 2010; Ketrez & Aksu-Koç, 2009; Maviş & Ege, 2002; Özcan & Topbaş, 2000; Topbaş *et al.*, 1997, 2012).

Studies on Atypical Language Development in Turkey

Although there is substantial research on phonological disorders (an extensive summary can be found in Topbaş and Yavaş [2006] and Topbaş [2007]), there are few linguistic descriptions of childhood language disorders pertaining to either SLI or other developmental disorders in Turkish-speaking children (Özcan & Topbaş, 1994; Topbaş & Özcan, 1995). In this section, we summarize the current findings from the limited research available on the language characteristics of Turkish-speaking children with LI.

Acarlar (2008) compared the use of verb and noun morphology in Turkish children with ALD and children with typical language development (TLD) who were matched by mean length of utterance in words (MLU-W). The ALD group consisted of three children with pervasive developmental disorders, five children with general language delay, one child with autism and one with SLI. Language samples were transcribed and coded for inflectional morphology using the Turkish-Systematic Analysis of Language Transcripts (T-SALT; Acarlar *et al.*, 2006) conventions and were analyzed for MLU-W, MLU in morphemes (MLU-M) and frequency and percentage use of a representative set of noun and verb affixes in obligatory contexts. The typically developing (TD) children made no morphological errors whereas the children with ALD at the same MLU level had difficulty with noun affixes, but not verb affixes. Both groups were error free in their use of verb morphology. An analysis of error patterns on noun affixes indicated a protracted course of development for children with ALD. Mastery of each affix seemed to occur at a later MLU than for the TLD group.

Güven *et al.* (2009) reported data on the morphosyntactic characteristics of children with SLI and TD children. The data of three children with SLI (mean age = 5;7) were compared with three age-matched and three language-matched TD children from the T-SALT database (mean MLU = 4.23). Spontaneous speech in conversational and narrative samples was analyzed using standard T-SALT measures, including MLU-W and MLU-M and accuracy of tense and non-tense morpheme use. The findings indicated that the productivity of Turkish children with SLI was delayed in that they used less complex sentences than the age- and language-matched children and they made more errors morphosyntactically. Turkish-speaking children with SLI used significantly fewer morphemes than both age-matched TD peers ($p = 0.05$) and language-matched children from the T-SALT database ($p = 0.05$). The authors also determined how often sentences of different lengths were used. Results indicated that children with SLI communicated mostly with short utterances (30% were one-word utterances and only 20% utterances were more than four words). In contrast, age-matched TD peers communicated mostly with sentences that consisted of more than three words (38.2%).

Next, the authors compared correct tense and non-tense morpheme use of the children to the age-matched and MLU-matched TD peers. Children with SLI produced more tense and non-tense morpheme errors (mean tense = 29.8%; mean non-tense = 26.2%) than the age-matched (mean tense = 0%; mean non-tense = 0%) and the MLU-matched (mean tense = 0%; mean non-tense = 1.3%) TD peers. The number and percentage of errors on tense and non-tense morpheme errors were very similar among the Turkish-speaking children with SLI. In addition, almost all the children in the group of typical language learners used many non-tense morphemes in complex sentences. Although some of the morphemes that the TD matches used in complex sentences were incorrect, the meaning was still clear in spite of the errors. In contrast, children with SLI used fewer morphemes than TD children.

In another study, Topbaş and Güven (2008) (cf. Topbaş, 2010a) focused on quantitative analyses of sentence repetition items on the TEDİL, the Turkish version of the Test of Early Language Development, Third Edition (TELD-3), to identify differences between TD ($n = 30$) and SLI children's ($n = 30$) capacity in repeating simple versus complex sentences and to identify any differences in error types. The number and type of errors in each sentence was analyzed in the following order: (a) the number of complete repetitions, incomplete repetitions and non-repetitions were compared to the target sentences; (b) specific error types in each incomplete sentence repetition (omission, addition of new elements, word-order inversion, errors of bound morphology and lexical substitutions); and (c) errors in simple versus complex types.

The results of the study indicated that children with SLI performed worse than their age-matched peers, with the majority of the errors consisting of omission of elements and errors of bound morphology. TD children and children with SLI were able to repeat many of the case markings but particular difficulties were observed with noun morphology in contrast to children learning other languages who have more trouble with verb morphology. When sentences required more processing, either omissions or lexical and morphological substitutions occurred. In general, the majority of children changed the structure of complex sentences to simpler constructions, either by omitting the whole subordinate clause or by deleting the non-obligatory constituents such as adverbial phrases, whereas some children's repetitions were totally ungrammatical. The analysis of errors in simple versus complex sentences yielded differences between the TD and SLI groups. Bound morphological errors were evident in both the simple and complex sentence repetitions of children with SLI while TD children had errors in only 3% of the complex sentences.

Acarlar and Johnston (2011) elaborated their earlier study of grammatical morphology with developmental disorders. Language samples were collected from 30 preschoolers: 10 children with developmental disorders, 10 TD children matched by age and 10 TD children matched by length of utterance. T-SALT then generated MLU-M, the total number of noun errors, the total number of verb errors and the percentage use in obligatory contexts for noun suffixes. The potential effects of input frequency on the order of acquisition were analyzed as well. Turkish children in the MLU-W control group, aged 3;4, used noun and verb suffixes with virtually no errors. Children in the group with atypical language showed more persistent morphological errors than either age or language matches, especially on noun suffixes. Children with ALD and children in the MLU-W-matched group were acquiring noun case suffixes in an order that was strongly related to input frequencies. The findings of Acarlar and Johnston seem to reflect the influence of salience, regularity and frequency on language learning.

A general conclusion can be inferred from the scarce evidence that Turkish children with SLI showed difficulties with grammatical morphology like children with SLI in other languages. At the same time, language patterns seen in children with SLI may differ from one language type to the next; for example, greater difficulty occurs with noun morphology in Turkish-speaking children with SLI in contrast with greater difficulty with verb morphology in English-speaking children with SLI. Children acquiring Turkish may have greater difficulty with those features of grammar that have higher cognitive processing costs. However, many aspects of TLD and ALD have yet to be investigated in depth in Turkish children before conclusions can be drawn. Other than those studies outlined above, there are ongoing studies on both monolingual and bilingual children with LIs mainly with SLI (COST Action Project IS0804; Maviş & Ölmez, n.d.; Topbaş, 2010a; Yarbay-Duman *et al.*, 2015; Yarbay-Duman & Topbaş, n.d.).

Language Assessment in Atypical Children

As mentioned above, the development of the SLT profession in Turkey and the inclusion of speech-language disorders within the legislation called for a need for valid and accurate diagnosis/assessment. This ultimately required comparison of a child's performance with a normative group (Merrell & Plante, 1997; Spaulding *et al.*, 2006). Consequently, a logical and timely first step was adapting tests from English to Turkish for normative assessment (cf. Topbaş, 2010b). Table 9.1 shows a list of some examples of language tests used in Turkey.

A challenge in the diagnosis of LI is that standardized language tests used to identify the condition may not work in translation, and they can only be interpreted if adequate norms exist for typical performance at different ages. In many countries, such data do not exist. Furthermore, even in English-speaking countries, there are difficulties in making international comparisons, because tests may be culturally specific (Parisse & Maillart, 2009). Standardized psychometric discrepancy criteria are more restrictive and perhaps less sensitive to LI than is clinical judgment based on a child's language performance in naturalistic contexts. While formal testing may ask children to engage in activities that are foreign to their experience, language sampling has the advantage of sampling a natural behavior of children. Due to the considerations discussed above, standardized tests are suggested to be only one aspect of a comprehensive assessment process (Šišková, 2012).

Measures of natural language samples

Measures derived from natural language samples require a significant investment of time; yet, they provide an index of the child's use of language in everyday informal settings and are especially useful for assessing a variety of pragmatic and discourse skills. Goffman and Leonard (2000) recommended using measures from natural language samples to assess language growth in children with SLI. Measures from natural language samples offer an assessment of a child's 'real-time language performance'. Such measures reveal a child's individual linguistic knowledge through verbal performance (Condouris *et al.*, 2003; Evans, 1996).

The use of objective measures from spontaneous language samples may provide a more clinically and ecologically valid approach to the

Table 9.1 Language tests used in Turkey

Tool	Age range	Author(s)	Norms
Test of Early Language Development-TELD-3: Turkish (Türkçe Erken Dil Gelişim Testi-TEDİL)	2;0– 6;11 years	Topbaş and Güven (2011)	+
Test of Language Development-TOLD-4: Turkish (Türkçe Okul Çağı Dil Gelişim Testi-TODİL)	4;0–9;11 years	Topbaş and Güven (in preparation)	+
CDI-MacArthur Communicative Inventory: Turkish (TİGE I and TİGE II-Türkçe İletişim Gelişim Envanteri)	08–18 months and 19–36 months	Aksu-Koç et al. (2012)	+
MLU as a Tool for Turkish Assessment	18–59 months	Ege (2010)	+
Preschool Language Scale (PLS-3): Turkish	2;0–6;0 years	Yalçınkaya and Belgin (2010)	Ongoing
T-SALT-Systematic Analysis of Language Transcripts-Turkish (Version 9) [computer software]	2;6–6;6	Acarlar et al. (2006)	+
TİFALDİ-Turkish Receptive & Expressive Language (Vocabulary) Test (Türkçe Alıcı ve İfade Edici Dil (Sözcük) Testi)	2;0–15 years	Güven and Berument (2010)	+
Sentence Repetition Test-Turkish (adaptation of SASIT by Marinis)	5;0–7;11 years	Topbaş et al. (in preparation within COST Action IS0804)	N/A
LDS-Turkish: Language Development Survey (DİLTAR-Dil Tarama Envanteri)	18–35 months	Topbaş et al. (in preparation)	+
LARSP for Turkish (TR-LARSP)	09 months–7;0 years	Topbaş et al. (2012)	N/A

identification of children with SLI than psychometric measures. A study by Dunn *et al.* (1996) compared the sensitivity of standardized test measures to measures derived from natural language samples for diagnosing SLI in English-speaking children. They found that measures from natural language samples, specifically MLU and percentage of utterances containing structural errors, were better at defining SLI than were the psychometric tests that had been given to the children in their study. These findings have important implications for clinicians and researchers who depend on these types of language measures for diagnostic purposes, assessment and investigations of language impairments in LI. However, few studies in Turkey have compared the use of spontaneous language measures of language in TD children and children with language difficulties due to different etiologies (Acarlar, 2008; Acarlar & Johnston, 2010, 2011; Ege & Erdem, 2008; Tüfekçioğlu, 2010) and SLI (Güven et al., 2009; Topbaş, 2010a).

Lexical measures

Measures of lexical diversity have been widely used in studies of language development and disorders. An intuitively straightforward measure of lexical diversity is the number of different words (NDW) used in a language sample. NDW has proved to be a potentially useful measure of child language development (Klee, 1992; Miller, 1991). However, NDW is dependent on the length of the language sample, and some form of standardization may be desired in comparing samples (e.g. using samples of fixed length, such as 50 or 100 utterances) (Lu, 2012).

Another traditional lexical diversity measure is the ratio of different words (types) to the total number of words (TNW; tokens), the so-called type-token ratio (TTR; e.g. Bates et al., 1988; Lieven, 1978). However, this measure has been criticized for its sensitivity to sample size since the ratio tends to decrease as the size of the sample increases (Hess et al., 1986; Richards, 1987 in Lu, 2012); that is, a longer text in general has a lower TTR value than a shorter text, which makes it especially complicated to use TTR in developmental comparisons between age groups, where the number of word tokens often increases with age.

Miller (1991) suggested that NDW might have better properties for investigating semantic development than TTR, which shows little developmental progression (Watkins et al., 1995). Normative data on NDW controlling for sample length are available in Systematic Analysis of Language Transcripts (SALT) databases including the Bilingual SE Version 2010 for English- and Spanish-speaking children (Miller & Iglesias, 2010) and the T-SALT database. Differences in NDW have been reported between normally developing and SLI groups up through the age of five years. Therefore, NDW is believed to show promise as a means of measuring lexical development both in the preschool years and beyond (Malvern & Richards, 1997).

Grammatical complexity

Grammatical complexity is another measurable property of language, and different scales of measurement have been used to quantify grammatical complexity. The best known and most widely used is MLU, a measure of utterance length used as an index of children's grammatical complexity. MLU has been used as a diagnostic measure to differentiate between TD children and language-impaired populations in English-speaking children (e.g. Klee *et al.*, 1989; Scarborough *et al.*, 1986, 1991). In TD children, MLU correlates significantly with age up to approximately MLU 2.5–3.0 (Klee, 1992; Rondal *et al.*, 1987). With MLUs greater than 3.0, the association between age and MLU is less reliable; however, it continues to be a valid predictor of syntactic complexity and diversity up to approximately MLU 4.0 (Rollins *et al.*, 1996).

Specific morphosyntactic structures

After three years of age, children with SLI usually exhibit morphological and syntactic deficits, which are evidenced by the use of lower complexity syntactic structures in their native tongue. Areas of significant morphosyntactic impairment include tense marking and agreement, omitted by English-speaking children with SLI through at least the early elementary years.

In summary, a variety of lexical and morphosyntactic language sample measures have been used for language assessment with English-speaking children with and without LI. The limited research available on the performance of Turkish-speaking children indicates these measures have potential for diagnostic use in Turkish. However, specific noun and verb morphological forms must also be considered in order to address important features of Turkish in language assessment. Therefore, we recently conducted a study in which we examined the language samples of children with LI on a variety of quantitative measures and on the use of specific noun and verb inflections.

The Study

We compared the language samples of 18 children with LI to normative data from TD children in the T-SALT database on commonly used language sample analysis measures: MLU-M and MLU-W, number of total and different words (TNW and NDW) and TTR. We also compared the children's use of specific noun and verb inflections.

The 18 children in the study (one girl and seven boys from Bursa and three girls and seven boys from Eskişehir) were 3–5 years of age, as shown in Table 9.2 (mean age was 4 years, 3 months). The children had been identified as having LI (possibly SLI) by SLTs. All of the children appeared to have normal motor and cognitive skills based upon the children's performance on the Ankara Development Test and the Denver Developmental Screening Test. Children with uncorrected hearing or vision impairment or multiple physical disabilities were excluded from the sample. They were all monolingual, speaking Turkish at home and at clinics. The children with LI had expressive language scores that were more than 1.5 SD below the mean for their age on the TEDİL (Topbaş & Güven, 2010). Most of the children had scores more than 1 SD below the mean on the TEDİL receptive scale as well, as shown in Table 9.2. As previously described, the TEDİL assesses expressive and receptive language in children from 2 to 7 years old.

Each child with LI was individually matched to the children of almost the same age group (±6 months) from the Turkish SALT (T-SALT) database, which includes data on 140 TD children aged 2;6–6;6 (Acarlar et al., 2006). We gathered 15-minute language samples, which included between 41 and 75 utterances, from the children with LI (Table 9.2).

Table 9.2 Children with LI and TD children selected from T-SALT database

	Age	Sex	No. of utterances (in 15 minutes)	TEDİL A raw score (SD)		Control group (T-SALT database)	
				Receptive	Expressive	Female	Male
1	3;1	M	65	9 (−1.80)	10 (−2.00)	15	18
2	3;4	F	59	10 (−1.60)	11 (−1.80)	17	19
3	3;7	M	41	8 (−2.00)	10 (−2.00)	22	18
4	3;7	M	63	9 (−1.80)	10 (−2.00)	22	18
5	3;9	M	42	8 (−2.00)	9 (−2.20)	20	18
6	3;9	F	44	12 (−1.20)	10 (−2.00)	20	18
7	3;10	M	47	11 (−1.40)	8 (−2.40)	18	20
8	3;11	M	71	14 (−0.80)	12 (−1.60)	20	20
9	4;1	M	60	12 (−2.40)	13 (−2.60)	19	19
10	4;1	M	45	13 (−2.20)	14 (−2.40)	19	19
11	4;2	F	53	11 (−2.60)	11 (−3.00)	19	17
12	4;5	M	59	11 (−2.60)	10 (−3.20)	18	16
13	4;7	F	75	9 (−3.00)	13 (−2.60)	18	15
14	4;9	M	46	14 (−2.00)	16 (−2.00)	17	18
15	5;2	M	71	18 (−1.83)	13 (−3.00)	17	16
16	5;3	M	56	13 (−2.66)	12 (−3.16)	17	17
17	5;8	M	54	20 (−1.50)	14 (−2.83)	20	18
18	5;9	M	46	19 (−1.66)	20 (−1.83)	25	22

Language sampling

A mother brought her child to the playroom. First, the child played with the toys alone, while the mother, the second author and an SLT with whom the child was not familiar, spoke quietly for 5 minutes. Then the mother left the room and the child played with the SLT for 15 minutes. The purpose of the play session was to elicit the highest level of play and language possible. The SLT was trained in language and play elicitation techniques, and had previous experience in interacting with preschoolers. Next, the child and his or her mother were given a standard set of toys provided that the child was able to participate for another 15–20 minutes interaction. Otherwise, this session was postponed to another day. The play set included toy cars, home furnishings, blocks, color markers and paper, a train set, puppets and picture-making booklets. The mothers were asked to play and interact with their children as they would at home.

We video and audio-recorded the sessions and an SLT student transcribed the speech samples. Ten transcripts were randomly selected for accuracy checks. If accuracy was judged inadequate, all the tapes done by that transcriber were rechecked by the graduate SLT. The percentage of agreement was rated word-for-word and morpheme-by-morpheme, and the interrater reliability for the transcriptions was 98.60%.

Language sample data

We derived the following measures from the language samples: grammatical complexity (MLU-M, MLU-W), lexical diversity (TNW, NDW and TTR) and morphosyntactic diversity (diversity of use of inflectional morphology and inflectional errors). The language samples of the children were 20–30 minutes long. Some of the samples of the language-impaired group included less than 50 utterances due to sparse production. Consequently, MLU-M, MLU-W, TNW, TTR and NDW were qualified as to time and utterance length. We selected these measures because of their sensitivity in indicating developmental changes in children's language abilities and their wide use in clinical practice and research on child language disorders.

We calculated the number of productive morphemes (excluding derivational morphemes) and words produced in intelligible utterances and determined the average number of morphemes/words per utterance (MLU-M and MLU-W).

NDW was calculated based on the NDW in language samples of a fixed length; in this work the sample lengths were (a) 50 utterances and, alternatively, (b) utterances produced in 15 minutes. Both methods of equalizing sample length have been shown to provide reliable measures of lexical diversity (Watkins et al., 1995).

TTR takes the NDW (or types) and compares it to the TNW (or tokens) to yield a ratio that serves as a measure of lexical diversity (Richards, 1987). Although TTR is widely used in both first and second language acquisition studies, Miller (1981) claimed that TTR for the first 50 utterances of a sample yielded a ratio of approximately 0.45, regardless of age, in the age range of 3–8 years. Similar results were reported (Klee, 1992) in a study of children ranging from 2 to 4 years old. However, because TTR may yield different results in Turkish-speaking children, we compared the TTR of children with LI with matches in the T-SALT database.

The findings

Spontaneous language measures were calculated for all of the children using T-SALT analyses. Data from 18 children with LI were compared to the data of TD children (±6 months of age) from language samples of equal length, based on utterances produced in 15 minutes. For NDW and TTR, comparisons were also made on an equal number of words (EW). Table 9.3 displays the overall performance of children with LI and TD children who were selected from the T-SALT database. We completed a series of group comparisons using *t*-test analyses to determine whether scores of the aforementioned language measures distinguished the two groups.

In our analyses, we compared the MLU-M, MLU-W, TNW, NDW and TTR ratios of typical children and children with LI in 15-minute samples. Children with LI performed significantly lower than control children on all grammatical and lexical measures based on *t*-test analyses, as shown in Table 9.3. Effect sizes were measured by calculating Cohen's *d* and EB *r* values, also shown in Table 9.3. Effect sizes for all measures except TTR were large and likely to be of clinical significance.

Table 9.3 Performance of LI and typically developing children in 15-minute language samples

Measure	15 minute samples							
	LI		TD SALT Database					
	Age mean 4;2		Age ±6 months					
	Mean	SD	Mean	SD	t	p	Cohen's d	EB r
MLU-M	1.76	0.33	4.59	0.45	−35.47	<0.001	−7.01	−0.96
MLU-W	1.30	0.10	2.53	0.22	−47.44	<0.001	−6.82	−0.95
TNW	72.5	16.8	140.3	30.2	−17.91	<0.001	−2.80	−0.81
NDW-EU	38.1	8.15	76.02	14.2	−19.69	<0.001	−3.26	−0.85
NDW-EW	38.3	8.13	47.9	8.61	−5.02	<0.001	−1.15	−0.49
TTR-EW	0.56	0.08	0.69	0.33	−1.50	<0.001	−0.54	−0.26

EU: equal number of utterances; EW: equal number of words.

Table 9.4 Performance of LI and typically developing children for noun and verb tense inflection types

Measure	50-utterance sample							
	LI		TD SALT database					
	Age mean 4;2		Age ±6 months					
	Mean	SD	Mean	SD	t	p	Cohen's d	EB r
Noun inflections								
Accusative	0.33	0.59	5.59	0.46	−37.56	<.001	−9.89	−0.98
Dative	0.22	0.54	6.28	0.86	−46.94	<.001	−7.27	−0.96
Locative	0.44	0.70	4.38	1.09	−23.74	<.001	−4.27	−0.90
Ablative	0.22	0.73	2.36	0.30	−12.42	<.001	−0.25	−0.12
Verb inflections								
Present progressive	4.72	4.84	17.76	3.90	−11.41	<.001	−2.96	−0.82
Past	4.38	3.08	8.44	1.00	−5.57	<.001	−1.76	−0.66
Perfect	0.38	0.60	3.26	0.47	−20.68	<.001	−5.28	−0.93
Present	0.50	0.70	1.95	1.91	−7.41	<.001	−1.41	−0.59
Future	1.11	1.49	1.95	0.19	−2.40	0.02	−0.79	−0.36

For analyses of noun and verb inflections we used group means, comparing the children with LI to the T-SALT data for children ages 3;8–4;10 (±6 months from the LI group mean age of 4;2). The children with LI used an average of 11.3 nouns and an average of 10.2 verbs in 50-utterance samples and a *t*-test indicated that there was no significant difference in the number of nouns versus verbs used. We examined the four most frequently occurring noun inflection types (case markings) and the five most frequently occurring verb (tense) inflection types. Among TD children, the mean use of dative and accusative case markings was the highest followed by locative inflections, as shown in Table 9.4. Among children with LI, the use of case markings was low. We found the present progressive and past to be the most frequently used of verb tense markings among the TD children, followed by the perfect. Although children with LI did not use verb tense markers as frequently as children in the T-SALT database, they did use present progressive and past markers more frequently than the other verb inflections. Overall, it seems that there is a very significant developmental lag in the use of noun and verb inflections among preschool children with LI.

Conclusions

The acquisition of language is critical to cognitive, social and emotional development throughout the lifespan and difficulty with language acquisition may have a far-reaching impact on those developmental areas. Thus, research on the identification of children at an early age who are at risk is important so that appropriate interventions can be provided. However, the identification and classification of a clinical population with LI who do not have other significant medical, sensory, environmental or developmental diagnoses (i.e. SLI) is still challenging.

Clinicians typically depend on measures of language to diagnose children with LIs, to assess a range of language skills and to design and monitor treatment programs. Researchers use language measures to define their participant populations, to document their participants' language status, to match groups of participants or to investigate aspects of LI in different populations. Typically, two classes of measures are used for these purposes: (a) standardized psychometric tests and (b) measures of spontaneous speech derived from natural language samples, which can be collected in a variety of ways in different contexts (Marinis, 2011). Thus, both for clinical and research purposes there is a need for a diversity of valid language measures. Children learning Turkish (a non-Indo-European agglutinating language) offer challenging opportunities to expand current views of LI and assessment tools.

In our work, we seek to gather evidence to support the validity of measures, namely, MLU and inflectional use for morphosyntactic complexity, and TTR and NDW for lexical diversity, by comparing the performance of TD children from the T-SALT database and children with LI on the basis of language samples of equal length. Generally, we have found that in all the measures, MLU-M and MLU-W, TNW, NDW and TTR, children with LI lag behind their typical peers. However, it is worth noting that TTR has shown less of a difference than the other measures, particularly for 50-utterance samples. This result is similar to the findings of Watkins *et al.* (1995), who reported that TTR did not differentiate TD children from children with SLI.

In a study by Leonard *et al.* (1999), NDW calculated from 100-utterance samples was compared for TD children and children with SLI ranging in age from 2;2 to 6;11. A significantly lower NDW was found for the children with SLI than for the TD children of the same age, as was true for the Turkish-speaking children with LI in our study. In a study of the growth of lexical diversity in nine preschoolers with SLI, Goffman and Leonard (2000) found that the NDW used by these children in a 50-utterance sample was equivalent to or exceeded by the number used by younger TD children at the same MLU levels. This proved true for the children with SLI who began the study with a low MLU, as well as for those who began with a higher MLU. However, Elin Thordardottir and Ellis Weismer (2001) reported no differences between children with SLI and a group of younger MLU-W-matched peers on measures of lexical diversity on both the number of different verbs and NDW in a 315-word sample.

From these studies, it can be inferred that children with SLI may have lexical deficits in addition to less complex morphosyntax compared to their peers when measures are taken from spontaneous speech. Morphosyntactic deficits are consistently found across studies. In the present study, MLU was lower than that of comparison children from the T-SALT database and the children with LI consistently used fewer noun and verb inflections than their peers. These results are compatible with the Acarlar and Johnston (2011) study.

Overall, the findings of our work support the evidence put forward by studies on Turkish children with LI (Acarlar, 2008; Acarlar & Johnston, 2010, 2011; Güven et al., 2009; Topbaş & Güven, 2008). If more normative information were to become available, these measures might show promise in providing norm-referenced yet ecologically valid means of identifying LI. However, sensitivity and specificity data are needed to further explore the measures as possible identifiers of LI. Nonetheless, the summary of our current work provides initial support for language sample analysis and the use of the linguistic measures to identify Turkish-speaking children suspected of LI.

Summary

Valid language measures for identifying LI among Turkish-speaking children and information on TLD and ALD are essential to providing appropriate assessment and intervention services. This chapter provided a brief review of research on TLD and ALD in Turkish-speaking children, information on Turkish standardized language tests and data on the performance of Turkish-speaking children with and without LI on a variety of language sample measures. Similar to findings for young children who speak other languages, language sample analyses reveal significant differences between Turkish-speaking children with TLD and with LI on MLU and vocabulary diversity indices as well as on the use of specific noun and verb inflections. From a clinical perspective, general indices used for language sample analysis, such as MLU and vocabulary diversity measures, capture broad areas of difficulty and analyses of particular inflections provide a more detailed picture of children's development of the forms specific to the language they speak. The use of broad indices along with more specific analyses of language forms and the contexts of their use hold promise for identifying LI and specific areas of difficulty in Turkish-speaking children.

Acknowledgments

Some of the results of this study are based on the MSc thesis of Şan (2010) (SLT) supervised by Maviş. We thank her for the efforts carried out in data collection and analysis. Part of the data for SLI children were taken from the project supported by TÜBİTAK, No. 109K001. We thank TÜBİTAK and the children who participated in this study.

References

Acarlar, F. (2008) Verb and noun morphology in atypical language development. Paper presented at The International Clinical Phonetics and Linguistics Association (ICPLA) 2008, Istanbul.

Acarlar, F. and Johnston, J. (2010) Turkish-SALT: Computer-assisted language sample analysis. In S. Topbaş and M. Yavas (eds) *Communication Disorders in Turkish* (pp. 119–136). Bristol: Multilingual Matters.

Acarlar, F. and Johnston, J. (2011) Acquisition of Turkish grammatical morphology by children with developmental disorders. *International Journal of Language & Communication Disorders* 46, 728–738.

Acarlar, F., Miller, J.F. and Johnston, J.R. (2006) Systematic Analysis of Language Transcripts (SALT), Turkish (Version 9) [computer software]. Language Analysis Lab, University of Wisconsin-Madison. (Distributed by the Turkish Psychological Association.)

Aksu-Koç, A. (2010) The course of normal language development in Turkish. In S. Topbaş and M. Yavaş (eds) *Communication Disorders in Turkish* (pp. 65–105). Bristol: Multilingual Matters.

Aksu-Koç, A., Acarlar, F., Küntay, A., Maviş, I., Sofu, H., Topbaş, S. and Turan, F. (2012) *CDI-MacArthur Communicative Inventory: Turkish (TİGE-Türkçe İletişim Gelişim Envanteri)*. Ankara: TUBİTAK Project.

Bates, E., Bretherton, I. and Snyder, L. (1988) *From First Words to Grammar: Individual Differences and Dissociable Mechanisms*. Cambridge: Cambridge University Press.

Condouris, K., Meyer, H. and Tager-Flusberg, H. (2003) Relationship between standardized measures of language and measures of spontaneous speech in children with autism. *American Journal of Speech Language Pathology* 12, 349–358.

COST Action IS0804 – Language Impairment in a Multilingual Society: Linguistic Patterns and the Road to Assessment. See www.bi-sli.org (accessed 24 August 2015).

Dunn, M., Flax, J., Sliwinski, M. and Aram, D. (1996) The use of spontaneous language measures as criteria for identifying children with specific language impairment: An attempt to reconcile clinical and research incongruence. *Journal of Speech and Hearing Research* 39, 643–654.

Ege, P. (2010) Mean length of utterance as a tool for morphological assessment in Turkish children. In S. Topbaş and M. Yavas (eds) *Communication Disorders in Turkish* (pp. 105–119). Bristol: Multilingual Matters.

Ege, P. and Erdem, R. (2008) The relationship between syntactic and semantic development in normal and mentally-retarded Turkish children. Paper presented at the 2nd International Conference on Special Education, Marmaris, Turkey.

Elin Thordardottir and Ellis Weismer, S. (2001) High frequency verbs and verb diversity in the spontaneous speech of school age children with specific language impairment. *International Journal of Language and Communication Disorders* 36, 221–244.

Erguvanlı, E.E. (1984) *The Function of Word Order in Turkish*. Berkeley, CA: University of California Press.

Evans, J. (1996) SLI subgroups: Interaction between discourse constraints and morphological deficits. *Journal of Speech and Hearing Research* 39, 655–660.

Goffman, L. and Leonard, J. (2000) Growth of language skills in preschool children with specific language impairment: Implications for assessment and intervention. *American Journal of Speech-Language Pathology* 9, 151–161.

Göksel, A. and Kerslake, C. (2005) *Turkish: A Comprehensive Grammar.* London: Routledge-Taylor & Francis.

Güven, A.G. and Berument, S.K. (2010) *TİFALDİ- Türkçe İfade Edici ve Alıcı Dil Testi (Sözcük Dağarcığı).* Ankara: Türk Psikologlar Derneği.

Güven, S., Topbaş, S. and Eroğlu, D. (2009) Comparison of morpho-syntactic characteristics of Turkish children with SLI and their typically developing peers. Paper presented at International Clinical Linguistics Conference, Madrid.

Hess, C.W., Sefton, K.M. and Landry, R.G. (1986) Sample size and type-token ratios for oral language of preschool children. *Journal of Speech and Hearing Research* 29, 129–134.

Klee, T. (1992) Developmental and diagnostic characteristics of quantitative measures of children's language production. *Topics in Language Disorders* 12, 28–41.

Klee, T., Schaffer, M., May, S., Membrino, I. and Mougey, K. (1989) A comparison of the age-MLU relation in normal and specifically language impaired preschool children. *Journal of Speech and Hearing Disorders* 54, 226–233.

Ketrez, F.N. and Aksu-Koç, A. (2009) Early nominal morphology: Emergence of case and number. In M. Voeikova and U. Stephany (eds) *The Development of Number and Case in the First Language Acquisition: A Cross-Linguistic Perspective* (pp. 15–48). Berlin: Mouton de Gruyter.

Kornfilt, J. (1997) *Turkish (Descriptive Grammar).* London & New York: Routledge.

Leonard, L.B., Miller, C. and Gerber, E. (1999) Grammatical morphology and the lexicon in children with specific language impairment. *Journal of Speech, Language and Hearing Research* 42, 362–378

Lieven, E.V.M. (1978) Conversations between mothers and young children: Individual differences and their possible implication for the study of child language learning. In N. Waterson and C.E. Snow (eds) *The Development of Communication* (pp. 173–187). Chichester: Wiley.

Lu, X. (2012) The relationship of lexical richness to the quality of ESL learners' oral narratives. *The Modern Language Journal* 96 (2), 190–208.

Malvern, D. and Richards, B. (1997) A new measure of lexical diversity. In A. Ryan and A. Wray (eds) *Evolving Models of Language* (pp. 58–71). Clevedon: Multilingual Matters.

Marinis, T. (2011) On the nature and cause of specific language impairment: A view from sentence processing and infant research. *Lingua* 121, 463–475.

Maviş, I. and Ege, P. (2002) The emergence of voice morphology in Turkish speaking children. Poster presentation at Symposium of International Association for the Study of Child Language (IASCL), July, Madison, WI.

Maviş, İ. and Ölmez, S. (n.d.) Vocabulary and grammar acquisition in Turkish assessed by CDI-TR: The comparison of typically developing (TD) & language delayed children (LD) (currently in review).

Merrell, A.W. and Plante, E. (1997) Norm-referenced test interpretation in the diagnostic process. *Language, Speech, and Hearing Services in Schools* 28, 50–58.

Miller, J.F. (1981) Procedures for analyzing free speech samples: Syntax and semantics. In J.F. Miller (ed.) *Assessing Language Production in Children: Experimental Procedures* (pp. 41–43). Baltimore, MD: University Park Press.

Miller, J. (1991) Quantifying productive language disorders. In J. Miller (ed.) *Research on Child Language Disorders: A Decade of Progress* (pp. 211–220). Austin, TX: Pro-Ed.

Miller, J. and Iglesias, A. (2010) Systematic Analysis of Language Transcripts (SALT, Bilingual SE Version 2010) [computer software]. Madison, WE: SALT Software.

Ministry of Health of Turkey (MoH, 2011) Bazı Kanun ve Kanun Hükmünde Kararnamelerde Değişiklil Yapılmasına Dair Kanun. Kanun No. 6225. *Resmi Gazete* 2796, 1–14.

Ministry of Education of Turkey (MoNE, 2014) Özel Eğitim Kurumları Yönetmeliği. *Resmi Gazete* 29014, 1–30.

Özcan, F.H. and Topbaş, S. (1994) Dil Ediniminde Adıl Kullanımı: Normal ve Özel Eğitim Gereksinimli Öğrenciler Arasında Bir Karşılaştırma (Pronominals in language acquisition: A comparison between typically developing children and children with special needs). *VIII. Dilbilim Kurultayı Bildiri Kitabı.* İstanbul Üniv. Yay.

Özcan, H.F. and Topbaş, S. (2000) Structural and semantic analysis of verbs in the acquisition of Turkish. In I. Barriere, G. Morgan, S. Chiat and B. Woll (eds) *Current Research in Language and Communication Science Vol 1* (pp. 57–67). London: City University.

Parisse, C. and Maillart, C. (2009) Specific language impairment as systemic developmental disorders. *Journal of Neurolinguistics* 22, 109–122.

Read, J. (2000) *Assessing Vocabulary.* Cambridge: Cambridge University Press.

Republic of Turkey Prime Ministry State Planning Organization, National Rural Development Strategy, 2002, Ankara: 2006, Retrieved from http:// ekutup.dpt.gov.tr/bolgesel/strateji/UKKS.pdf

Richards, B. (1987) Type-token ratios: What do they really tell us? *Journal of Child Language* 14, 201–209.

Rollins, P.R., Snow, C. and Willett, J. (1996) Predictors of MLU: Semantic and morphological developments. *First Language* 16, 243–259.

Rondal, J.A., Ghiotto, M., Bredart, S. and Bachelet, J.F. (1987) Age-relation, reliability, and grammatical validity of measures of utterance length. *Journal of Child Language* 14, 433–446.

Scarborough, H.S., Rescorla, L., Tager-Flusberg, H. and Fowler, A.E. (1991) The relation of utterance length to grammatical complexity in normal and language-disordered groups. *Applied Psycholinguistics* 12, 23–45.

Scarborough, H., Wyckoff, J. and Davidson, R. (1986) A reconsideration of the relation between age and mean utterance length. *Journal of Speech and Hearing Research* 29, 394–399.

Spaulding, T.J., Plante, E., Farinella, K.A. (2006) Eligibility criteria for language impairment: Is the low end of normal always appropriate? *Language, Speech, and Hearing Services in Schools* 37, 61–72.

Şan, A. (2010) 3-6 yaş arası özgül dil bozukluğu olan çocuklarla normal gelişim gösteren çocukların dil özelliklerinin analizi ve karşılaştırılması. Unpublished MSc thesis, Anadolu Üniversitesi.

Šišková, Z. (2012) Lexical richness in EFL students' narratives. In C. Ciarlo and D.S. Giannoni (eds) *Language Studies Working Papers.* Vol. 4. Reading: University of Reading, 26–36.

Topbaş, S. (2006) A Turkish perspective on communication disorders. *Logopedics Phoniatrics Vocology* 31, 76–88.

Topbaş, S. (2007) Turkish speech acquisition. In S. McLeod (ed.) *The International Guide to Speech Acquisition* (pp. 566–579). Clifton Park, NY: Thomson Delmar Learning.

Topbaş, S. (2010a) Specific language impairment in Turkish: Adapting the Test of Early Language Development (TELD-3) as a first step in measuring language impairments. In S. Topbaş and M. Yavaş (eds) *Communication Disorders in Turkish* (pp. 137–160). Bristol: Multilingual Matters.

Topbaş, S. (2010b) A closer look at the developing profession of speech and language pathology. In S. Topbaş and M. Yavaş (eds) *Communication Disorders in Turkish* (pp. 3–27). Bristol: Multilingual Matters.

Topbaş, S. and Güven, S. (2008) Assessing language impairments in Turkish by TELD-3: Implications for SLI. Paper presented at 12th International Clinical Phonetics and Linguistics Association (ICPLA) Congress, Istanbul, Turkey.

Topbaş, S. and Güven, S. (2011) *Test of Early Language Development (TELD-3): Turkish version.* TEDİL: Türkçe Erken Dil Gelişim Testi. Project research supported by TUBİTAK No. 109K001. Ankara: Detay Pub.

Topbaş, S. and Güven, S. (in preparation) *Test of Language Development-TOLD-P:4-Turkish (Türkçe Okul Çağı Dil Gelişim Testi-TODİL).* Project research supported by TUBİTAK No. 109K001.

Topbaş, S. and Özcan, F.H (1995) Anlatılarda Bağlaç Kullanımı: Normal ve Özel Eğitim Gereksinimli Öğrenciler Arasında Karşılaştırma (Conjunction use in narratives: A comparison between typically developing children and children with special needs). *XI. Dilbilim Kurultayı Bildiri Kitabı.* Bolu: Abant İzzet Baysal Üniversitesi Yayınları (pp 82–96).

Topbaş, S. and Yavaş, M. (2006) Phonological acquisition and disorders in Turkish. In Z. Hua and B. Dodd (eds) *Phonological Development and Disorders in Children: A Multilingual Perspective* (pp. 233–264). Cleavdon: Multilingual Matters.

Topbaş, S., Maviş, I. and Başal, M. (1997) Acquisition of bound morphemes: Nominal case morphology in Turkish. In K. İmer and N.E. Uzun (eds) *Proceedings of the 8th International Conference on Turkish Linguistics* (pp. 127–137). Ankara: Ankara University.

Topbaş, S., Cangökçe-Yaşar and Ball, M. (2012) LARSP for Turkish (TR-LARSP). In M.J. Ball, D. Crystal and P. Fletcher (eds) *Assessing Grammar: The Languages of LARSP* (pp. 282–302). Bristol: Multilingual Matters.

Topbaş, S., Göçümen, G. and Rescorla, L. (in preparation) Language Development Survey: Turkish Version. Supported by Anadolu University Project No. 1203E042, Eskisehir.

Topbaş, S., Aydın, A., Kazanoğlu, D. and Tadıhan-Ozkan, E. (in preparation) Turkish Sentence Repetition Test. In Project: COST Action IS0804 – Language Impairment in a Multilingual Society: Linguistic Patterns and the Road to Assessment. See www.bi-sli.org (accessed 24 August 2015).

Tüfekçioğlu, U. (2010) Speech Characteristics of hearing impaired Turkish children. In S. Topbaş and M. Yavas (eds) *Communication Disorders in Turkish* (pp. 160–186). Bristol: Multilingual Matters.

Watkins, R., Kelly, D., Harbers, H. and Hollis, W. (1995) Measuring children's lexical diversity: Differentiating typical and impaired language learners. *Journal of Speech and Hearing Research* 38, 1349–1355.

World Health Organization and the World Bank (2011) World Report on Disability. Geneva: World Health Organization. See www.who.int (accessed 7 June 2011).

Yalçınkaya F. and Belgin E. (2010) *Preschool Language Scale-Turkish Version.* Ankara: Hacettepe University.

Yarbay-Duman, T., Blom, E. and Topbaş, S. (2015) At the intersection of cognition and grammar: Deficits comprehending counterfactuals in Turkish children with specific language impairment. *Journal of Speech and Hearing Research* 58, 410–421. DOI: 10.1044/2015_JSLHR-L-14-0054

Yarbay-Duman, T. and Topbaş, S. (n.d.) Children's understanding of epistemic certainty: Comprehension of tense and aspect inflections in Turkish children with specific language impairment (currently in review).

Yavaş, M. (2010) Some structural characteristics of Turkish. In S. Topbaş and M. Yavaş (eds) *Communication Disorders in Turkish* (pp. 48–62). Bristol: Multilingual Matters.

10 Linguistic Variation and Assessment Implications for Spanish-Speaking Children in the United States

Barbara L. Rodríguez

Introduction

Speech-language pathologists (SLPs) in the United States work with children from increasingly diverse linguistic, cultural and socioeconomic backgrounds due to demographic changes in the United States. The changing landscape of the population living in the United States over the past several years is similar to that seen in many areas throughout the world due to increasing globalization and migration. These changes result in the need for SLPs to be knowledgeable about the linguistic variability characterizing the populations they serve. The Hispanic/Latino population in the United States is a prime example of an increasing demographic with significant within-group variability.

Over the last several decades, the US Hispanic population has demonstrated dramatic growth. The US Census Bureau reported that in 1970 approximately 9.6 million individuals were of Hispanic descent and in 2013 there were 54 million (Ryan, 2013). Current projections indicate that by 2060, 128.8 million individuals in the United States will identify themselves as of Hispanic background (Ryan, 2013), and according to this projection, the Hispanic population will constitute 31% of the nation's population by that date. Not only is the Hispanic population increasing in number, it is also becoming quite diverse in its composition with individuals arriving to the United States from Mexico, Puerto Rico and Cuba, as well as Central and South America. In 2010, 63% of the Hispanic population in the United States was of Mexican background, 9.4% of Puerto Rican background and 3.7% of Cuban descent (Ennis *et al.*, 2011).

Languages spoken at home are not evenly distributed throughout the country. Some regions in the United States have high percentages of non-English speakers, while others have lower percentages. For example, in the state of West Virginia, only 2% of individuals 5 years of age and over report speaking a language other than English at home (Ryan, 2013). Conversely, in the state of California, 44% reported the same. Spanish is overwhelmingly the most common non-English language spoken in the United States. The number of US residents 5 years of age and older who spoke Spanish at home in 2012 totaled 38.3 million (US Census Bureau, 2012). This represents a 121% increase since 1990 when it was 17.3 million. Those who speak Spanish in the home constituted 13% of U.S. residents 5 years of age and older with more than half (58%) of Spanish speakers reporting that they speak English 'very well' (Ryan, 2013).

The increase in Spanish speakers observed over the last several decades reflects the arrival of new immigrants from Latin America and growth in the nation's Hispanic population. Variability within the Hispanic population, often as a result of differences in country of origin, is realized in the linguistic characteristics observed. Within a single language group, differences in linguistic features are apparent, including distinctions in a speaker's semantics and syntax. These differences, often reflecting one's country of origin, constitute a specific variety or dialect of the language spoken. Cardenas (1970) described the major varieties of Spanish spoken in the United States – Mexican Spanish, Puerto Rican Spanish, Cuban Spanish and Peninsular Spanish.

The American Speech, Language and Hearing Association (ASHA) requires that all SLPs exhibit clinical competence when serving children from diverse backgrounds, including Spanish-speaking Latino children (ASHA, 2013). Unfortunately, research has shown that SLPs have limited training in providing SLP services to bilingual children and their families, lack confidence in their abilities when assessing and preparing intervention plans for Spanish-speaking children with communication disorders and desire continuing education in this area (Hammer Scheffner et al., 2004). Clinical competence in assessment and intervention with an increasingly diverse clinical population is critically important to improve the quality of services and outcomes. When providing speech and language services to children from Spanish-speaking communities, SLPs must be familiar with the linguistic features of Spanish, as well as the Mexican and Puerto Rican Spanish dialects, the most commonly spoken dialects of Spanish in the United States (Brown & Patten, 2014).

The purpose of this chapter is to address this need by: (a) reviewing the features of standard Spanish, with the focus on morphosyntactic rules; (b) discussing the morphosyntactic features of the Mexican and Puerto Rican dialects of Spanish; (c) describing the morphosyntactic characteristics of Spanish-speaking children with specific language impairment (SLI); and (d) outlining considerations that need to be made when assessing the language skills of Spanish-speaking children. Although this chapter focuses on Mexican and Puerto Rican dialects of Spanish, there are other dialects of Spanish spoken by Spanish-speaking immigrants, including Salvadoran, Guatemalan and Cuban dialects, described by Lipski (1994, 2008), Otheguy *et al.* (2007) and Guitart (1976). Note that throughout the chapter, the term *Hispanic* is used when referring to information collected by US governmental agencies such as the Census Bureau and the US Department of Education; the term *Latino* is used to refer to Spanish-speaking populations that trace their ancestry to Latin America and the Caribbean islands (Suárez-Orozco & Páez, 2009).

Linguistic Varieties of Spanish Employed by US Latinos

Although Latinos living in the United States share many linguistic and sociocultural experiences, differences in cultural traditions and practices exist between the various groups as a result of socioeconomic factors, diverse political histories, immigration experiences, cultural sensibilities and social dilemmas (Rodriguez & Olswang, 2002; Suárez-Orozco & Páez, 2009; Zentella, 2009). In addition, differences are found in the variety or dialect of Spanish that is spoken with variation in the pronunciation, grammatical patterns and vocabulary used by the speaker. Dialects are typically associated with a geographic region, including country of origin, and are considered to be symbolic representations of the speakers' historical, social and cultural backgrounds (Penny, 2004).

Knowledge about the various dialects of Spanish is particularly important when determining whether or not a child has a language impairment. Several years ago, ASHA (1983) issued a position statement concerning social dialects, which clearly stated that no dialectal variety of English is a disorder or pathological form of speech or language. Although the focus of this position paper highlighted varieties of English, the fundamental position applies to any language spoken, including Spanish. Without knowledge of the characteristics of the various dialects, SLPs risk diagnosing a child as having a language impairment when he or she may not. Although a rich body of literature describing the phonological variants of Spanish exists (e.g. Goldstein, 2004; Goldstein & Iglesias, 1996; Iglesias & Goldstein, 1998; McLeod & Goldstein, 2011), there is little information describing the morphosyntactic features of Spanish dialects. The focus of the following section is on the morphosyntactic features of 'standard' Spanish and the two principle dialects of Spanish used in the United States: Mexican and Puerto Rican. These dialects share the basic structures of 'standard' Spanish but possess unique grammatical features that diverge from the standard forms.

Features of standard forms of Spanish

Spanish, like English, is part of the Indo-European family of languages, and is further classified as a Romance language, meaning that it is descended from Latin (Ruhlen, 1991). It is a language with a rich verbal morphology that marks tense, mood, aspect, person and number, leaving the speaker the option to express or omit subject personal pronouns (Penny, 2002). A description of the basic verb, noun and syntax features of Spanish follows.

Spanish verb inflections

Spanish verbs are comprised of a root and an inflection. The root denotes the verb being used, and the inflection signifies tense, number and subject pronoun (Zagona, 2002). Spanish regular verbs are divided, according to the infinitive ending, into three main conjugations: (a) *–ar* as in the verb *trabajar* (to work); (b) *–er* as in the verb *aprender* (to learn); or (c) *–ir* as in the verb *escribir* (to write). The inflections added to the verb root identify two features: (a) the tense – when the action of the verb is taking place; and (b) person – who is performing the action of the verb. For example, to form the present tense of a verb ending in *–ar*, the *–ar* is dropped and an inflection that corresponds to the personal subject pronoun is added to the root (*trabajar: Yo trabajo* [I work]). In contrast, adding an inflection to the infinitive forms the future verb tense. For instance, to express an action that will occur, a Spanish speaker will add an ending to the infinitive form of the verb (*trabajar: Yo trabajaré mañana* [I will work tomorrow]).

The mood of a verb indicates what type of role the verb plays in a sentence and/or the speaker's attitude toward it. The most common verb mood is the indicative mood that indicates action and state of being (e.g. *Emma está enferma* [Emma is sick]). The subjunctive mood is used to express an action or state of being in the context of the speaker's reaction to it. Most commonly, the subjunctive verb is used in a clause that starts with the relative pronoun *que* (which, that or who). Frequently, sentences that contain a subjunctive verb are used to express doubt, uncertainty, denial, desire, commands or reactions. An example of the subjunctive mood is '*Estoy triste que Emma esté enferma* (I am sad that Emma is sick)'.

Copular verbs

The Spanish verbs *ser* and *estar* both translate to the English form 'to be'; however, the difference between them is crucial. *Ser* denotes being, nature, identity or possession, while *estar* means condition, state or place. For example, *ser* would be used in the following sentence '*Ella es mi hija* (She is my daughter)'. *Ser* can also be used with adjectives or adjectival phrases to refer to identity or nature. For example, *Somos mexicanos* (We are Mexicans), *Es callado* (He's the quiet type) and *Esa maestra es excelente* (That teacher is excellent). *Ser* is used to denote possession as indicated in the following sentence, '*La casa es de mi yerno* (The house belongs to my son-in-law)'. In contrast, *estar* is used to indicate state (*Estoy feliz* [I'm happy]) and is used with adjectives to indicate emotional, physical and mental states of being (*está triste* [he is sad]; *está sano* [is healthy]; and *estuvo nervioso* [he was nervous]). *Estar* is also used to indicate place (*no está en casa* [he's not at home]) or location (*Miguel está en México* [Miguel is in Mexico]).

Spanish nouns

In Spanish, a noun (person, thing, place or quality) is either masculine or feminine. Gender is a grammatical property that applies to animate and inanimate notions alike (Corbett, 1991). Moreover, the elements of a noun phrase (adjectives, articles, possessives and demonstratives) must agree in gender with the noun or pronoun to which they relate. Gender is an inherent grammatical feature of any noun, and it serves to trigger agreement in the articles and adjectives in the noun phrase (Zagona, 2002). The noun phrase, '*las casas bonitas* (the pretty houses)' illustrates gender agreement in the article *las* (the, plural), noun *casas* (houses) and modifier *bonitas* (pretty, plural). Nouns that describe masculine persons or animals usually end in –*o*, while nouns that describe feminine persons or animals generally end in –*a*. Nouns that end in –*sión*, –*ción*, –*tad*, –*tud*, –*umbre* are feminine, and those that end in –*ma* are usually masculine. There is no perfect correspondence between word ending and gender; nouns that end in –*a* are not automatically feminine nouns. Words like *día* (day), *problema* (problem), *sistema* (system) and other words of Greek origin that end in –*a* are masculine in gender in Spanish (Martinez-Gibson, 2011).

In Spanish, there are two types of articles, definite and indefinite. Definite articles *el/la* (the), *los/las* (the, plural) indicate reference to a specific noun or nouns, whereas indefinite articles *uno/una* (one), *unos/unas* (some) are used when the speaker is not referring to a specific noun or nouns. Articles are feminine or masculine, and their gender is dependent upon the noun.

To form plural nouns in Spanish, a speaker adds either –*s* or –*es*. If a noun ends in a vowel, the plural noun is formed by adding –*s*. For example, the singular noun *el chico* (the boy) becomes *los chicos* (the boys) and *la clase* (the class) becomes *las clases* (the classes). In contrast, if a noun ends in a consonant, the plural noun is formed by adding –*es*. For example, *la flor* (the flower) becomes *las flores* (the flowers) and *la ciudad* (the city) becomes *las ciudades* (the cities). When the noun ends in –*z*, changing the –*z* to –*ces* forms the plural. For example, *el juez* (the judge) becomes *los jueces* (the judges) and *una vez* (once) becomes *dos veces* (twice). When a noun ends in a stressed –*é*, the plural is formed by simply adding –*s*, and words that end in other stressed vowels have –*es* added, as in *el café* (the coffee) becomes *los cafés* (the coffees).

Spanish speakers frequently use diminutive suffixes to indicate size, quantity and short duration. For example, the diminutive of *un vaso* (a drinking glass) is *un vasito* (a little drinking glass). The most common Spanish diminutive suffixes are *–ito* and *–cito* along with their feminine equivalents, *–ita* and *–cita*. Generally, words ending in *–a, -o* or *–te* form the diminutive by dropping the final vowel and adding *–ito* or *–ita*, while *–cito* or *–cita* are added to words ending in consonants. For example, the diminutive of *un pájaro* (a bird) is *un pajarito* (a little bird) and the diminutive of *el cajón* (the drawer) is *el cajoncito* (the little drawer).

Spanish syntax
Word order of sentences
Spanish has many word order possibilities (Zagona, 2002); however, in Spanish, a typical statement consists of a noun followed by a verb followed by an object (if the verb has an object). For example, *'Marcos compró el libro* (Marcos bought the book)'. However, a statement can also be formed with the subject followed by an object pronoun and then a verb. For example, *'Marcos lo compró* (Marcos bought it)'. Finally, a statement can be formulated by placing a verb ahead of the noun, which can have the effect of placing more emphasis on the verb. For example, *'Duermen los niños* (The children are sleeping)'.

Word order of questions
In Spanish, questions may be formulated using one of two options: (a) using intonation while preserving the word order of a simple statement (e.g. *¿Marcos compró el libro?* [Marcos bought the book?]) or (b) using a question word followed by a verb and subject. For example, *'¿Dónde está el libro?* (Where is the book?)'. It is not obligatory to express a subject pronoun overtly, since the information regarding person and number is reflected by the morphological markings of the verb (Zagona, 2002). For example, the question *'¿Qué dices?* (What do you say?)'* is expressed without overtly marking person and number. The verb's morphological marking *dices* (say) indicates the person and number *tú* (you, singular). When the subject is overtly expressed (i.e. *¿Qué dices tú?* [What do you say?]), usually in a post-verbal position, the effect is to call special attention to the subject. Generally speaking, to form a question, the verb and its subject are inverted (i.e. *¿Lees tú?* [Do you read?]).

Use of subject pronouns
The subject of a sentence is the person, place or thing, which performs the action. When a new topic is introduced in conversation, the subject is initially established through the explicit use of a noun. Once the referent has been established, speakers of English replace the noun with a subject pronoun; however, in Spanish, subject pronouns may or may not be overtly

expressed. Spanish is a 'pro-drop' language, which means that the pronoun can be dropped. The overt expression of a pronoun is not necessary for comprehension because the subject of the verb is evident from the conjugated verb; for example, the English expression 'I go' can be expressed in Spanish as '*Yo voy*' or simply '*voy*'. There are a few instances in Spanish where the subject pronouns are overtly expressed. First, subject pronouns are generally used when the pronoun stands alone. For example, in response to a question, '*¿Quién ha venido?* (Who has come?) *Ellos.* (They did)'. Subject pronouns are also overtly expressed when there is a change of subject within a sentence. In the following statement, the pronouns are expressed because of the change of subject, '*Tú estás cansada, pero ella está descansada* (You are tired, but she is rested)'. Finally, Spanish speakers may also overtly express the subject pronoun to stress the polite tone of an utterance as in the following statement, '*¿A dónde van ustedes?* (Where are you going?)'.

Summary

Spanish, a Romance language, is heavily inflected with a subject-verb-object sentence structure. Verbs have three infinitive endings (*–ar, –er* and *–ir*) and are conjugated to form the various present, preterite and future verb tenses. Spanish in the United States is highly diverse and exhibits a wide array of regional variation, including the Mexican and Puerto Rican varieties which are considered the most notable (Lipski, 2008). A brief description of the features of these two commonly spoken Spanish dialects follows.

Characteristics of Mexican and Puerto Rican Dialects of Spanish

The Mexican and Puerto Rican dialects of Spanish differ from the characteristics of standard Spanish previously described. The unique features of these dialects might be indicative of linguistic simplification and restructuring, a phenomenon that commonly occurs in language contact situations (e.g. Lipski, 1996; Mougeon & Beniak, 1991). The unique features of the two dialects are discussed in the following sections along with explanations from the linguistics literature about how these features are thought to have developed.

The Mexican dialect of Spanish

Features of the Mexican dialect of Spanish are reflected in differences in verb morphology, mood, gender agreement and use of pronouns and prepositions (Martínez, 2006).

Verb morphology

In the Mexican varieties of Spanish, the three conjugation groups have been reduced to two groups, with infinitive verb forms ending in *–ir* often treated like verbs ending in *–er* (Sanchez, 1994). For example, speakers of Mexican Spanish may be observed to use *salemos* instead of *salimos* (we leave). In effect, Mexican Spanish speakers use the first-person plural form for verbs ending in *–er* with verbs ending in *–er* and *–ir*. Therefore, the verbs *salir* (to leave) and *comer* (to eat) are treated similarly when formulating the first-person plural form.

Another feature of the Mexican varieties of Spanish observed in verb morphology is in the use of the first-person plural verb ending. Speakers of Mexican Spanish change the first-person plural verb ending *–mos* to *–nos* when it appears in a verb form with the stress on the antepenultimate (or third to the last) syllable of a word (Sanchez, 1994). For example, in Mexican Spanish the first-person plural imperfect indicative verb form of *vivir* (to live) is *vivíanos* (we lived) rather than *vivíamos*. In standard Spanish, these forms are typically stressed on the antepenultimate syllable of the word. This feature is also evident in other verb tenses, including the conditional tense *comeríanos* (we would eat) and the imperfect subjunctive *estuviéranos* (we were), when the stress is on the antepenultimate syllable of the verb.

Speakers of Mexican Spanish varieties often extend the person-number morphological rule in the preterite verb tense (Hidalgo, 1990; Sanchez, 1994). The second-person singular morpheme is typically *–s* in all verb tenses, except in the preterite where the morpheme is *–ste*. For example, the second-person singular verb form for the word *comer* (to eat) in the present tense is *comes* (you eat), the imperfect tense is *comías* (you used to eat) and the preterite tense is *comiste* (you ate). Speakers of Mexican Spanish will add *-s* in the second-person singular of the preterite. As a result, *comiste* becomes *comistes*. In some southwestern regions of the United States (e.g. Texas, New Mexico), the preterite morpheme is *–tes* rather than *–ste* and as a result the preterite of *comer* is *comites* for some Spanish speakers.

Verb mood

A characteristic of the Mexican Spanish dialect is verb simplification when speakers use the indicative rather than the subjunctive verb mood (Ocampo, 1990). The simplification process has been observed to occur in categorical and variable contexts. The categorical contexts only allow the presence of indicative or subjunctive forms, while the variable contexts allow the presence of either the subjunctive or indicative forms. In the Mexican dialect, the subjunctive mood is used mainly in categorical or obligatory contexts and less frequently in variable or optional contexts. The result is the replacement of the subjunctive with the indicative mood as in the following example: *'Lo siento que tienes frío'* instead of *'Lo siento que tengas frío'* (I'm sorry that you are cold).

Use of ser and estar

The Spanish copulas *ser* and *estar*, when used with an adjective, relate a quality expressed by the adjective to the subject. *Ser* is used to indicate that a group shares a particular quality. For example, in the sentence, '*Pedro es alto* (Pedro is tall)', the speaker indicates that Pedro belongs to a group whose members share the same quality. In contrast, *estar* is used to express a quality of the subject as an individual. For instance, in the sentence '*Pedro está alto* (Pedro is tall)', the speaker assigns a quality to Pedro as an individual rather than a quality that is shared by members of a group. Gutiérrez (2003) discussed the notion that speakers of Mexican Spanish use the *estar* form in ways that do not conform to this distinction, by choosing *estar* where speakers of other varieties would use *ser*, which results in an extension of the semantic domain of *estar* toward *ser*. For example, speakers of Mexican varieties of Spanish may say, '*Pedro está alto* (Pedro is tall)' instead of '*Pedro es alto* (Pedro is tall)' when communicating that Pedro belongs to a group of individuals who share the same quality of height (Sanchez, 1994).

Nouns and gender agreement

Much of the literature describing Mexican varieties of Spanish suggests that gender agreement with nouns is being lost, resulting in the simplification of this grammatical category. The tendency is to assign feminine gender word ending to nouns ending in *–ma* and *–ta* following the principle of transparency (Sanchez, 1982). The principle of transparency is the tendency for speakers to make things as easy as possible by reducing dissimilar forms to similar forms (Wolfram & Schilling-Estes, 1998). As a result, Mexican Spanish speakers tend to assign feminine rather than masculine gender to nouns of Greek origin ending in *–ma* and *–ta* (e.g. *idioma* [language], *clima* [climate], *planeta* [planet]). In addition, gender agreement is often violated within a noun phrase and in copulative sentences; in such cases, the masculine form of the adjective is used with a feminine gender noun.

Plural forms of nouns

Speakers of Mexican varieties of Spanish form plural nouns by applying two rules simultaneously. The *–s* plural morpheme, in standard Spanish, is used after a stressed *–á* and *–é*, as in *sofás* (couches). For nouns ending with a consonant, the *–es* plural morpheme is applied, as in *papeles* (papers). In contrast, speakers of Mexican Spanish apply both rules to nouns ending in stressed *–á* and *–é* resulting in the use of *–ses*, as in *pie/pieses* (foot/feet) and *café/cafeses* (coffee/coffees) (Sanchez, 1982). In addition, in nouns ending in an unstressed vowel and *–s* with stress on the penultimate syllable, speakers of the Mexican variety of Spanish don't overtly mark the plural form on the noun. For example, for the word *lápiz* (pencil), pronounced /lapis/ (pencil), the singular form is *el lápiz* and the plural form is *los lápiz* (the pencils), rather than *los lápices*.

Pronouns

The use of the personal pronouns *tú* (you, informal) and *usted* (you, formal) is associated with role relationships, attitudinal or affective postures and stylistic considerations. The use of *tú* occurs more frequently in informal domains of interaction, while the use of *usted* appears in formal domains of interaction. The pronoun system has undergone change in the Mexican variety of Spanish (Jaramillo, 1990; Sanchez, 1994). Regional differences within the Mexican Spanish dialect occur in the use of *tú* and *usted* when addressing individuals who occupy status-laden positions. Mexican Spanish speakers in the southwestern United States (i.e. New Mexico) tend to maintain this distinction and use *usted* to address individuals who occupy status-laden positions (Jaramillo, 1990), while Mexican Spanish speakers in the Western United States (i.e. California) rarely use *usted* and tend not to maintain the informal and formal distinctions (Sanchez, 1994).

The Puerto Rican dialect of Spanish

The primary characteristics of the Puerto Rican dialect of Spanish include final –*s* deletion across a variety of grammatical categories, frequent use of overt pronouns, preferred verb tenses, distinction between formal and informal modes of address and placement of subjects in a preverbal position in questions.

Final –s deletion

In Puerto Rican Spanish, final –*s* deletion is a highly prominent feature of the dialect (Hochberg, 1986). This characteristic occurs frequently and affects a number of grammatical categories, including verb morphology, the plural marking of nouns, pronouns, articles, descriptive adjectives and demonstratives. The importance of such deletion in Spanish lies in the crucial morphological role that /s/ plays.

Puerto Rican Spanish speakers may delete the final –*s* of the second-person form of verbs resulting in morphological ambiguity. Morphological ambiguity occurs when finite verbs in the first- and third-person singular share the same form (Gili Gaya, 1970). The second- and third-person present and conditional verb forms become ambiguous or impossible to differentiate. For example, in standard Spanish, the second-person present tense of the verb *comer* (to eat) is *comes* (you eat) and the third-person present tense is *come* (he/she eats). Speakers of Puerto Rican Spanish may delete the final –*s* in the second-person present tense and use *come* for *comes*; thus, creating ambiguity with the third-person present tense (*come*). The second- and third-person present tense verbs share the same form '*come*' and are virtually indistinguishable from one another. Similarly, –s deletion in the second-person conditional verb tense *estudiarías* (you would study) renders it indistinguishable from the third-person conditional verb *estudiaría* (he/she would study).

Final –s is also a critical feature that distinguishes between plural and singular forms across a number of grammatical categories including articles, nouns and demonstratives. Speakers of Puerto Rican Spanish tend to delete the final –s in definite and indefinite articles and the corresponding nouns. For example, '*las pelotas*' (the balls) becomes '*la pelota*' (the ball). Thus, ambiguity in the noun phrase is created when the final –s is deleted in the article and the noun rendering the plural form '*las pelotas*' and the singular form '*la pelota*' identical.

Deletion of –s is also observed in Puerto Rican Spanish speakers' use of a singular predicate adjective to describe a plural noun phrase subject (Hidalgo, 1990). For example, in the sentence '*Los niños están agradecido por sus libros.* (The children are grateful for their books.)', the singular predicate adjective '*agradecido*' (grateful) is used to describe the plural subject '*niños*' (children). Similarly, in a coordinate noun phrase containing two or more plural nouns, the plural marker /s/ is normally maintained only in the first noun (Hidalgo, 1990). For example, the plural /s/ is retained for the first plural noun but not for the second plural noun in the following sentence, '*Los niños leen libros y periódico en español.* (The children read books and newspaper in Spanish.)'. Similar ambiguity results when Puerto Rican Spanish speakers delete the final –s in plural demonstrative adjectives and pronouns. For example, the plurality expressed in the following sentence '*Estos son grandes.* (These are big.)' may be expressed as '*Esto son grande.* (This are big.)'. In standard Spanish, the plural demonstratives and pronouns, '*estos, estas, esos, esas, aquellos* and *aquellas*' (these, those, those over there), end with an –s. When final –s is deleted, ambiguity between the singular and plural forms results.

Deletion of final –s is a core feature of Puerto Rican Spanish that is realized across grammatical categories. In Penny's (2002) historical account of the Spanish language, the deletion of final –s was described as a weakening process with different levels of intensity. The least intense weakening occurs when /s/ is realized as the fricative [h] before /d/ as in *desde* (since), while the most intense form of weakening occurs when /s/ is eliminated in all phonetic environments. When final –s is eliminated, its grammatical function is transferred to other phonemes, typically the preceding vowel which becomes elongated (or lengthened).

Use of subject pronouns

The Puerto Rican variety of Spanish is characterized by the frequent use of subject pronouns. Several years ago, Hochberg (1986) suggested a link between /s/ deletion and subject pronoun usage and contended that since the inflectional morpheme –s is omitted, personal pronouns are used more frequently to compensate for the ambiguity in person that might arise. Hochberg (1986) found a higher frequency of personal pronoun expression for subjects in those verb classes where potential ambiguity of form may occur, lending support to the notion that personal pronouns functionally compensate for information missing from the verb form as a result of the –s deletion. In an /s/-deleting dialect like Puerto Rican Spanish, a speaker's choice of a pronominal or null subject is influenced by the inflected form of a finite verb, so verbs with no potential ambiguity of person will less frequently receive an expressed subject pronoun. Those verb tenses in which ambiguity in marking is possible, given the sameness of form, will have a higher rate of expressed pronominal subjects.

Verb tense and mood

The verb system characteristic of Puerto Rican Spanish speakers remains relatively unchanged when compared to standard Spanish. Several years ago, Pousada and Poplack (1982) noted that the most frequently used verb tenses of Puerto Rican Spanish speakers include the present, imperfect and preterite, and they argued that the verbal paradigm had remained stable. However, the subjunctive mood is giving way to the indicative in presuppositions over time (e.g. Bookhamer, 2013; Guitart, 1987). In addition, Puerto Rican Spanish speakers often delete the word final /r/ in infinitives (e.g. *trabajar* [to work] becomes *trabaja*), as detailed by Hidalgo (1990).

Word order

Another feature of Puerto Rican Spanish is the word order used to form questions. In Spanish, questions are typically formed by shifting the subject to a post-verbal position (*'¿Que quieres tú?* [What do want you?]'). In Puerto Rican Spanish, the subject is often not shifted to the post-verbal position (e.g. *'¿Que tú quieres?* [What you want?]'; Quirk *et al.*, 1972) and this commonly occurs with the second-person singular subject pronoun *tú* (Lantolf, 1980; Zentella, 1997). The order of preference, from most to least common, for subject pronouns that appear in a preverbal position in questions is as follows: *tú* (you, informal), *yo* (I), proper name, *usted* (you, formal), *nosotros* (us), *ustedes* (you all) and *él* (him).

Summary

The Mexican and Puerto Rican dialects of Spanish spoken in the United States are characterized by a number of morphosyntactic features. The morphosyntactic characteristics of Puerto Rican and Mexican Spanish are the result of diverse regional, social and cultural realities. Thus, each dialect is distinguishable by a set of key linguistic features that involve verb and noun morphology, verb tense and mood and the use of personal pronouns. Knowledge of these linguistic features will guide SLPs in making well-informed clinical decisions when differentiating between a language impairment and a language difference.

Specific Language Impairment in Spanish-Speaking Children

SLI is characterized as a significant deficit in spoken language in children who have no hearing loss or other developmental delays (Leonard, 2014). It is one of the most common childhood learning disabilities, affecting approximately 7%–8% of children in kindergarten (Tomblin et al., 1997). The exact cause of SLI is unknown; however, recent studies suggest that SLI has a genetic link (e.g. Bishop, 2002; Bishop et al., 1995). Studies examining Spanish-speaking children with a variety of measures indicate that deficits in morphology and linguistic processing characterize SLI in this population.

Spanish-speaking children with language impairment show more limited use of several different grammatical morphemes when compared to same-age peers and typically developing children with similar mean length of utterance (MLU; Bedore & Leonard, 2001). Spanish-speaking children with SLI performed more poorly than their peers on their use of the grammatical morpheme types related to the noun phrase and three of the nine verb morpheme types. Noun-related morphemes, such as adjective-agreement inflections and omission of direct object clitics, were most notable. The children with SLI showed significantly lower scores than age-matched control children for third-person singular and plural. The majority of the verbal inflection errors observed consisted of the production of third-person singular present indicative verb form when a different person, number and tense were required. They found that Mexican Spanish-speaking children living in the United States omitted the plural marker on plural nouns at very high levels. Later, Bedore and Leonard (2005) analyzed the language transcripts gathered from the same group of children and found that the children with SLI were significantly worse than the age-matched control participants in their use of third-person plural present tense.

Instead of relying solely on spontaneous measures, researchers have also utilized elicited production tasks to identify clinical markers of SLI in Spanish-speaking children. Grinstead et al. (2009) tested 42 monolingual Spanish-speaking children, 21 of whom were diagnosed with SLI and 21 of whom were typically developing, age-matched controls. Using an elicited production task, they found that the children with SLI performed significantly below the controls in producing finite verb forms. Recently, they have also argued that tense can be used to distinguish children with

SLI from those without because six of seven of their spontaneous measures (number of different words, MLU in words, MLU in morphemes, MLU of verb phrase and mean length of T-unit) distinguished children with SLI from those without (Grinstead *et al.*, 2013).

Production difficulties in definite article production have also been observed in Spanish-speaking children with SLI. For example, Restrepo and Gutiérrez-Clellen (2001) found difficulties in the production of the singular masculine form (*el*) in a sample of Spanish-speaking children with SLI. The errors consisted of substitution and omission errors. Similarly, Anderson and Souto (2005) evaluated patterns of article use in a group of monolingual Puerto Rican Spanish-speaking children with SLI. Three different spontaneous speech samples were gathered from 11 children with SLI and 11 age-matched peers and an experimental task was also administered to assess the children's use of articles with a variety of nouns. The results for both spontaneous speech and experimental data indicated that children with SLI performed poorer in their use of Spanish articles than did their age-matched peers. The majority of errors observed consisted of the omission of the target articles.

Spanish-speaking children with SLI appear to be less effective in using various cues to assign gender to nouns. Anderson and Lockowitz (2009) designed a study to identify how Spanish-speaking children with and without SLI employed cues to assign gender to new nouns. Using an invented word task, four types of cues were presented: noun-internal cues (semantic transparency and word ending) and noun external cues (article gender and adjective gender). For both groups of children, semantic transparency did not appear to be a strong cue in identifying a noun's gender. In contrast, noun word endings (masculine *–o* and feminine *–a*) appeared to be a stronger cue for identifying gender, especially for children with SLI. The children with typical language development outperformed the children with SLI in their use of article cues. Article gender appeared to be a strong cue for typically developing children but not for children with SLI. These results are similar to earlier work by Pérez-Pereria (1991), which indicated that children more effectively used morphophonological cues, such as word ending, than semantic cues, suggesting that children rely on structural information in assigning gender. Anderson and Lockowitz (2009) further examined individual children's responses and noted that children with SLI did not benefit from the presentation of a cue to a word's inherent gender, such as use of the word in a phrase with either the definite feminine '*las*' or definite masculine '*los*' (the) plural article.

Grammatical features along with parent report information appear to be accurate identifiers of SLI in Spanish speakers. For instance, Restrepo (1998) examined the performance of 31 predominately Spanish-speaking children with normal language and 31 children with language impairment across measures of vocabulary, novel bound-morpheme learning skills, language form and information reported by parents. Parents also responded to questions about their perceptions of their children's speech and language skills and family history of speech and language problems. She found that parental report of the child's speech and language skills and the number of grammatical errors per T-unit were most accurate in classifying children with language impairment.

Linguistic processing deficits are also considered to be a clinical marker of SLI. Recently, several investigations have sought to determine whether language-based processing tasks, such as non-word repetition (NWR), accurately separate children with SLI from children with typical language development. For example, Girbau and Schwartz (2007) evaluated the performance of 11 Spanish-speaking children with SLI and 11 age-matched children with typical language development on the repetition of non-words that were consistent with the phonotactic patterns of Spanish. The task included 20 non-words, four at each syllable length (one, two, three, four and five syllables). The children with SLI performed more poorly on their production of three-, four- and five-syllable non-words. Substitutions were observed to be the most frequent error type for both groups of children. Children's NWR was also highly correlated with the standardized language measures, and likelihood ratios indicated that NWR performance was a highly accurate identifier of language status.

Similarly, Guiberson and Rodriguez (2013) tested the NWR skills of a group of preschool children with language impairment and children with typical language development. Using the NWR task developed by Ebert et al. (2008), which consisted of 20 non-word stimuli that follow Spanish phonotactic constraints and phoneme frequency patterns, they found that the children with language impairment scored significantly lower than the children with typically developing language skills. Two scoring procedures, an item-level (right or wrong) and a percent phoneme correct (PPC) scoring approach, were compared to evaluate differences in the classification accuracy values associated with each approach. Item-level scoring yielded adequate sensitivity and specificity values, while the PPC yielded unacceptable sensitivity and adequate specificity. These results provided preliminary evidence that an item-level scoring procedure may yield better results than a PPC scoring approach when applied to Spanish NWR measures. Moreover, a developmental pattern in Spanish-speaking preschoolers was observed with young children having more difficulty with NWR, especially with longer stimulus items. Although these findings were promising, NWR should not be used by itself to identify SLI in Spanish-speaking children.

In summary, there is mounting evidence detailing the linguistic and processing characteristics in Spanish-speaking children suspected to have an SLI. Researchers have employed a variety of methods to examine morphosyntactic and linguistic processing abilities, which provide direction for clinicians in designing language assessments for this population.

Implications for Language Assessment

Children from Spanish-speaking environments are subject to the problems of over- or underidentification for language impairment in the United States due in part to the variability in children's language learning environments. The accurate identification of SLI in this population is further complicated by the limited availability of psychometrically sound Spanish language assessment tools. However, the recent emergence of data on clinical markers of SLI in Spanish-speaking children should help guide clinicians in accurately identifying children with SLI. Hence, SLPs should base their diagnostic decisions on the results of multiple data sources, including a detailed case history, spontaneous language samples, elicited production tasks and linguistic processing tasks.

Detailed case history information must be gathered from the family during the initial phase of language assessment. The case history should include questions to probe the nature of parental concern regarding the child's speech and language skills (Restrepo, 1998). In addition, it is critically important that the case history include information detailing the child's language learning environment by asking about both parents' (or other significant adults in the child's life) countries of origin and dialects spoken. Gathering this information will help the SLPs identify characteristics of the child's Spanish due to dialect and minimize the misinterpretation of dialect features from features of SLI.

Information about how long the family and child have been living in the United States mainland can also be helpful, as the dialect of the country of origin may differ from the dialect of the US community in which the family resides. Language patterns change over time, and changes vary between communities (Wolfram & Schilling-Estes, 1998). Therefore, information about the length of time in the United States will assist the SLP in anticipating the linguistic features the child may use during the assessment. Also, if the SLP is not a speaker of Spanish or is not knowledgeable about the child's dialect, the case history information will inform the clinician about the types of resources, such as an interpreter, that will be needed to complete the language assessment process.

If an interpreter is needed during the assessment, it is essential that this individual either speaks or has knowledge of the features of the child's dialect. A knowledgeable interpreter can inform the SLP about which characteristics of the child's language are typical for his or her dialectical community, thereby reducing the probability of misdiagnosis based on dialectical or non-standard features of Spanish. One cannot assume, however, that all speakers of Spanish have explicit knowledge of the rules of Spanish or the differences between all Spanish dialects. Therefore, interpreters must be carefully selected and trained to make certain that the assessment yields accurate information (Langdon, 2002).

A detailed case history should be complemented with a series of language tasks to examine the child's morphosyntactic and linguistic processing skills. A spontaneous language sample should be collected for the careful analysis of the child's use of noun- and verb-related morphology (Bedore & Leonard, 2001, 2005), number of errors per T-unit (Restrepo, 1998) and definite article production (Restrepo & Gutierrez-Clellen, 2001). The language sample, combined with the case history information, provides the clinician with the data needed to disentangle features of the child's dialect from identifiers of SLI. However, clinicians must keep in mind that the language sample may not have provided the child with ample opportunities to produce the targeted structures (e.g. gender). Therefore, elicited production tasks could be added to the assessment protocol to ensure that a complete portrait of the child's language skills is obtained. Elicited production tasks could target the child's production of gender agreement in nouns (Anderson & Lockowitz, 2009) and finite verb forms (Grinstead et al., 2009).

Finally, a child's linguistic processing skills should be examined. NWR tasks have been used with Spanish-speaking preschool (Guiberson & Rodriguez, 2013) and school-age children (Girbau & Schwartz, 2007). The non-word items must follow the phonotactic constraints of Spanish and include items of increasing syllable length. Preliminary evidence suggests that item-level scoring procedures result in adequate sensitivity and specificity values. However, the research in this area cautions clinicians to avoid using this task as the only measure to identify SLI.

In summary, multiple sources of information, which include language samples, elicitation tasks, linguistic processing measures and detailed case history/parental report data, are recommended as sources that should be considered by clinicians when evaluating Spanish-speaking children. The accurate diagnosis of SLI in Spanish-speaking children relies on the identification of the grammatical features of SLI while simultaneously taking into account the linguistic features of Mexican and Puerto Rican varieties of Spanish. Although this chapter focuses on aspects of linguistic variability within the US Spanish-speaking Latino population, the cultural variability within this population is also an important clinical consideration. When assessing Spanish-speaking children's language skills, clinicians are also encouraged to be cognizant of the variability in US Latinos' cultural values and beliefs and consider how they impact language assessment results and the development of culturally relevant intervention programs (e.g. Rodriguez & Olswang, 2002, 2003).

References

American Speech-Language Hearing Association (1983) Social dialects [Position Statement]. See www.asha.org/policy (accessed 24 July 2014).

American Speech-Language Hearing Association (2013) Cultural and linguistic competence [Issues in Ethics]. See www.asha.org/Practice/ethics/ (accessed 24 July 2014).

Anderson, R.T. and Souto, S.M. (2005) The use of articles by monolingual Puerto Rican Spanish-speaking children with language impairment. *Applied Psycholinguistics* 26, 621–647.

Anderson, R.T. and Lockowitz, A. (2009) How do children ascribe gender to nouns? A study of Spanish-speaking children with and without specific language impairment. *Clinical Linguistics & Phonetics* 23, 489–506.

Bedore, L.M. and Leonard, L.B. (2001) Grammatical morphology deficits in Spanish-speaking children with specific language impairment. *Journal of Speech, Language, and Hearing Research* 44, 905–924.

Bedore, L.M. and Leonard, L.B. (2005) Verb inflections and noun phrase morphology in the spontaneous speech of Spanish-speaking children with specific language impairment. *Applied Psycholinguistics* 26, 195–225.

Bishop, D.V.M. (2002) Motor immaturity and specific speech and language impairment: Evidence for a common genetic basis. *American Journal of Medical Genetics* 114, 56–63.

Bishop, D.V.M., North, T. and Donlan, C. (1995) Genetic basis of specific language impairment: Evidence from a twin study. *Developmental Medicine & Child Neurology* 37, 56–71.

Bookhamer, K. (2013) The variable grammar of the Spanish subjunctive in second-generation bilinguals in New York City. Dissertation Abstracts International.

Brown, A. and Patten, E. (2014) *Statistical Portrait of Hispanics in the United States, 2012.* Washington, DC: Pew Research Center.

Cardenas, D.N. (1970) *Dominant Spanish Dialects Spoken in the United States.* Washington, DC: Center for Applied Linguistics.

Corbett, G.G. (1991) *Gender.* Cambridge: Cambridge University Press.

Ebert, K.D., Kalanek, J., Cordero, K.N. and Kohnert, K. (2008) Spanish nonword repetition: Stimuli development and preliminary results. *Communication Disorders Quarterly* 29, 67–74.

Ennis, S.R., Ríos-Vargas, M., and Albert, N.G. (2011) *The Hispanic Population: 2010.* Washington, DC: U.S. Census Bureau.

Gili Gaya, S. (1970) *VOX Curso Superior de Sintaxis Española* (9th edn). Barcelona: Bibliograf.

Girbau, D. and Schwartz, R.G. (2007) Non-word repetition in Spanish-speaking children with specific language impairment (SLI). *International Journal of Communication Disorders* 42, 59–75.

Goldstein, B. (2004) Speech issues in children from Latino backgrounds. In R. Kent (ed.) *MIT Encyclopedia of Communication Disorders* (pp. 210–213). Cambridge, MA: MIT Press.

Goldstein, B. and Iglesias, A. (1996) Phonological patterns in normally developing Spanish-speaking 3- and 4-year-olds of Puerto Rican descent. *Language Speech and Hearing Services in Schools* 27, 82–90.

Grinstead, J., De la Mora, J., Vega-Mendoza, M. and Flores, B. (2009) An elicited production test of the optional infinitive stage in child Spanish. In J. Crawford, K. Otaki and M. Takahashi (eds) *Proceedings of the 3rd Conference of Generative Approaches to Language Acquisition – North America* (pp. 36–45). Somerville, MA: Cascadilla Press.

Grinstead, J., Baron, A., Vega-Mendoza, M., De la Mora, J., Cantú-Sánchez, M. and Flores, B. (2013) Tense marking and spontaneous speech measures in Spanish specific language impairment: A discriminant function analysis. *Journal of Speech, Language, and Hearing Research* 56, 352–363.

Guiberson, M. and Rodriguez, B. (2013) Classification accuracy of nonword repetition when used with preschool-age Spanish-speaking children. *Language, Speech, and Hearing Services in Schools* 44, 121–132.

Guitart, J.M. (1976) *Markedness and a Cuban Dialect of Spanish*. Washington, DC: Georgetown University Press.

Guitart, J.M. (1987) On the use of the Spanish subjunctive in two Caribbean dialects: A pragmatic analysis. *Thesaurus* 42, 141–148.

Gutiérrez, M.J. (2003) Simplification and innovation in U.S. Spanish. *Multilingual* 22, 169–184.

Hammer Scheffner, C., Detwiler, J.S., Detwiler, J., Blood, G.W. and Qualls, C. (2004) Speech language pathologists' training and confidence in serving Spanish-English bilingual children. *Journal of Communication Disorders* 37, 91–108.

Hidalgo, M. (1990) The emergence of standard Spanish in the American continent: Implications for Latin American dialectology. *Language Problems & Language Planning* 14, 47–63.

Hochberg, J.G. (1986) Functional compensation for /s/ deletion in Puerto Rican Spanish. *Language* 62, 609–621.

Iglesias, A. and Goldstein, B. (1998) Language and dialectal variations. In J. Bernthal and N. Bankson (eds) *Articulation and Phonological Disorders* (4th edn; pp. 148–171). Needham Heights, MA: Allyn & Bacon Publishing Co.

Jaramillo, J.A. (1990) Domain constraints on the use of *tú* and *usted*. In J. Bergen (ed.) *Spanish in the United States: Sociolinguistic Issues* (pp. 14–22). Washington, DC: Georgetown University Press.

Langdon, H.W. (2002) *Collaborating with Interpreters and Translators: A Practitioner's Handbook*. Austin, TX: Pro-Ed Publishing Company.

Lantolf, J.P. (1980) Constraints on interrogative word order in Puerto Rican Spanish. *The Bilingual Review* 7, 113–122.

Leonard, L.B. (2014) *Children with Specific Language Impairment* (2nd edn). Cambridge, MA: The MIT Press.

Lipski, J.M. (1994) *Latin American Spanish*. New York: Longman Linguistics Library.

Lipski, J.M. (1996) Los dialectos vestigiales del español en los Estados Unidos: Estado de la cuestión. *Signo & Seña* 6, 459–489.

Lipski, J.M. (2008) *Varieties of Spanish in the United States*. Washington, DC: Georgetown University Press.

Martínez, G.A. (2006) *Mexican Americans and Language: Del Dicho al Hecho*. Tucson, AZ: The University of Arizona Press.

Martinez-Gibson, E.A. (2011) A comparative study on gender agreement errors in the spoken Spanish of heritage speakers and second language learners. *Porta Linguarum* 15, 177–193.

McLeod, S. and Goldstein, B. (2011) *Multilingual Aspects of Speech Sound Disorders in Children*. Bristol: Multilingual Matters.

Mougeon, R. and Beniak, É. (1991) *Linguistic Consequences of Language Contact and Restriction: The Case of French in Ontario*. Oxford: Oxford University Press.

Ocampo, F. (1990) El subjuntivo en tres generaciones de hablantes bilingues. In J. Bergen (ed.) *Spanish in the United States: Sociolinguistic Issues* (pp. 39–48). Washington, DC: Georgetown University Press.

Otheguy, R., Zentella, A.C. and Livert, D. (2007) Language and dialect contact in Spanish is New York: Toward the formation of a speech community. *Language* 83, 770–802.

Penny, R. (2002) *A History of the Spanish Language* (2nd edn). Cambridge: Cambridge University Press.

Penny, R. (2004) *Variation and Change in Spanish*. Cambridge: Cambridge University Press.

Pérez-Pereira, M. (1991) The acquisition of gender: What Spanish children can tell us. *Journal of Child Language* 18, 571–590.

Pousada, A. and Poplack, S. (1982) No case for convergence: The Puerto Rican Spanish verb system in a language contact situation. In G. Keller and J. Fishman (eds) *Bilingual Education for Hispanic Students in the United States* (pp. 206–236). New York: Columbia University Teachers College Press.

Quirk, R., Greenbaum, S., Leech, G. and Svartvik, J. (1972) *A Grammar of Contemporary English*. London: Longman.

Restrepo, M.A. (1998) Identifiers of predominantly Spanish-speaking children with language impairment. *Journal of Speech, Language, and Hearing Research* 41, 1398–1411.

Restrepo, M.A. and Gutiérrez-Clellen, V.F. (2001) Article production in bilingual children with specific language impairment. *Journal of Child Language* 28, 433–452.

Rodriguez, B. and Olswang, L.B. (2002) Cultural diversity is more than group differences: An example from the Hispanic community. *Contemporary Issues in Communication Science and Disorders* 29, 154–164.

Rodriguez, B. and Olswang, L.B. (2003) Mexican-American and Anglo-American mothers' beliefs and values about child rearing, education, and language impairment. *American Journal of Speech-Language Pathology* 12, 452–462.

Ruhlen, M. (1991) *A Guide to the World's Languages. Volume 1: Classification*. Palo Alto, CA: Stanford University Press.

Ryan, C. (2013) *Language use in the United States: 2011. American Community Survey reports*. U.S. Census Bureau, Washington, DC.

Sánchez, R. (1982) Our linguistic and social context. In J. Amastae and L. Elías-Olivares (eds) *Spanish in the United States: Sociolinguistics Aspects* (pp. 9–46). Cambridge: Cambridge University Press.

Sánchez, R. (1994) The Spanish of Chicanos. In R. Sanchez (ed.) *Chicano Discourse: Socio Historic Perspectives* (pp. 98–138). Houston, TX: Arte Público Press.

Suárez-Orozco, M. and Páez, M. (2009) *Latinos: Remaking America*. Berkley, CA: University of California Press.

Tomblin, J.B., Records, N.L., Buckwalter, P., Zhang, X., Smith, E. and O'Brien (1997) Prevalence of specific language impairment in kindergarten children. *Journal of Speech, Language, and Hearing Research* 40, 1245–1260.

Wolfram, W. and Schilling-Estes, N. (1998) *American English: Dialects and Variation*. Malden, MA: Blackwell Publishers.

Zagona, K. (2002) *The Syntax of Spanish*. Cambridge: Cambridge University Press.

Zentella, A.C. (1997) *Growing Up Bilingual: Puerto Rican Children in New York*. Oxford: Blackwell Publishers.

Zentella, A.C. (2009) Latina/o languages and identities. In M. Suarez-Orozco and M. Paez (eds) *Latinos: Remaking America* (pp. 321–338). Berkeley, CA: University of California Press.

Index